THE HOME APOTHECARY FULL COLLECTION

Your In-Depth Holistic Guide with Natural Herbal Remedies for Long-Lasting Wellness and Optimal Health

Megan Morren

GET YOUR BONUS NOW!

THE BONUS IS 100% FREE

1500 NATURAL REMEDIES

**TO GET IT SCAN
THE QR CODE BELOW OR GO TO**

skybonusbook.com/megan-morren-fc

TABLE OF CONTENTS

BOOK 1: THE FOUNDATIONS OF HERBAL MEDICINE

CHAPTER 1: THE HISTORY OF HERBAL HEALING

The roots of herbal healing stretch back to the dawn of civilization, where ancient texts and archaeological findings reveal the use of plants for medicinal purposes. The earliest recorded evidence comes from the Sumerians, around 5000 years ago, who compiled lists of plants on clay tablets. These civilizations understood the importance of plants not just for food but for their healing properties. Moving forward in time, the Egyptians further advanced herbal medicine, as evidenced by the Ebers Papyrus, dating back to 1550 BCE. This document contains over 700 remedies, including garlic for heart conditions and aloe vera for skin care.

In ancient China, the discovery and use of medicinal herbs were methodically documented in texts such as the "Shennong Bencao Jing," attributed to the mythical emperor Shennong. This text categorizes hundreds of medicinal plants and their uses, laying the groundwork for Traditional Chinese Medicine. Similarly, in India, the Ayurvedic system of medicine was developed over 3000 years ago, with texts like the "Charaka Samhita" detailing the medicinal properties of over 500 herbs. The Greeks and Romans also made significant contributions to herbal medicine. Hippocrates, often called the father of medicine, emphasized the healing power of nature and the importance of dietary and herbal treatments. His contemporary, Theophrastus, is known as the father of botany for his extensive work on plant classification. Dioscorides, a Greek physician in the Roman army, compiled the "De Materia Medica," an encyclopedia of medicinal plants that remained a central reference for over 1500 years.

During the Middle Ages in Europe, monasteries preserved and expanded upon ancient herbal knowledge, cultivating medicinal plants in their gardens. The Islamic world also played a crucial role in preserving and enhancing the knowledge of herbs. Scholars like Avicenna, in his "Canon of Medicine," integrated the herbal traditions of the Greeks with the findings of Arabic physicians, further enriching the global tapestry of herbal medicine.

The Age of Exploration in the 15th and 16th centuries brought European settlers into contact with the rich herbal traditions of the Americas, Africa, and Asia, leading to the exchange of medicinal plants and knowledge. This period saw the introduction of many new herbs into Europe, such as cinchona bark from South America, used to treat malaria. In the 19th century, with the rise of chemical analysis, scientists began isolating active compounds from plants, leading to the development of modern pharmaceuticals. However, this shift towards synthetic drugs did not diminish the importance of plants in medicine. Many of today's pharmaceuticals are derived from plants, and the World Health Organization estimates that a significant portion of the world's population still relies on traditional herbal remedies as their primary form of healthcare.

In recent decades, there has been a resurgence of interest in herbal medicine in the Western world, driven by a desire for natural and holistic approaches to health. This has led to increased scientific research into the efficacy and safety of medicinal herbs, as well as a greater integration of herbal therapies into mainstream healthcare. Understanding the history of herbal healing offers a profound appreciation for the knowledge passed down through generations and the enduring power of plants to heal and nurture the human body. This rich tradition forms the foundation upon which modern herbal medicine continues to build, blending ancient wisdom with contemporary science to promote health and wellness.

The Evolution of Herbal Medicine

The evolution of herbal medicine through time is a testament to humanity's enduring relationship with the natural world. This intricate history showcases a progression from intuitive, empirical practices to a more structured and scientific approach, reflecting broader shifts in human understanding and societal development. Initially, herbal medicine was deeply entwined with spiritual and ritualistic practices, with healers and shamans using plants in ceremonies believed to invoke healing powers. These early practitioners relied on a profound knowledge of their local flora, passed down orally from one generation to the next, to treat ailments and maintain health within their communities.

As civilizations advanced, the empirical knowledge of herbs began to be documented, leading to the creation of the first materia medica in various cultures. These texts, such as the "Shennong Bencao Jing" in China and the "Ebers Papyrus" in Egypt, were pivotal in transitioning herbal medicine from an oral tradition to a codified science. This documentation allowed for the sharing of herbal knowledge across cultures and geographies, facilitating a rich exchange of medicinal plant uses and preparations.

The scientific revolution of the 16th and 17th centuries marked a significant turning point in the evolution of herbal medicine. The development of botanical gardens and the practice of systematic botany helped standardize plant names and properties, making herbal knowledge more accessible and reliable. This period also saw the advent of chemical analysis, enabling researchers to isolate and identify the active compounds in medicinal plants. This analytical approach laid the groundwork for modern pharmacology but also led to a decline in the holistic use of plants, as the focus shifted towards single, active ingredients.

Despite the rise of synthetic pharmaceuticals, the 20th and 21st centuries have witnessed a resurgence in the interest and use of herbal medicine. This revival is fueled by a growing body of scientific research validating the efficacy of many traditional remedies, alongside a broader cultural shift towards natural and holistic health practices. Today, herbal medicine bridges ancient wisdom and contemporary science, offering a complementary approach to health and wellness that honors the complexity of both plants and human health.

CHAPTER 2: UNDERSTANDING MEDICINAL HERBS

Medicinal herbs, often referred to as the backbone of traditional and holistic medicine, possess a wide array of chemical compounds that interact with the body in complex ways. These compounds, including alkaloids, flavonoids, and glycosides, are responsible for the herbs' therapeutic effects. To harness these benefits effectively, it's crucial to understand the active constituents of herbs, their mechanisms of action within the human body, and how to prepare and use these plants safely and effectively.

Active Constituents of Herbs: Each medicinal herb contains a unique set of chemical compounds that define its therapeutic properties. For example, alkaloids, found in herbs like echinacea and goldenseal, have potent immune-boosting and antimicrobial effects. Flavonoids, present in chamomile and hawthorn, are known for their antioxidant and anti-inflammatory properties. Understanding these constituents is key to selecting the right herb for the desired health benefit.

Mechanisms of Action: The way these compounds interact with the human body can vary greatly. Some, like the salicylic acid found in willow bark, act similarly to synthetic aspirin by reducing inflammation and pain. Others, such as the saponins in ginseng, boost energy levels and improve immune function by influencing hormonal pathways. Recognizing these mechanisms helps in crafting effective herbal remedies tailored to specific conditions.

Preparation and Usage: The method of preparing an herb can significantly affect its potency and efficacy. Infusions and decoctions are common methods for extracting the active compounds from softer parts and harder materials of the plant, respectively. Tinctures, made by soaking herbs in alcohol or vinegar, offer a concentrated and long-lasting form of herbal medicine. The choice of preparation method should consider the herb's active constituents and the desired therapeutic effect.

Dosage and Administration: Determining the correct dosage is critical for safety and effectiveness. Factors such as the individual's age, health condition, and the potency of the herb must be considered. For instance, potent herbs like valerian root, used for sleep disorders, require careful dosing to avoid side effects such as drowsiness or dizziness.

Safety and Precautions: While medicinal herbs offer numerous health benefits, they can also pose risks if not used correctly. It's essential to be aware of potential side effects and interactions with other medications. Herbs like St. John's Wort can interact with prescription medications, including antidepressants and birth control pills, leading to adverse effects. Consulting with a healthcare professional before starting any herbal regimen is advisable, especially for individuals with pre-existing conditions or those taking other medications.

Quality and Sourcing: The therapeutic value of an herb is largely dependent on its quality and purity. Factors such as the herb's growing conditions, harvesting methods, and storage can all impact its potency. Opting for organically grown herbs and reputable sources can help ensure the highest quality and safety.

Incorporating medicinal herbs into health and wellness routines requires a foundational understanding of these key aspects. By recognizing the active constituents, understanding their effects on the body, choosing the appropriate preparation and dosage, and being mindful of safety precautions, individuals can make informed decisions about using herbal remedies to support their health and well-being.

How Herbs Work in the Human Body

When discussing **how herbs work in the human body**, it's essential to delve into the biochemical interactions that occur upon ingestion or application of these natural substances. The human body is a complex system, and the way it responds to herbal compounds is both fascinating and intricate. Medicinal herbs contain a variety of **bioactive compounds** that can influence physiological processes, offering therapeutic benefits or, in some cases, presenting risks.

Bioactive Compounds and Their Actions: Medicinal herbs are rich in a variety of compounds such as **alkaloids, terpenoids, flavonoids, and glycosides**. Each of these compounds interacts with the body in specific ways. For instance, alkaloids, which are nitrogen-containing compounds found in plants like belladonna and opium poppy, can significantly affect the nervous system and pain perception. Flavonoids, on the other hand, are known for their antioxidant properties, helping to neutralize harmful free radicals in the body.

Interaction with Cellular Pathways: Upon entering the body, the active compounds in herbs can interact with cellular pathways. They may bind to receptors on the surface of cells or interact with enzymes within cellular processes. For example, the compound **curcumin**, found in turmeric, is known to inhibit certain enzymes involved in inflammation, thereby exerting anti-inflammatory effects. This interaction with cellular pathways is crucial for the therapeutic effects of herbs.

Absorption and Metabolism: The body's ability to absorb and metabolize herbal compounds is a critical factor in their effectiveness. Factors such as the herb's form (e.g., tea, tincture, capsule), the presence of other substances (e.g., food in the stomach), and individual differences in metabolism can all influence the bioavailability of herbal compounds. For instance, **piperine** in black pepper can enhance the absorption of curcumin by the body, making the combination more effective than curcumin alone.

Herbal Synergy: The concept of synergy plays a significant role in herbal medicine. Many herbs contain multiple active compounds that can work together to produce a more potent effect than any single compound alone. This synergy can enhance the desired therapeutic effects or reduce potential side effects. A well-known example is the combination of **echinacea** and **goldenseal**, where echinacea's immune-boosting properties complement goldenseal's antimicrobial activity.

Dosage and Efficacy: The efficacy of an herb is closely tied to its dosage. Too little may not produce the desired effect, while too much can lead to adverse reactions. The optimal dosage can vary widely depending on the herb, the condition being treated, and the individual's characteristics such as age, weight, and overall health. Precise dosing instructions, often based on empirical evidence and clinical studies, are crucial for maximizing benefits and minimizing risks.

Individual Responses: It's important to note that individuals can respond differently to the same herb due to genetic variations, existing health conditions, and concurrent use of medications. What works well for one person may not work for another, or may even cause adverse effects. Personalized herbal therapy, taking into account an individual's unique circumstances and health status, is therefore a key aspect of effective herbal treatment.

Safety and Interactions: While many herbs are safe for general use, some can interact with prescription medications, over-the-counter drugs, and other herbs. These interactions can alter the effectiveness of the drugs or lead to unexpected side effects. For example, **St. John's Wort** can interfere with the metabolism of many pharmaceuticals, potentially reducing their efficacy. Awareness and understanding of these interactions are essential for anyone using herbal remedies, especially those who are also taking other medications.

Incorporating herbs into one's health regimen involves more than just choosing a plant with a long history of use for a particular ailment. It requires an understanding of how these herbs work within the body, how they are absorbed and metabolized, and how they interact with other substances. By paying close attention to these factors, individuals can better harness the healing power of herbs in a safe and effective manner.

CHAPTER 3: HERBAL SAFETY AND PRECAUTIONS

When considering the use of herbal remedies, it's paramount to prioritize safety and take necessary precautions to avoid potential risks. Herbs, though natural, are potent substances that can interact with medications, affect physiological conditions, and cause allergic reactions in some individuals. The following guidelines are designed to help users navigate the safe use of herbal remedies:

1. **Consult with a Healthcare Professional**: Before incorporating any new herbal remedy into your regimen, especially if you are pregnant, nursing, or have existing health conditions, consulting with a healthcare professional is crucial. This step is vital for individuals on medication, as some herbs can interact with drugs, potentially altering their effectiveness or leading to adverse effects.

2. **Accurate Identification**: Ensure that the herbs you use are correctly identified. Misidentification can lead to the use of a potentially harmful plant. Purchasing herbs from reputable sources or consulting with a professional herbalist can mitigate this risk.

3. **Understand Proper Dosage**: The effectiveness and safety of an herbal remedy are closely tied to its dosage. Adhering to recommended dosages on product labels or those provided by a healthcare provider is essential. Starting with the lowest possible dose and gradually increasing it can help minimize the risk of adverse effects.

4. **Be Aware of Side Effects**: Like any medication, herbs can cause side effects. Researching and being aware of possible side effects associated with an herb will prepare you to recognize and respond to any adverse reactions promptly.

5. **Consider Age and Health Conditions**: Children, the elderly, and individuals with specific health conditions may be more susceptible to the effects of certain herbs. Adjusting dosages accordingly or avoiding some herbs altogether may be necessary for these populations.

6. **Pregnancy and Nursing**: Many herbs should be avoided during pregnancy and while nursing, as they can affect both the mother and the baby. Herbs such as comfrey and pennyroyal, for example, are known to pose risks during pregnancy.

7. **Allergic Reactions**: Be mindful of potential allergic reactions, especially if you have a history of allergies. Testing a small amount of a new herb on the skin or starting with a low oral dose can help identify any allergic response.

8. **Interactions with Medications**: Some herbs can interact with prescription or over-the-counter medications, either enhancing or inhibiting their effects. For instance, St. John's Wort is known to interact with a wide range of medications, including antidepressants and birth control pills.

9. **Quality and Purity**: Opt for high-quality, organically grown herbs to ensure they are free from contaminants such as pesticides, heavy metals, and microbial contaminants. Reputable suppliers will often provide information on the sourcing and testing of their products.

10. **Preparation and Storage**: Proper preparation and storage of herbs are vital to maintain their potency and safety. Dried herbs should be stored in airtight containers away from light and moisture, while tinctures and extracts should be kept in dark glass bottles. Following preparation instructions carefully, whether making teas, tinctures, or salves, ensures that the final product is both effective and safe.

By adhering to these guidelines, individuals can safely explore the benefits of herbal remedies while minimizing potential risks. Remember, the goal of using herbal medicine is to support health and wellness, which requires a careful and informed approach to both selection and use.

Toxic Herbs Identification Guide

Identifying toxic herbs and avoiding dangerous plants is a critical aspect of practicing herbal medicine safely. While many plants offer significant health benefits, others can be harmful or even deadly if ingested or used improperly. This guide aims to equip you with the knowledge to distinguish between safe and toxic herbs, focusing on visual identification, understanding plant families known for toxicity, recognizing common toxic herbs, and adhering to safety practices when foraging or purchasing herbs.

Visual identification is your first line of defense against toxic herbs. Many toxic plants have distinct characteristics that can alert you to their potential danger. For example, the presence of milky sap, which is found in plants like the common milkweed (Asclepias syriaca) and the giant hogweed (Heracleum mantegazzianum), can indicate toxicity. However, it's crucial to note that some beneficial herbs also exhibit this trait, necessitating further investigation. Another visual clue is the plant's coloration; certain toxic berries are brightly colored, such as the red berries of the deadly nightshade (Atropa belladonna), serving as a warning sign in nature. Additionally, the shape and arrangement of leaves can provide hints; plants in the Apiaceae family, like poison hemlock (Conium maculatum), have finely divided, feathery leaves that resemble those of harmless culinary herbs like parsley but are highly toxic.

Understanding plant families known for toxicity can further aid in avoiding dangerous herbs. The Apiaceae family, for instance, includes both edible plants like carrots and toxic ones like water hemlock (Cicuta maculata), one of the most poisonous plants in North America. Familiarizing yourself with these families and their distinguishing features is essential for safe foraging and herbal practice. The Solanaceae family is another group with notorious members, including belladonna and mandrake (Mandragora officinarum), which contain tropane alkaloids responsible for their toxic effects.

Recognizing common toxic herbs by their names and appearances is another crucial skill. For example, foxglove (Digitalis purpurea), while used in heart medication, is deadly in improper doses, easily recognizable by its tall spikes of purple flowers. Learning to identify such plants and understanding their toxic components will help prevent accidental ingestion or misuse.

When foraging for herbs, always adhere to the following safety practices: never harvest plants from areas that may be contaminated with pesticides or heavy metals, such as roadsides or industrial areas; avoid picking plants that you cannot positively identify with 100% certainty, using multiple sources for identification when possible; and be wary of look-alikes, as many safe herbs have toxic doppelgangers. For instance, the beneficial herb queen anne's lace (Daucus carota) closely resembles the deadly poison hemlock, but they can be distinguished by the hairy stems of queen anne's lace, which poison hemlock lacks.

Purchasing herbs from reputable sources is equally important. Ensure that the supplier provides detailed information about the herb's origin, proper identification, and purity. This is particularly crucial for less common herbs or those with known toxic relatives. Suppliers should adhere to rigorous testing standards to ensure their products are free from contamination and correctly identified.

In summary, the ability to identify toxic herbs and avoid dangerous plants is a foundational skill in herbal medicine. By developing a keen eye for visual identification, understanding the characteristics of plant families known for toxicity, recognizing common toxic herbs, and adhering to safe foraging and purchasing practices, you can protect yourself and others from the potential dangers of toxic plants. Remember, when in doubt, consult with a professional herbalist or botanist, and always err on the side of caution when dealing with unfamiliar plants.

BOOK 2: BUILDING YOUR HOME APOTHECARY

Creating an effective herbal workspace requires careful consideration of several key factors to ensure that your home apothecary is both functional and conducive to the preparation of herbal remedies. The first step is to select an appropriate location. Ideally, this space should be away from direct sunlight to prevent the degradation of herbs' therapeutic properties, yet well-lit enough to comfortably work in. Natural light is preferable, but if it's not available, install full-spectrum LED lights to mimic sunlight, which is essential for examining the quality of herbs and for detailed work.

The workspace should be equipped with a sturdy table or countertop that is resistant to stains and easy to clean. Materials like stainless steel or sealed wood are excellent choices due to their durability and ease of maintenance. Ensure the surface is spacious enough to accommodate your tools, herbs, and preparation processes without clutter. An ergonomic chair that supports a comfortable sitting posture during long hours of work is also crucial.

Storage is another critical aspect of setting up your herbal workspace. Use glass jars with airtight lids to store dried herbs and protect them from moisture and air, which can diminish their potency. Label each jar with the herb's name, date of acquisition or harvest, and any other pertinent details. For tinctures, extracts, and oils, amber or cobalt blue bottles are recommended to block out damaging light, further preserving the preparations' effectiveness.

Organize your tools thoughtfully within arm's reach for efficiency. Essential tools include a mortar and pestle for grinding herbs, a digital scale for precise measurements, measuring spoons and cups, a selection of sieves and strainers, and a variety of spoons and spatulas. Consider also having a small stove or hot plate for decoctions and infusions, along with a selection of pots and pans dedicated solely to herbal preparation to avoid contamination from food flavors or residues.

Ventilation is paramount to ensure that the workspace remains free from dust and that any fumes or strong aromas from herbal processing are adequately dissipated. If natural ventilation is insufficient, install a small exhaust fan or use an air purifier to maintain air quality.

By meticulously selecting the location, furnishing the space with the appropriate furniture and storage solutions, organizing tools and materials for easy access, and maintaining a clean and ventilated environment, you can create an herbal workspace that enhances your ability to craft effective remedies and supports your journey in herbalism.

Essential Tools for Home Herbalism

In the realm of home herbalism, the selection and use of the right tools can significantly enhance the quality and efficacy of the remedies you create. Each tool serves a specific purpose, from precise measurement to the fine grinding of herbs, ensuring that your herbal preparations are both potent and consistent. Let's delve into the essential tools required for home herbalism, focusing on their functions and offering recommendations for materials and types that best suit these purposes.

A mortar and pestle are indispensable for grinding herbs into powders or making pastes. Opt for a mortar and pestle made of ceramic or granite for durability and ease of cleaning. The rough interior of a granite mortar and pestle, for example, is ideal for efficiently breaking down herbs, releasing their full flavor and medicinal properties without absorbing them into the material.

Digital scales are crucial for ensuring accurate measurements of herbs, oils, and other components of your remedies. Look for a digital scale that measures in both grams and ounces, with a precision of at least 0.01 grams, to accommodate the varying quantities needed for different preparations. A scale with a tare function allows you to subtract the weight of containers easily, ensuring precise measurements of the ingredients alone.

Measuring spoons and cups are necessary for adding the correct volumes of liquids or semi-solids. Stainless steel measuring tools are recommended for their longevity and ease of sterilization. Ensure you have a complete set that includes measurements from 1/4 teaspoon up to 1 cup, as herbal recipes often require small and precise amounts of various ingredients.

Storage jars with airtight lids are essential for preserving the potency and freshness of both dried herbs and finished products. Glass jars are preferable, as they do not interact chemically with their contents and allow you to see the stored herbs. Amber glass jars offer the added benefit of protecting light-sensitive materials from degradation. Label each jar with the name of the herb, the date of storage, and any other pertinent details such as origin or specific uses.

For the preparation of tinctures, extracts, and syrups, a selection of sieves and strainers is necessary to separate solids from liquids. Stainless steel or food-grade nylon mesh strainers of various mesh sizes allow for the filtration of different consistencies, ensuring a smooth final product. Additionally, cheesecloth can be used for straining finer particles or for wrapping herbs during the infusion process.

Spoons and spatulas are needed for mixing and transferring ingredients. Silicone or stainless steel options are preferred for their resistance to staining and absorption of flavors and odors. Having a variety of sizes on hand, from small spatulas for scooping out salves to large spoons for stirring decoctions, will facilitate ease of preparation.

For the heating of ingredients, a small stove or hot plate, along with a set of stainless steel pots and pans, is beneficial. This equipment should be dedicated solely to herbal preparation to prevent contamination from food flavors or residues. Stainless steel is recommended for its even heat distribution and ease of cleaning.

Lastly, consider the environment of your workspace. Good ventilation is key to ensuring that any dust from dried herbs or fumes from heating processes does not accumulate. If natural ventilation is not sufficient, a small exhaust fan can help maintain air quality, while an air purifier can remove particulates from the air.

By equipping your home apothecary with these essential tools, you create a foundation for the effective and safe preparation of herbal remedies. Each tool not only aids in the creation of these remedies but also ensures that the process is as precise and beneficial as possible, honoring the tradition of herbalism and the natural potency of the plants you work with.

CHAPTER 2: GROWING MEDICINAL HERBS

To successfully grow your own medicinal herbs, it's essential to understand the specific needs of each plant, from soil type to sunlight exposure. Begin by selecting herbs that are well-suited to your climate. Research the USDA Hardiness Zone for your area to ensure the herbs you choose can thrive. For herbs that prefer well-drained soil, such as lavender and rosemary, incorporate sand or gravel into the planting area to improve drainage. Conversely, for moisture-loving herbs like mint, consider adding organic matter to retain moisture.

Sunlight is crucial for the growth of most medicinal herbs. Aim for a location that receives at least six hours of direct sunlight daily. However, some herbs, such as lemon balm and mint, can tolerate partial shade.

Watering needs vary among herbs. While drought-tolerant herbs like thyme and oregano require minimal watering once established, others, including basil and cilantro, need consistently moist soil. Implement a watering schedule based on the specific needs of each herb, checking the soil moisture at a depth of one inch to determine if watering is necessary.

Soil pH is another critical factor. Most herbs thrive in a pH range of 6.0 to 7.0. Test your soil using a pH testing kit available at garden centers. If the pH is too low, incorporate lime to raise it. If it's too high, adding sulfur can help lower it to the desired range.

Fertilization should be approached with caution. Over-fertilizing can lead to lush foliage with diminished flavor and medicinal properties. Opt for a balanced, slow-release organic fertilizer applied sparingly in the spring and possibly again in mid-summer for herbs that show signs of nutrient deficiency.

Propagation can be done through seeds, cuttings, or division. For seeds, start indoors in trays with seed starting mix six to eight weeks before the last frost date, then transplant outdoors when the weather stabilizes. Cuttings from established plants can be rooted in water or a moist soil mix. Division involves separating mature plants into smaller sections and replanting them to give more room for growth.

Pest and disease management is vital for maintaining healthy herbs. Regularly inspect plants for signs of distress. Implement natural pest control methods such as introducing beneficial insects, using neem oil, or making homemade insecticidal soaps. For fungal diseases, ensure adequate air circulation around plants and avoid overhead watering to keep foliage dry.

Harvesting should be done judiciously to ensure plants remain vigorous. Harvest leaves and flowers in the morning after the dew has dried but before the sun is at its peak, as this is when the concentration of active compounds is highest. Never harvest more than one-third of the plant at a time to allow it to recover.

By adhering to these guidelines, you can cultivate a thriving medicinal herb garden that will enhance your home apothecary. Each herb offers unique benefits, and growing them yourself ensures you have access to the freshest, most potent remedies right at your fingertips. Remember, the key to successful herb gardening is understanding and catering to the specific needs of each plant, from soil conditions and sunlight to watering and harvesting practices.

Choosing the Right Herbs for Your Climate

Selecting the appropriate herbs for your climate is a foundational step in establishing a successful and sustainable medicinal herb garden. This process involves understanding your local weather patterns, soil conditions, and the specific needs of each herb you wish to grow. To begin, familiarize yourself with the USDA Hardiness Zone of your area. This system divides North America into 13 zones based on the average annual minimum winter temperature. Knowing your zone helps in identifying which herbs are most likely to thrive in your local climate.

For those residing in cooler climates, zones 3-6, focus on hardy perennial herbs such as sage (Salvia officinalis), thyme (Thymus vulgaris), and mint (Mentha spp.). These herbs can withstand cold winters. It's crucial to provide them with well-draining soil and mulch for winter protection. In contrast, warmer climates, zones 7-11, offer a conducive environment for a broader range of herbs including basil (Ocimum basilicum), rosemary (Rosmarinus officinalis), and lavender (Lavandula spp.), which prefer hot, sunny conditions. These herbs require soil that allows for quick drainage to prevent root rot and should be placed in areas receiving full sun exposure for the majority of the day.

Soil quality and pH level play a significant role in the health and productivity of your herb garden. Most culinary and medicinal herbs prefer a soil pH between 6.0 and 7.5, indicating slightly acidic to neutral soil. Conduct a soil test using a pH testing kit available at garden centers to determine your soil's current state. If your soil is too acidic (pH below 6.0), incorporate garden lime to raise the pH. For alkaline soil (pH above 7.5), mix in sulfur or aluminum sulfate to lower the pH to the desired level.

In addition to pH, consider the soil's texture and drainage capabilities. Herbs generally do not thrive in heavy, compacted soil. Improve clay-rich soil by adding organic matter such as compost or aged manure, which enhances soil structure and drainage while providing essential nutrients. For sandy soil, which drains quickly but retains fewer nutrients, increase water and nutrient retention by incorporating organic matter.

Watering practices must be tailored to the specific needs of each herb. Mediterranean herbs such as oregano (Origanum vulgare) and lavender require less water and can suffer from overwatering, which leads to root diseases. On the other hand, herbs like cilantro (Coriandrum sativum) and parsley (Petroselinum crispum) prefer consistently moist soil. Implement a watering schedule that meets the needs of each herb, generally providing more water during hot, dry periods and reducing frequency as temperatures cool or during rainy spells.

When selecting herbs, also consider their lifecycle. Annual herbs, such as basil and cilantro, complete their lifecycle in one growing season and must be replanted each year. Perennials, like rosemary and thyme, survive winter in suitable climates and return year after year, offering a more permanent fixture in your garden. Biennials, such as parsley, have a two-year lifecycle, growing foliage the first year and flowering the second year before dying.

Understanding the growth habits of herbs is essential for garden planning. Some herbs, like mint, are known for their aggressive growth and can quickly take over a garden space. To prevent this, plant mint in containers or confined spaces. Conversely, herbs like basil are more contained and suitable for planting in garden beds or mixed borders.

By carefully selecting herbs suited to your climate, soil, and water conditions, you can create a vibrant, productive herb garden. Paying attention to the specific requirements of each herb ensures not only their survival but also their flourishing, providing you with a bountiful supply of fresh herbs for culinary, medicinal, and aromatic uses.

CHAPTER 3: ORGANIZING YOUR APOTHECARY

Organizing your apothecary is a crucial step in ensuring that your herbal remedies are both effective and safe to use. The organization not only helps in locating herbs and supplies quickly but also in maintaining the potency and freshness of your herbs. Here are detailed steps and recommendations for organizing your home apothecary:

1. **Categorize Your Herbs and Supplies**: Begin by categorizing your herbs and supplies. You might categorize herbs based on their use (digestive, respiratory, etc.), form (dried, tincture, oil), or alphabetically. Supplies can be categorized by type (containers, preparation tools, labeling supplies).

2. **Use Appropriate Storage Containers**: For dried herbs, use airtight glass jars to prevent moisture and air from degrading the herbs. Amber or cobalt blue bottles are ideal for tinctures and oils to protect them from light. Ensure containers are clearly labeled with the herb's name, date of acquisition or harvest, and any other pertinent details.

3. **Implement a Labeling System**: Labels should include the common name and Latin name of the herb, the date of harvest or purchase, and the part of the plant used. If you've made a tincture or oil, include the solvent used and the date of preparation. Waterproof labels are recommended to withstand cleaning or any spills.

4. **Create a Dedicated Workspace**: Allocate a specific area in your home as your apothecary workspace. This should be a clean, well-lit area away from direct sunlight, with easy access to your organized herbs and supplies. The workspace should include a sturdy table or countertop and an ergonomic chair.

5. **Shelving and Storage Solutions**: Install shelves at a comfortable height to store your categorized and labeled containers. Use drawer organizers or small storage bins to keep smaller items like measuring spoons, pipettes, and labels organized. Consider a magnetic board or hooks for hanging tools that are frequently used.

6. **Maintain an Inventory List**: Keep a detailed inventory list of all your herbs and supplies, including quantities and expiration dates. This can be in a digital format or a physical binder. Regularly update this list as you use supplies and acquire new ones.

7. **Establish a First-In, First-Out System**: Organize your herbs and supplies so that the oldest stock is used first. This is particularly important for herbs and products with a limited shelf life to ensure they are used while at their peak potency.

8. **Designate Areas for Different Processes**: If space allows, designate specific areas for different processes such as drying herbs, preparing tinctures, and packaging finished products. This helps prevent cross-contamination and keeps your workspace organized.

9. **Use Lighting Effectively**: Ensure your apothecary and workspace are well-lit with natural light or full-spectrum LED lights. Good lighting is essential for accurately identifying herbs and for tasks requiring precision.

10. **Implement Safety Measures**: Store any toxic or potentially harmful herbs and substances in a locked cabinet or out of reach of children and pets. Clearly label these substances and ensure they are stored in containers that are distinct from those used for safe herbs.

11. **Regular Cleaning and Maintenance**: Schedule regular cleaning sessions to keep your apothecary area and tools clean and organized. Use natural cleaning agents to avoid introducing chemicals into your preparation area.

12. **Accessibility and Ergonomics**: Organize your space so that frequently used items are within easy reach and that you can work comfortably without straining. Adjust shelving and work surfaces to suit your height and ensure a comfortable posture while working.

By meticulously organizing your apothecary following these detailed steps, you create an efficient, safe, and pleasant environment for preparing herbal remedies. This organization not only enhances the quality of your preparations but also deepens your connection to the healing power of herbs.

Labeling and Storing Herbal Supplies

When it comes to **labeling**, precision and clarity are paramount. Each label should include the **common name** of the herb, its **Latin name** to avoid any confusion with similarly named herbs, the **date of harvest** or purchase to track freshness, and the **part of the plant** used (e.g., leaf, root). For preparations like tinctures or oils, also note the **solvent** (e.g., alcohol, glycerin) and the **date of preparation**. Utilize waterproof, smudge-proof labels to ensure that information remains legible even in a working apothecary environment. A fine-tip permanent marker is recommended for writing on labels to ensure legibility and durability of the text.

Storing herbs properly is crucial to maintaining their potency and freshness. Dried herbs are best kept in **airtight glass jars** to protect them from moisture and air, which can lead to degradation. **Amber or cobalt blue bottles** are ideal for storing liquids like tinctures and oils, as these colored containers block harmful UV light, preserving the preparations' effectiveness. Store these containers in a cool, dark place — a cupboard away from direct sunlight or a pantry is ideal. Ensure that the storage area is dry to prevent any moisture from compromising the herbs' quality.

For **maintaining** herbal supplies, regular checks are necessary to ensure that herbs and preparations have not surpassed their **expiration dates** or lost their potency. Dried herbs generally maintain their potency for 1-3 years, while tinctures can last up to 5 years if stored correctly. Any signs of mold, unusual odors, or color changes can indicate that an herb or preparation has deteriorated and should be discarded.

Implementing a **first-in, first-out** system ensures that older stock is used before newer stock, minimizing waste. This can be facilitated by organizing herbs and preparations so that those with earlier dates are positioned in front of or above those with later dates, ensuring they are selected first during use.

Ventilation plays a critical role in maintaining an optimal environment for storing herbs. Ensure that the storage area is well-ventilated to prevent any buildup of humidity which could potentially harm the herbs. If the area is prone to dampness, consider using a dehumidifier to maintain a dry environment.

Accessibility is another important factor in organizing your apothecary. Arrange herbs and supplies in a manner that makes them easy to find and reach. Grouping herbs by their use (e.g., digestive aids, respiratory herbs) or alphabetically can facilitate this. Utilize shelving units, drawer organizers, and storage bins to maximize space and keep smaller items organized. For tools and frequently used items, magnetic boards, hooks, or pegboards can offer convenient access.

By adhering to these detailed steps for labeling, storing, and maintaining your herbal supplies, you ensure that your home apothecary remains a well-organized, efficient, and safe space for crafting herbal remedies. This meticulous approach not only extends the shelf life of your herbs and preparations but also supports the integrity and efficacy of your healing practices.

BOOK 3: EVERYDAY HERBAL REMEDIES

CHAPTER 1: HERBS FOR COMMON AILMENTS

In addressing common ailments, herbs have been a cornerstone of natural health practices for centuries. Their application ranges from soothing digestive issues to alleviating respiratory conditions. This section delves into specific herbs that are beneficial for everyday health concerns, providing detailed recipes and usage instructions to harness their healing properties effectively.

Digestive Health: Ginger and Peppermint

Ginger is renowned for its ability to ease nausea and improve digestion. For quick relief from indigestion or motion sickness, a simple ginger tea can be made by slicing 1 inch of fresh ginger root and steeping it in boiling water for 10 minutes. Strain and enjoy warm, adding honey if desired for taste. Peppermint, on the other hand, is excellent for soothing bloating and gas. A peppermint tea can be prepared by steeping 1 tablespoon of dried peppermint leaves in 1 cup of boiling water for 5-7 minutes. This tea can be consumed after meals to aid digestion.

Respiratory Health: Eucalyptus and Thyme

Eucalyptus is a powerful herb for clearing congestion, thanks to its cineole content which acts as an expectorant. For a homemade eucalyptus steam inhalation, add 2-3 drops of eucalyptus essential oil to a bowl of hot water, cover your head with a towel, and inhale deeply for 5-10 minutes. Thyme is beneficial for coughs and sore throats due to its antispasmodic and antibacterial properties. A thyme tea can be made by steeping 2 teaspoons of dried thyme in 1 cup of boiling water for 10 minutes, then strain. Drink warm with honey to soothe a sore throat.

Stress and Anxiety: Chamomile and Lavender

Chamomile is widely used for its calming effects, making it an ideal choice for stress and anxiety relief. To prepare chamomile tea, steep 1 tablespoon of dried chamomile flowers in 1 cup of boiling water for 5-7 minutes. Lavender also has a soothing effect on the nervous system. For a relaxing lavender tea, mix 1 teaspoon of dried lavender flowers with 1 cup of boiling water and steep for 5 minutes. This tea is perfect for unwinding before bedtime.

Skin Irritations: Calendula and Aloe Vera

Calendula is known for its healing properties, especially for cuts, scrapes, and other skin irritations. A calendula poultice can be made by grinding dried calendula flowers into a paste with a small amount of water and applying it directly to the affected area. Aloe Vera is another excellent herb for skin health, particularly for burns and sunburns. Fresh aloe vera gel can be applied directly to the skin for immediate cooling relief.

Immune Support: Echinacea and Elderberry

Echinacea is a powerful immune booster, best taken at the first sign of illness. For an echinacea tincture, soak 1 part dried echinacea root in 5 parts alcohol (vodka or brandy) for 6 weeks, shaking daily. Strain and take 1 teaspoon up to three times daily at the onset of cold or flu symptoms. Elderberry is known for its antiviral properties, making it effective against colds and flu. An elderberry syrup can be made by simmering 1 cup of dried elderberries in 4 cups of water until reduced by half, then strain. Add 1 cup of honey, stir until dissolved, and take 1 tablespoon daily for immune support.

Each of these herbs offers a natural way to address common health concerns, from digestive discomfort to immune support. By incorporating these herbal remedies into your daily routine, you can harness the power of nature to maintain and improve your health.

Digestive Health: Herbs for Gut Support

Fennel and ginger stand out as key herbs in the management of digestive health issues, ranging from mild bloating to more chronic conditions like Irritable Bowel Syndrome (IBS). Both herbs have been utilized for centuries due to their therapeutic properties, offering natural and effective relief for various gastrointestinal complaints.

Fennel (Foeniculum vulgare) is renowned for its carminative properties, which means it can help in the reduction of gas in the gastrointestinal tract and alleviate bloating. To harness the benefits of fennel for digestive health, you can prepare a simple fennel tea. Start by crushing 1 teaspoon of fennel seeds to release their oil, which is where the digestive benefits lie. Boil 1 cup of water and pour it over the crushed seeds in a mug. Cover and steep for 10 minutes to ensure the volatile oils do not escape. Strain the tea and drink it warm. For those experiencing chronic digestive discomfort, consuming fennel tea after meals can help facilitate digestion and prevent gas formation.

Ginger (Zingiber officinale), on the other hand, is widely recognized for its ability to soothe the digestive tract, reduce nausea, and promote the proper movement of food through the intestines. To make a ginger digestive aid, begin by peeling and thinly slicing a 2-inch piece of fresh ginger root. Add the ginger slices to 2 cups of water in a small pot and bring to a boil. Lower the heat and simmer for 20 minutes to allow the ginger compounds to infuse into the water. Strain the liquid and consume it warm. Adding a teaspoon of honey not only enhances the flavor but also provides additional soothing properties. Drinking ginger tea 20 minutes before meals can stimulate digestion and prevent common digestive issues like bloating and discomfort.

For individuals dealing with IBS, incorporating these herbs into their daily routine can offer significant relief. It's important to note that while both fennel and ginger are generally safe for most people, those with specific health conditions or pregnant women should consult with a healthcare provider before adding these herbs to their regimen.

To ensure optimal freshness and potency of these herbs, store fennel seeds in an airtight container in a cool, dark place, and keep fresh ginger root in the refrigerator. When selecting ginger at the store, look for a root with smooth, taut skin, which indicates freshness.

Incorporating fennel and ginger into your diet can be a simple yet effective way to support digestive health. Whether used individually or together, these herbs offer a natural approach to mitigating digestive discomfort and promoting overall gastrointestinal wellness.

Ginger Tonic for Indigestion Relief A warming tonic for stomach discomfort.

Beneficial effects

Ginger tonic is renowned for its ability to soothe indigestion, reduce nausea, and promote healthy digestion. The active compounds in ginger, such as gingerol, have anti-inflammatory and antioxidant properties that can help alleviate stomach discomfort and support overall gastrointestinal health.

Portions

Serves 2

Preparation time

10 minutes

Cooking time

5 minutes

Ingredients

- 2 inches of fresh ginger root, peeled and thinly sliced
- 2 cups of water
- 1 tablespoon of honey, or to taste
- Juice of half a lemon
- A pinch of cayenne pepper (optional)

Instructions

1. In a small saucepan, combine the sliced ginger and water. Bring the mixture to a boil over high heat.
2. Once boiling, reduce the heat to low and simmer the ginger for about 5 minutes. This allows the ginger's beneficial compounds to infuse into the water.
3. After simmering, remove the saucepan from the heat and let it sit for a couple of minutes to cool slightly.
4. Strain the ginger pieces from the water using a fine mesh strainer or cheesecloth, pouring the infused water into a heat-resistant pitcher or jar.
5. Stir in the honey until it is fully dissolved. Honey not only adds sweetness but also has its own soothing properties for the digestive system.
6. Add the lemon juice to the ginger infusion. Lemon juice can enhance the tonic's flavor and add vitamin C, aiding digestion and boosting immunity.
7. If you're using cayenne pepper, add a small pinch now. Cayenne pepper can stimulate digestion and improve circulation, but it's optional depending on your taste and tolerance for spice.
8. Serve the tonic warm or allow it to cool completely and serve it chilled, based on personal preference.

Variations

- For a caffeine-free energy boost, add a slice of fresh turmeric root during the simmering process. Turmeric contains curcumin, which has potent anti-inflammatory and antioxidant properties.
- Replace honey with maple syrup for a vegan alternative that still adds a touch of sweetness.
- Add a stick of cinnamon while simmering the ginger for a warming spice flavor that also has digestive benefits.

Storage tips

This ginger tonic can be stored in an airtight container in the refrigerator for up to 5 days. Reheat gently on the stove or enjoy cold for a refreshing drink.

Tips for allergens

For those with allergies to honey, using maple syrup or agave nectar are suitable alternatives that do not compromise the soothing effects of the tonic.

Scientific references

- "Ginger in gastrointestinal disorders: A systematic review of clinical trials," published in Food Science & Nutrition, highlights ginger's effectiveness in treating gastrointestinal issues.

CHAPTER 2: RESPIRATORY HEALTH & ALLERGIES

Eucalyptus and Thyme are two potent herbs that have been traditionally used to support respiratory health. Their properties can be harnessed through various methods to alleviate symptoms associated with colds, coughs, and seasonal allergies. Here, we detail how to effectively use these herbs for respiratory relief.

Eucalyptus (Eucalyptus globulus) is renowned for its cineole content, a compound that acts as an expectorant to help clear congestion. To create a eucalyptus steam inhalation, you will need:
- 2-3 drops of eucalyptus essential oil
- A bowl of boiling water

Pour the boiling water into a bowl and add the eucalyptus essential oil. Drape a towel over your head and the bowl, ensuring no steam escapes. Inhale deeply for 5-10 minutes. This method helps to loosen mucus and clear the nasal passages, providing relief from congestion.

Thyme (Thymus vulgaris) possesses antispasmodic and antibacterial properties, making it effective for treating coughs and sore throats. To prepare thyme tea:
- 2 teaspoons of dried thyme
- 1 cup of boiling water

Steep the dried thyme in boiling water for 10 minutes. Strain the mixture and drink warm. Adding honey not only improves the taste but also offers additional throat-soothing benefits. Thyme tea can be consumed two to three times daily to relieve cough and sore throat symptoms.

For those suffering from seasonal allergies, incorporating **Nettles (Urtica dioica)** and **Goldenrod (Solidago virgaurea)** into your herbal regimen can be beneficial. Both herbs are known to possess natural antihistamine properties, which can help reduce the body's allergic response.

Nettles and Lemon Allergy Relief Tea:
- 1 tablespoon of dried nettle leaves
- 1 teaspoon of dried goldenrod
- 1 slice of lemon
- 1 cup of boiling water

Combine the nettle leaves and goldenrod in a tea infuser and place it in a mug. Add the slice of lemon. Pour boiling water over the herbs and lemon, then cover and steep for 10-15 minutes. Strain and enjoy this tea once daily during allergy season to help manage symptoms.

It's important to source your herbs from reputable suppliers to ensure they are free from contaminants and have been properly identified. Store your dried herbs in airtight containers away from direct sunlight and moisture to preserve their potency.

For individuals with existing health conditions or those currently taking medication, it's advisable to consult with a healthcare provider before incorporating these herbal remedies into your routine. While eucalyptus and thyme are generally safe for most adults, they may interact with certain medications or be contraindicated in specific medical conditions.

By integrating eucalyptus and thyme into your health care practices, you can take advantage of their natural healing properties to support respiratory health and alleviate symptoms associated with seasonal allergies. Remember, consistency and quality of herbs are key to achieving the best results.

Herbs for Colds and Sinus Relief

Eucalyptus, thyme, and elderberry stand as pillars in the natural treatment of colds, coughs, and sinus congestion, each bringing its unique properties to the forefront of herbal remedies. Eucalyptus, known scientifically as Eucalyptus globulus, is celebrated for its cineole or eucalyptol content, a compound that acts as an expectorant, helping to clear mucus from the airways, making breathing easier. To harness the benefits of eucalyptus for respiratory relief, one can employ eucalyptus essential oil in a steam inhalation method. Begin by boiling a pot of water and transferring it to a heat-resistant bowl. Add 3-5 drops of eucalyptus essential oil to the hot water. Lean over the bowl, drape a large towel over your head and the bowl to trap the steam, and inhale deeply for 5-10 minutes. This method facilitates the loosening of mucus and opens up the nasal passages, providing relief from congestion. Thyme, or Thymus vulgaris, is revered for its antispasmodic, antibacterial, and expectorant properties, making it an effective remedy for coughs and sore throats. A simple thyme tea can be prepared by adding 2 teaspoons of dried thyme leaves to a cup of boiling water. Cover and steep for 10-15 minutes to allow the volatile oils to infuse into the water, then strain. Drinking this tea three times a day can provide soothing relief for coughs and sore throats. For an enhanced effect, one might add honey, which brings its own antibacterial properties and can make the tea more palatable. Elderberry, scientifically known as Sambucus nigra, is widely recognized for its immune-boosting and antiviral properties, making it particularly effective in the treatment and prevention of colds and flu. Elderberry works by inhibiting the replication of viruses, thus shortening the duration of illness and alleviating symptoms. To create an elderberry syrup, combine 1 cup of dried elderberries with 4 cups of water in a saucepan. Bring to a boil, reduce heat, and simmer until the liquid is reduced by half, about 45 minutes. Strain the mixture using a fine mesh sieve, pressing the berries to extract all the liquid. While the liquid is still warm, stir in 1 cup of honey until fully dissolved. Store the syrup in a sealed glass bottle in the refrigerator. For cold and flu prevention, adults can take 1 tablespoon daily, and children over the age of one can take 1 teaspoon daily. At the first sign of illness, the dosage can be increased to every 3-4 hours.

When utilizing these herbs, it's crucial to source high-quality, organic (when possible) materials to ensure the absence of contaminants and the presence of high levels of beneficial compounds. Additionally, while these herbal remedies can offer significant relief and support during illness, they should not replace medical treatment when necessary. Individuals with specific health conditions, pregnant women, or those on medication should consult with a healthcare professional before beginning any new herbal regimen. Incorporating eucalyptus, thyme, and elderberry into one's herbal medicine cabinet provides a robust toolkit for addressing the symptoms of colds, coughs, and sinus congestion. Whether used individually or in combination, these herbs offer a natural, effective way to support respiratory health and enhance overall well-being during the cold and flu season.

Elderberry Syrup for Immune Support A tried-and-true recipe to boost immunity.

Beneficial effects

Elderberry syrup is celebrated for its immune-boosting properties. Rich in antioxidants and vitamins that can help fight colds and flu, elderberry syrup acts as a natural remedy to enhance the body's immune response. Studies have shown that elderberry can shorten the duration of colds and lessen the severity of symptoms.

Portions

Makes approximately 16 ounces

Preparation time

15 minutes

Cooking time

45 minutes

Ingredients

- 3/4 cup of dried elderberries
- 3 cups of water
- 1 teaspoon of ground cinnamon or 1 cinnamon stick
- 1/2 teaspoon of ground cloves
- 1 tablespoon of fresh ginger, grated
- 1 cup of raw honey

Instructions

1. Combine the dried elderberries, water, cinnamon, cloves, and grated ginger in a medium saucepan. If you're using a cinnamon stick, add it whole.
2. Bring the mixture to a boil over high heat, then reduce the heat to low, allowing it to simmer for about 45 minutes. This slow simmer helps to extract the beneficial compounds from the elderberries and spices.
3. Once the mixture has reduced by almost half, remove the saucepan from the heat and let it cool until it's safe to handle.
4. Mash the elderberries gently using the back of a spoon to release any remaining juice.
5. Strain the mixture through a fine mesh sieve or cheesecloth into a large bowl, pressing on the elderberry solids to extract as much liquid as possible. Discard the solids.
6. After the liquid has cooled to lukewarm, add the raw honey and stir until it's completely dissolved. It's important to wait until the mixture is not too hot to preserve the beneficial enzymes and nutrients in the raw honey.
7. Transfer the elderberry syrup to a sterilized glass bottle or jar.

Variations
- For an extra immune boost, add 1/2 teaspoon of ground turmeric during the simmering process.
- If you prefer a thicker syrup, reduce the water to 2 cups instead of 3.

Storage tips
Store the elderberry syrup in an airtight container in the refrigerator. It will keep for up to two months. For longer storage, you can freeze the syrup in an ice cube tray and then transfer the frozen cubes to a freezer bag, keeping them frozen until needed.

Tips for allergens
If you're allergic to honey, you can substitute it with maple syrup. However, this will alter the flavor and the preservative qualities of the syrup, potentially reducing its shelf life.

Scientific references
- "Randomized study of the efficacy and safety of oral elderberry extract in the treatment of influenza A and B virus infections" published in the Journal of International Medical Research, which supports elderberry's effectiveness in reducing the duration and severity of cold symptoms.

CHAPTER 3: EMOTIONAL WELLBEING WITH HERBS

In the realm of emotional wellbeing, herbs play a pivotal role in managing stress, anxiety, and mood fluctuations. The natural compounds found in certain herbs interact with the body's nervous system in a way that can promote relaxation, reduce stress responses, and enhance mood. Here, we delve into specific herbs known for their calming and uplifting properties, providing detailed instructions on how to incorporate them into daily routines for emotional balance and resilience.

Valerian (Valeriana officinalis) is renowned for its sedative qualities, making it an excellent choice for those struggling with insomnia or anxiety. To prepare a valerian root tea, take 1 teaspoon of dried valerian root and steep it in 1 cup of boiling water for 10 minutes. It's best consumed in the evening, about 30 minutes before bedtime, to facilitate a restful night's sleep. Due to its potent effects, valerian should be used with caution and not combined with other sedative medications.

St. John's Wort (Hypericum perforatum) has been widely studied for its potential to alleviate mild to moderate depression. For a St. John's Wort infusion, use 2 teaspoons of the dried herb per cup of boiling water, steeping for 15 minutes. This tea can be drunk two to three times a day. It's important to note that St. John's Wort can interact with a variety of medications, including antidepressants, so consulting with a healthcare provider before use is crucial.

Holy Basil (Ocimum sanctum), also known as Tulsi, is an adaptogen that helps the body cope with stress. To enjoy Holy Basil, add 1 tablespoon of the fresh or dried leaves to a cup of boiling water, steep for 5 minutes, and then strain. Drinking Holy Basil tea once in the morning and once in the evening can help modulate stress responses throughout the day.

Lemon Balm (Melissa officinalis) is celebrated for its ability to elevate mood and improve cognitive function. A refreshing lemon balm tea can be made by steeping 1-2 teaspoons of dried lemon balm leaves in boiling water for 10 minutes. This herb is gentle enough to be enjoyed throughout the day and is particularly beneficial during moments of heightened stress or when concentration is needed.

Passionflower (Passiflora incarnata) is effective in reducing anxiety and promoting sleep. For a passionflower tea, steep 1 teaspoon of dried passionflower in 1 cup of boiling water for 10 minutes. This tea is best consumed in the evening to prepare the body and mind for sleep.

When selecting herbs for emotional wellbeing, choosing high-quality, organic sources whenever possible is essential to ensure the absence of pesticides and contaminants. Dried herbs should be stored in airtight containers away from light and moisture to preserve their potency.

Incorporating these herbs into your daily routine requires mindfulness and consistency. Start with small doses to see how your body responds, and adjust accordingly. Always consult with a healthcare professional before beginning any new herbal regimen, especially if you are pregnant, nursing, or taking other medications.

Calming Herbs for Stress and Anxiety

In addressing the critical issue of stress and anxiety, the use of nervine herbs such as chamomile, valerian, and lemon balm presents a natural and effective approach to fostering emotional wellbeing. These herbs, known for their calming and uplifting properties, interact with the nervous system in a way that can significantly alleviate symptoms of stress and anxiety, promoting a sense of calm and relaxation.

Chamomile (Matricaria chamomilla), with its gentle sedative effects, is particularly beneficial for those experiencing difficulty sleeping or constant feelings of restlessness. To prepare a chamomile infusion, add 2 to 3 teaspoons of dried chamomile flowers to 1 cup of boiling water. Cover and steep for 10 minutes to ensure the volatile oils, which contribute to its soothing effects, are not lost to evaporation. Straining the tea and consuming it 30 minutes before bedtime can help ease the mind and prepare the body for a restful sleep. For those with a busy lifestyle, incorporating chamomile tea into the evening routine can serve as a simple yet powerful ritual to reduce stress and anxiety levels.

Valerian (Valeriana officinalis), another potent nervine, is renowned for its ability to improve sleep quality and reduce the time it takes to fall asleep. Unlike chamomile, valerian root has a more pronounced effect on severe insomnia and anxiety due to its interaction with gamma-aminobutyric acid (GABA), a neurotransmitter that regulates nerve impulses in your brain and nervous system. To harness valerian's full potential, take 1 teaspoon of dried valerian root and steep it in 1 cup of hot water for 15 minutes. It is recommended to drink valerian root tea 1 hour before bedtime. Given its strong flavor, mixing valerian root tea with honey or blending it with other herbs like chamomile and lemon balm can make it more palatable. Lemon balm (Melissa officinalis), with its uplifting and mood-enhancing properties, stands out as a versatile herb for combating anxiety and boosting cognitive function. For a refreshing lemon balm tea, use 1 to 2 teaspoons of dried lemon balm leaves per cup of boiling water, steeping for about 5 to 10 minutes. Lemon balm tea can be enjoyed throughout the day, especially during moments of heightened stress, to provide a calming effect without inducing drowsiness. Additionally, lemon balm can be combined with other herbs like chamomile and valerian to create a comprehensive herbal blend targeting both stress and sleep disturbances. When selecting herbs, opting for organic sources is crucial to avoid the intake of pesticides and chemicals that could undermine their health benefits. Dried herbs should be stored in airtight containers and placed in a cool, dark area to maintain their potency and effectiveness. Starting with small doses allows for monitoring the body's response, and adjustments can be made accordingly to achieve the desired therapeutic effect. Incorporating chamomile, valerian, and lemon balm into one's daily routine offers a holistic and integrative approach to managing stress and anxiety. Whether used individually or in combination, these nervine herbs provide a natural pathway to enhancing emotional wellbeing, underscoring the power of herbal medicine in supporting the body's inherent ability to heal and maintain balance.

Lavender and Lemon Balm Relaxation Tea A tea blend for calming the nerves.

Beneficial effects
Lavender and lemon balm tea is a soothing herbal blend known for its calming effects on the nervous system, making it an excellent choice for reducing stress and anxiety. Lavender is widely recognized for its ability to promote relaxation and improve sleep quality. Lemon balm, on the other hand, has been used traditionally to ease symptoms of stress, help with anxiety, and boost cognitive function. Together, these herbs create a powerful tea that can help calm the nerves and promote a sense of well-being.

Portions
Serves 2

Preparation time
5 minutes

Cooking time
10 minutes

Ingredients
- 1 tablespoon dried lavender flowers
- 2 tablespoons dried lemon balm leaves
- 2 cups boiling water
- Honey or stevia to taste (optional)
- Lemon slice for garnish (optional)

Instructions
1. Boil 2 cups of water in a kettle or a pot.
2. While the water is boiling, measure out 1 tablespoon of dried lavender flowers and 2 tablespoons of dried lemon balm leaves. Combine them in a tea infuser or teapot.
3. Once the water has reached a rolling boil, pour it over the lavender and lemon balm in the infuser or teapot.
4. Cover the teapot or infuser and let the herbs steep for about 5 to 10 minutes, depending on how strong you prefer your tea. The longer it steeps, the more potent the calming effects will be.
5. After steeping, remove the infuser or strain the tea to remove the loose herbs.
6. If desired, sweeten the tea with honey or stevia to taste. This step is optional and can be adjusted based on personal preference.
7. Serve the tea in cups and, if you like, garnish each cup with a slice of lemon for an extra touch of flavor and a hint of vitamin C.
8. Enjoy the tea in a quiet, comfortable setting for the maximum relaxation effect.

Variations
- For a cooler, refreshing version, allow the tea to cool completely and serve it over ice. This makes for a soothing summer beverage.
- Add a cinnamon stick to the pot while steeping for a warming, slightly spicy flavor that complements the floral notes of the lavender and the citrusy undertones of the lemon balm.

- Combine with chamomile flowers for an even more potent nighttime tea blend that can help improve sleep quality.

Storage tips

Any leftover tea can be stored in a sealed container in the refrigerator for up to 2 days. Reheat gently on the stove or enjoy cold for a refreshing drink.

Tips for allergens

For those with allergies or sensitivities to honey, stevia serves as a great alternative sweetener that does not trigger common allergic reactions.

Scientific references

- "Lavender and the Nervous System," published in Evidence-Based Complementary and Alternative Medicine, highlights lavender's anxiolytic (anxiety-reducing) effects.
- "Melissa officinalis L. (Lemon balm) – A Review on its Cognitive and Neuroprotective Effects," published in Phytotherapy Research, discusses lemon balm's positive impact on cognitive function and stress relief.

BOOK 4: ADVANCED HERBAL TECHNIQUES

CHAPTER 1: CRAFTING TINCTURES AND EXTRACTS

Alcohol and Glycerin Tincture Basics

Creating alcohol and glycerin tinctures involves a precise process of extracting the therapeutic compounds from herbs. This method preserves the active constituents, offering a long-lasting and convenient way to utilize herbal remedies. Here's a detailed guide to crafting your own tinctures.

Selecting Your Solvent: For alcohol-based tinctures, use a high-proof alcohol like vodka or brandy, ideally 80-100 proof (40-50% alcohol by volume) for optimal extraction and preservation. Glycerin, a non-alcoholic solvent, is a sweet, syrupy liquid ideal for those avoiding alcohol. It's less effective at extracting certain compounds but is excellent for creating child-friendly remedies.

Preparing the Herbs: Start with dried herbs, as water content in fresh herbs can dilute the tincture and encourage spoilage. Finely chop or grind your herbs to increase the surface area for better extraction.

Jar Selection: Choose a clean, dry glass jar with a tight-fitting lid. The size depends on the volume of tincture you wish to make, but a pint-sized mason jar is a good starting point.

Herb-to-Solvent Ratio: For dried herbs, a 1:5 herb-to-alcohol ratio by weight (e.g., 20 grams of herb to 100 milliliters of alcohol) is standard. For glycerin, a 1:8 ratio is recommended due to its lower solvency.

Mixing: Place your herbs in the jar, then pour the solvent over them, ensuring the herbs are completely submerged. If they float to the top, add more solvent, or gently stir to ensure all parts are in contact with the solvent.

Sealing and Storing: Seal the jar tightly to prevent evaporation. Label the jar with the herb name, type of solvent, and the date. Store the jar in a cool, dark place, shaking it daily to mix the herbs with the solvent.

Maceration Time: Allow the mixture to macerate for 4-6 weeks. This time allows the solvent to extract the active compounds from the herbs.

Straining: After maceration, strain the mixture through a fine mesh strainer or cheesecloth into another clean jar. Press or squeeze the herb material to extract as much liquid as possible.

Bottling: Transfer the strained tincture into dark glass dropper bottles for easy use. Label each bottle with the herb name, solvent type, and date of production.

Dosage: Tincture dosage can vary widely based on the herb, the condition being treated, and the individual. As a general guideline, 1-2 ml (20-40 drops) three times a day for adults is a common starting point. Consult with a healthcare professional for specific recommendations.

Storage: Store your tinctures in a cool, dark place. Alcohol-based tinctures have a shelf life of several years, while glycerin-based tinctures should be used within 1-2 years.

By following these steps, you can create potent and personalized herbal tinctures. This method allows you to harness the benefits of medicinal herbs in a concentrated, easy-to-use form, providing a valuable addition to your home apothecary.

Echinacea Immune-Boosting Tincture A recipe for creating a long-lasting extract.

Beneficial effects

Echinacea is renowned for its immune-boosting properties, making it a popular choice for preventing and fighting off colds and flu. It's believed to increase the body's production of white blood cells, which fight infections. This tincture, when taken at the onset of cold symptoms, can help reduce the severity and duration of the illness.

Portions

Makes about 1 cup (8 ounces)

Preparation time

10 minutes (plus 4-6 weeks for steeping)

Ingredients

- 1/2 cup dried echinacea purpurea (flowers and roots)
- 1 cup high-proof alcohol (such as vodka or brandy, at least 80 proof)
- 1 clean glass jar with a tight-fitting lid
- Cheesecloth or a fine mesh strainer
- Amber dropper bottles for storage

Instructions

1. Place the dried echinacea in the clean glass jar.
2. Pour the alcohol over the echinacea, ensuring the herbs are completely submerged. If they float to the top, use a clean spoon to press them down and release any trapped air bubbles.
3. Seal the jar tightly with the lid. Label the jar with the contents and the date.
4. Store the jar in a cool, dark place for 4-6 weeks. The back of a cupboard or a closet shelf away from direct sunlight is ideal. This allows the active compounds in the echinacea to infuse into the alcohol.
5. Shake the jar gently every few days to mix the contents and promote extraction.
6. After 4-6 weeks, open the jar and strain the tincture through a cheesecloth or fine mesh strainer into a clean bowl. Squeeze or press the cheesecloth to extract as much liquid as possible.
7. Transfer the strained tincture into amber dropper bottles for easy use and dosage. Label the bottles with the contents and the date of straining.
8. Discard the spent echinacea solids.

Variations

- For a non-alcoholic version, glycerin can be used in place of alcohol, though the extraction process may differ slightly and the shelf life will be shorter.
- Add other immune-supporting herbs such as elderberry, astragalus, or ginger to the tincture for added benefits. Adjust the proportions to ensure the primary focus remains on echinacea.

Storage tips

Store the echinacea tincture in a cool, dark place. Amber bottles help protect the tincture from light, preserving its potency. Properly stored, the tincture can last for several years.

Tips for allergens

For those with allergies to alcohol, a glycerin-based tincture offers a viable alternative. Ensure any additional herbs used in variations are also free from allergens specific to the individual's needs.

Scientific references

- "Echinacea for preventing and treating the common cold." This systematic review and meta-analysis, published in The Cochrane Database of Systematic Reviews, supports the use of echinacea in managing cold symptoms and reducing the duration of the illness.

CHAPTER 2: INFUSIONS, DECOCTIONS, SYRUPS

Infusions, decoctions, and syrups are foundational techniques in herbal medicine, each offering unique benefits and applications. Understanding how to properly prepare these can significantly enhance the potency and efficacy of your herbal remedies.

Infusions are akin to making tea but are often steeped for a longer period. They are ideal for extracting the volatile oils and other delicate constituents from softer plant parts like leaves, flowers, and aromatic herbs. To prepare an infusion, you'll need about one ounce of dried herb or two ounces of fresh herb per pint of boiling water. Place the herb in a heat-proof container, pour boiling water over it, and cover to prevent the escape of volatile oils. Steep for 15 to 20 minutes for leaves or flowers, and up to 4 hours for roots. Strain and consume or use as directed.

Decoctions involve simmering tougher plant materials such as roots, bark, and seeds to extract their active compounds. Begin by crushing or coarsely chopping the plant material to increase the surface area. Use one ounce of dried herb or two ounces of fresh herb per pint of water. Place the herb in a pot, add cold water, and slowly bring to a boil. Reduce heat and simmer gently, covered, for 20 to 45 minutes, depending on the toughness of the material. The liquid should reduce by about one-third. Strain and use as needed.

Syrups offer a palatable way to administer herbal remedies, especially beneficial for children or those averse to the taste of herbal preparations. To make a syrup, start with an infusion or decoction as your herbal base. Strain the liquid and measure its volume, then add an equal volume of honey or, for vegans, a suitable plant-based sweetener. Gently heat the mixture, stirring constantly, until the sweetener is fully dissolved. Do not boil. For preservation, add a small amount of brandy or vegetable glycerin—about one ounce for every ten ounces of syrup. Bottle in sterilized glass containers, label, and store in a cool, dark place or refrigerate for extended shelf life.

For all these preparations, it's crucial to use purified or distilled water to avoid contaminants that could affect the remedy's quality. Additionally, always label your creations with the date, ingredients, and dosage instructions. Proper storage is essential to maintain the potency of your herbal remedies. Infusions and decoctions are best used fresh but can be stored for a short period in the refrigerator, typically up to 48 hours. Syrups, due to their sugar content, have a longer shelf life and can be kept for several weeks to months when refrigerated.

By mastering these techniques, you can create a wide range of herbal remedies tailored to specific needs, ensuring you have the tools at hand to support health and wellness naturally.

Choosing the Right Method for Each Herb

When selecting the appropriate method for preparing herbal remedies, it's crucial to consider the specific properties and constituents of each herb. This decision impacts the effectiveness of the final product, whether it be an infusion, decoction, or syrup. Here, we'll delve into how to choose between water, alcohol, or honey as the solvent based on the herb in question.

Water is the most commonly used solvent for making infusions and decoctions. It's ideal for extracting water-soluble compounds such as flavonoids, vitamins, and minerals. For herbs with delicate parts like leaves and flowers, an **infusion** is best. Use one ounce of dried herb (or two ounces of fresh) per pint of boiling water. Steep leaves or flowers for 15 to 20 minutes, and roots for up to 4 hours to ensure all beneficial compounds are extracted. In contrast, **decoctions** are suited for tougher plant materials like roots, barks, and seeds. These require simmering in water for 20 to 45 minutes to break down hardy cell walls and release their active ingredients.

Alcohol serves as a powerful solvent for creating tinctures, capable of extracting both water-soluble and alcohol-soluble compounds, including alkaloids, terpenes, and resins. This makes it exceptionally versatile for a wide range of herbs. The ideal alcohol concentration is 40-50% (80-100 proof) for most herbs. When preparing a tincture, a general guideline is a 1:5 herb-to-alcohol ratio by weight for dried herbs. Alcohol-based tinctures are long-lasting, with a shelf life of several years, making them a convenient and effective way to preserve and consume herbal remedies.

Honey is not only a sweetener but also acts as a mild preservative and solvent, particularly in the preparation of syrups. It's best suited for herbs that are primarily used for their soothing properties, such as those targeting the throat and respiratory system. To make a syrup, begin with an herbal infusion or decoction as the base. After straining the liquid, measure its volume and add an equal amount of honey, warming the mixture just enough to blend the ingredients without boiling. Honey-based syrups are especially beneficial for children or anyone who might find the taste of other herbal preparations unpalatable. Adding a small amount of brandy or vegetable glycerin can extend the shelf life of your syrup.

In choosing the right solvent, consider the herb's key constituents and the desired effect of the remedy. **Water** is universally accessible and excellent for extracting a broad range of compounds, but it may not preserve the remedy as long as alcohol. **Alcohol** is unparalleled for its extraction capabilities and preservation qualities, making it ideal for tinctures that require long shelf lives. **Honey**, while not as potent a solvent, offers a sweet, palatable means to administer and preserve herbal remedies in the form of syrups. For each preparation, ensure to use purified or distilled water to avoid any contaminants that might affect the quality of your herbal remedy. When using alcohol, opt for high-proof vodka or brandy for the best preservation and extraction efficiency. And when choosing honey, select raw, organic varieties to maximize the therapeutic benefits.

Cough-Soothing Thyme and Honey Syrup A recipe for creating a syrup for respiratory health.

Beneficial effects
Thyme and honey syrup is a traditional remedy known for its cough-soothing and antimicrobial properties. Thyme contains compounds like thymol and carvacrol, which have been shown to relax the tracheal muscles (involved in coughing) and reduce inflammation. Honey, on the other hand, is well-regarded for its soothing effect on sore throats and its ability to suppress coughing, making it an excellent natural cough suppressant. Together, they create a powerful syrup that can alleviate coughs associated with colds and respiratory infections.

Portions
Makes about 1 cup

Preparation time
5 minutes

Cooking time
20 minutes

Ingredients
- 1 cup of water
- 2 tablespoons of dried thyme leaves
- 1 cup of raw honey

Instructions
1. Pour 1 cup of water into a small saucepan and bring it to a boil over medium-high heat.
2. Once the water is boiling, add 2 tablespoons of dried thyme leaves to the saucepan.
3. Reduce the heat to low and let the thyme simmer in the water for about 15 minutes. This process extracts the medicinal compounds from the thyme leaves.
4. After simmering, remove the saucepan from the heat and allow it to cool slightly, just enough so it's safe to handle but still warm.
5. Strain the thyme-infused water through a fine mesh sieve or cheesecloth into a heat-resistant bowl or measuring cup, pressing on the thyme leaves to extract as much liquid as possible. Discard the thyme leaves.
6. While the thyme infusion is still warm (but not hot, to preserve the beneficial enzymes in honey), add 1 cup of raw honey to the bowl.
7. Stir the mixture gently until the honey is completely dissolved into the thyme infusion.
8. Pour the finished syrup into a clean, dry glass bottle or jar with a tight-fitting lid.

Variations
- For added respiratory benefits, include a tablespoon of freshly grated ginger or a few slices of lemon during the simmering process. Both ginger and lemon have additional antimicrobial and immune-boosting properties.
- If you prefer a thinner syrup, you can adjust the water to honey ratio, using up to 1 1/4 cups of water for a less viscous consistency.

Storage tips

Store the thyme and honey syrup in the refrigerator in a tightly sealed container. It will keep for up to 2 months. For best results, label the container with the date it was made to keep track of its freshness.

Tips for allergens

For individuals with allergies to honey, a suitable alternative is agave syrup, although this may alter the flavor and medicinal properties slightly. Always ensure that the thyme used is free from contaminants and is sourced from a reputable supplier to avoid any potential allergic reactions.

Scientific references

- "Antibacterial and antifungal activities of thymol: A brief review of the literature" published in the Food Chemistry journal, which discusses thymol's antimicrobial properties.
- "Honey: A Therapeutic Agent for Disorders of the Upper Respiratory Tract" published in the Phytotherapy Research journal, highlighting honey's effectiveness in cough suppression and throat soothing.

CHAPTER 3: TOPICAL APPLICATIONS AND SKINCARE

Salves, Lotions, and Creams for Healing

Turning herbs into effective topical treatments such as salves, lotions, and creams for healing and hydration involves a meticulous process that harnesses the therapeutic properties of medicinal plants. These topical applications can provide relief for a variety of skin conditions, promote healing, and offer deep hydration. The key to creating potent and beneficial herbal skincare products lies in selecting the right herbs, understanding the base materials, and following precise preparation methods.

To begin, select herbs known for their skin-healing and hydrating properties. Calendula, for instance, is renowned for its ability to soothe and repair the skin, making it an excellent choice for salves aimed at healing cuts, burns, and rashes. Chamomile, with its anti-inflammatory properties, is ideal for lotions designed to calm irritated skin. For creams that moisturize and protect, shea butter and cocoa butter provide a rich, emollient base that deeply nourishes the skin, while herbs like aloe vera and lavender can add hydrating and soothing benefits.

The preparation of herbal oils is the foundational step in creating salves, lotions, and creams. Begin by infusing your chosen herbs in a carrier oil such as olive oil, coconut oil, or almond oil. This can be done through a slow infusion method, where herbs and oil are combined in a jar and left to infuse at room temperature for 4-6 weeks, or a quick infusion method, where the mixture is gently heated for a few hours on a low heat source to expedite the process. Strain the herbs from the oil using a fine mesh sieve or cheesecloth, ensuring all plant material is removed, leaving behind the infused oil rich in the plant's medicinal properties.

For salves, the next step involves combining the infused oil with beeswax, which acts as a thickening agent. A general guideline is to use approximately 1 ounce of beeswax per cup of infused oil. Gently heat the infused oil and beeswax together until the beeswax is completely melted, stirring to ensure a uniform mixture. At this point, essential oils can be added for additional therapeutic benefits and fragrance. Pour the mixture into containers and allow it to cool and solidify.

Creating lotions requires an emulsion of water and oil. With your herbal infused oil prepared, combine it with distilled water at a ratio that suits your desired consistency, typically starting with equal parts oil and water. To bind the oil and water together, an emulsifier such as emulsifying wax is necessary. Heat the oil and emulsifying wax together until the wax is melted, then slowly add the heated water phase while vigorously mixing until the lotion begins to thicken and cool. Essential oils and preservatives can be added to enhance the lotion's properties and extend its shelf life.

Creams follow a similar process to lotions but typically have a higher oil content, creating a thicker, more luxurious product. The process of heating and combining the oil, water, and emulsifying wax is the same, but with a greater proportion of oil to water. This results in a richer cream that is especially beneficial for dry or damaged skin.

Throughout the preparation of salves, lotions, and creams, maintaining cleanliness and preventing contamination is crucial. Use sterilized equipment, work in a clean environment, and consider incorporating natural preservatives such as vitamin E oil or grapefruit seed extract to extend the shelf life of your products. By carefully selecting herbs with specific healing properties, understanding the roles of base materials, and adhering to precise preparation techniques, you can create effective topical herbal treatments. These salves, lotions, and creams not only offer therapeutic benefits but also provide a natural and holistic approach to skin care and hydration.

Calendula and Comfrey Healing Salve A DIY salve for wounds and rashes.

Beneficial effects

Calendula and comfrey are both renowned for their healing properties, particularly when it comes to skin care. Calendula is celebrated for its anti-inflammatory, antimicrobial, and astringent qualities, making it an excellent choice for soothing cuts, wounds, and rashes. Comfrey, on the other hand, contains allantoin, a compound that promotes cell regeneration and can significantly speed up the healing process of the skin. Together, these herbs create a powerful salve that can reduce healing time, soothe irritated skin, and prevent infection.

Portions

Makes approximately 8 ounces
Preparation time
15 minutes
Cooking time
1 hour
Ingredients
- 1/2 cup dried calendula flowers
- 1/2 cup dried comfrey leaves
- 1 cup coconut oil
- 1/2 cup beeswax pellets
- 10 drops lavender essential oil (optional for added antimicrobial and soothing properties)
- 1 teaspoon vitamin E oil (optional for added skin nourishment and preservative qualities)
- Cheesecloth or fine mesh strainer
- Clean, dry jars or tins for storage
Instructions
1. Begin by combining the dried calendula flowers and comfrey leaves with the coconut oil in a double boiler. If you don't have a double boiler, you can place a heat-safe bowl over a pot of simmering water.
2. Heat the mixture over low heat for about 1 hour to allow the herbs to infuse into the oil. Stir occasionally to ensure even heating and prevent burning.
3. After the infusion process, remove the mixture from heat and let it cool slightly for a few minutes.
4. Place the cheesecloth or fine mesh strainer over a clean bowl and pour the mixture through it to strain out the plant material. Press or squeeze the herbs to extract as much oil as possible. Discard the used herbs.
5. Return the infused oil to the double boiler and add the beeswax pellets. Heat gently, stirring constantly, until the beeswax is completely melted and combined with the oil.
6. Remove from heat and let the mixture cool for a couple of minutes before adding the optional lavender essential oil and vitamin E oil. Stir well to ensure all ingredients are evenly distributed.
7. Carefully pour the liquid salve into clean, dry jars or tins. Allow the salve to cool and solidify completely before sealing with lids.
8. Label your containers with the contents and date made.
Variations
- For a vegan version, replace beeswax with an equal amount of candelilla wax or soy wax.
- Add other healing essential oils like tea tree or chamomile for different therapeutic effects.
Storage tips
Store the salve in a cool, dark place. The shelf life will be approximately 1-2 years if stored properly. If the salve shows any signs of spoilage, discard it.
Tips for allergens
For those with coconut oil sensitivities, olive oil or almond oil can be used as a substitute. Always patch test before applying to larger areas of skin, especially if you have sensitive skin or are prone to allergies.
Scientific references
- "Anti-inflammatory and wound healing activity of a growth substance in Aloe vera," published in the Journal of the American Podiatric Medical Association, highlights the healing properties of herbal ingredients similar to those found in calendula and comfrey.
- "Comfrey: A Clinical Overview," published in Phytotherapy Research, discusses the efficacy of comfrey in skin regeneration and wound healing.

BOOK 5: HERBAL REMEDIES FOR DIGESTIVE HEALTH

CHAPTER 1: CARMINATIVES AND DIGESTIVE TONICS

Carminatives and digestive tonics play a crucial role in maintaining digestive health by soothing the digestive tract, reducing gas, and stimulating digestion. Understanding how to incorporate these herbs into your daily regimen can significantly enhance your digestive wellness. Here, we delve into the specifics of selecting, preparing, and utilizing these powerful natural remedies.

Carminatives are herbs that help reduce gas and bloating in the digestive system. They work by relaxing the digestive tract muscles, which facilitates the release of trapped gas and eases discomfort. Common carminative herbs include **Peppermint**, **Fennel**, **Ginger**, and **Chamomile**. These herbs can be used in various forms, such as teas, tinctures, or capsules, depending on your preference and the specific herb's properties.

To prepare a **Peppermint Tea**, which is renowned for its soothing effect on the digestive system, you'll need:
- 1-2 teaspoons of dried peppermint leaves
- 8 ounces of boiling water

Steep the peppermint leaves in boiling water for 5-10 minutes, depending on the desired strength. Strain the leaves and enjoy the tea either hot or cold. This tea is particularly beneficial after meals to aid digestion and prevent gas and bloating.

Fennel Seeds are another excellent carminative that can be chewed directly after meals or used to make a digestive tea. To make **Fennel Tea**:
- Crush 1 teaspoon of fennel seeds to release their oil.
- Pour 8 ounces of boiling water over the crushed seeds.
- Allow the tea to steep for 10-15 minutes before straining.

This tea is effective in relieving gas and bloating and can be consumed 2-3 times a day as needed.

Ginger is a potent digestive aid that can be used fresh, dried, or in powdered form. To make a simple **Ginger Digestive Tonic**:
- Slice 1 inch of fresh ginger root.
- Boil the slices in 2 cups of water for 10 minutes.
- Strain the ginger pieces from the water and add honey or lemon to taste if desired.

This tonic can be consumed before meals to stimulate digestion or after meals to ease discomfort.

Digestive Tonics are formulations designed to strengthen and tone the digestive system, improving overall digestive function. They often contain a blend of herbs that work synergistically to enhance digestion, absorption, and elimination. Common ingredients in digestive tonics include **Bitter Herbs** such as **Dandelion Root**, **Gentian Root**, and **Burdock Root**. These herbs stimulate digestive secretions and promote the body's natural digestive processes.

To create a **Basic Digestive Tonic**:
- Combine equal parts of dried dandelion root, gentian root, and burdock root.
- Use 1 teaspoon of this herbal blend per cup of boiling water.
- Steep for 15-20 minutes and strain.

This tonic can be consumed 15-30 minutes before meals to prepare the digestive system for food intake.

Incorporating carminatives and digestive tonics into your daily routine can significantly improve digestive health and comfort. Always start with small doses to assess your body's response, and adjust accordingly. For those with chronic digestive issues, consulting with a healthcare professional before adding new herbal remedies to your regimen is advisable. Remember, the key to effective herbal treatment is consistency and patience, as the benefits accumulate over time.

How Carminative Herbs Soothe the Gut

Carminative herbs play a pivotal role in soothing the gut by facilitating the expulsion of gas from the intestines, thereby alleviating bloating and discomfort. These herbs contain specific compounds that relax the gastrointestinal tract's muscles, enhancing digestion and preventing the formation of gas. The mechanism through which carminative herbs exert their effects involves several key actions, including the stimulation of digestive enzymes, calming of the digestive tract, and reduction of spasms in the gut muscles.

One of the primary ways carminative herbs soothe the gut is through their volatile oils. These oils, found in herbs such as **peppermint**, **fennel**, and **ginger**, are released during digestion. They act directly on the smooth muscle of the digestive tract, causing relaxation and reducing spasms that can trap gas and cause discomfort. For instance, peppermint oil contains menthol, which has a relaxing effect on the gut's smooth muscle. To harness this benefit, one might prepare a peppermint tea by steeping 1 teaspoon of dried peppermint leaves in 1 cup of boiling water for 10 minutes, then straining and drinking the tea 20 minutes before meals to aid digestion and gas expulsion.

Furthermore, carminative herbs stimulate the production of digestive enzymes, which play a crucial role in breaking down food more efficiently, thus reducing the likelihood of gas formation. Fennel, for example, not only helps in expelling gas but also in the production of gastric enzymes. A simple way to incorporate fennel into the diet is by chewing on half a teaspoon of fennel seeds after meals or preparing a fennel tea by steeping 1 to 2 teaspoons of crushed fennel seeds in boiling water.

Another aspect of how carminative herbs aid in soothing the gut is through their anti-inflammatory properties. Inflammation in the gastrointestinal tract can lead to discomfort and impaired digestion, leading to gas buildup. Herbs like **ginger** contain compounds such as gingerols, which have been shown to reduce inflammation in the gut. A ginger tea can be made by slicing a 1-inch piece of fresh ginger and steeping it in boiling water for 5 to 10 minutes, which can be consumed before meals to aid digestion and reduce inflammation.

In addition to their direct effects on the gut, carminative herbs also have a calming effect on the nervous system, which can indirectly benefit digestion. Stress and anxiety can disrupt normal digestive processes, leading to issues like gas and bloating. Herbs such as **chamomile** are known for their soothing properties on the nervous system, which can, in turn, promote healthier digestive function. A chamomile tea made by steeping 1 tablespoon of dried chamomile flowers in 1 cup of boiling water for 5 minutes can be consumed in the evening to promote relaxation and support digestive health.

Fennel and Mint Digestive Tea

Beneficial effects

Fennel and mint digestive tea combines the soothing properties of mint with the digestive support of fennel seeds. Mint is known for its ability to ease digestive discomfort and reduce symptoms of irritable bowel syndrome, such as bloating and indigestion. Fennel seeds, on the other hand, have been traditionally used to treat various digestive ailments, including gas, bloating, and cramps. This tea serves as a natural remedy to promote healthy digestion and provide relief from digestive discomfort.

Portions

Serves 2

Preparation time

5 minutes

Cooking time

10 minutes

Ingredients

- 1 tablespoon dried mint leaves
- 1 tablespoon fennel seeds
- 2 cups boiling water
- Honey or lemon (optional, for taste)

Instructions

1. Begin by boiling 2 cups of water in a kettle or a saucepan.
2. While the water is heating, take a tablespoon of dried mint leaves and a tablespoon of fennel seeds. If you have a mortar and pestle, lightly crush the fennel seeds to release their oils and flavor, enhancing the tea's digestive benefits.
3. Place the mint leaves and crushed fennel seeds into a teapot or a heat-resistant pitcher.
4. Once the water has reached a rolling boil, pour it over the mint leaves and fennel seeds in the teapot or pitcher.
5. Cover the teapot or pitcher with a lid or a small plate to retain the heat and allow the herbs to steep. Let them infuse for about 10 minutes. The longer you steep, the stronger the flavor and therapeutic properties will be.
6. After steeping, strain the tea into two cups, removing the mint leaves and fennel seeds.

7. If desired, add honey or a squeeze of lemon to each cup for additional flavor. Honey can soothe the throat and add a natural sweetness, while lemon adds a refreshing citrus note and vitamin C.

Variations
- For a cooler, refreshing version, allow the tea to cool completely and then refrigerate. Serve over ice for a soothing summer beverage.
- Add a slice of fresh ginger during the steeping process for an extra digestive boost and a warming flavor.
- Combine with chamomile flowers for an even more relaxing and digestive-friendly tea blend.

Storage tips
If you have leftover tea, it can be stored in a sealed container in the refrigerator for up to 2 days. Enjoy it cold, or gently reheat on the stove or in a microwave.

Tips for allergens
For those with allergies or sensitivities to honey, stevia or maple syrup can serve as sweetener alternatives. Always ensure that the herbs used are sourced from reputable suppliers to avoid contamination with allergens.

Scientific references
- "Peppermint Oil for the Treatment of Irritable Bowel Syndrome: A Systematic Review and Meta-analysis," published in the Journal of Clinical Gastroenterology, highlights the benefits of peppermint (mint) in digestive health.
- "Effect of Fennel (Foeniculum Vulgare) Used in the Treatment of Gastrointestinal Disorders: A Systematic Review," found in the World Journal of Gastrointestinal Pharmacology and Therapeutics, discusses the digestive benefits of fennel seeds.

Detoxifying Herbs for Digestive Health

Detoxifying herbs play a crucial role in supporting digestive health by aiding the liver and gallbladder in their essential functions of cleansing and bile production, respectively. These organs are pivotal in the detoxification process, breaking down toxins and facilitating their safe elimination from the body. Incorporating specific herbs into your wellness routine can enhance this natural detoxification, contributing to improved digestive health and overall well-being.

Milk Thistle (Silybum marianum) is renowned for its hepatoprotective properties, primarily due to the active compound silymarin. Silymarin acts as an antioxidant, protecting liver cells from damage by toxins and facilitating the regeneration of damaged liver tissue. For optimal benefits, look for a standardized extract containing 70% to 80% silymarin. The recommended dosage is 100 to 200 mg, taken twice daily with meals. Ensure the product is encapsulated or in tablet form to protect the active compounds from degradation.

Dandelion Root (Taraxacum officinale) supports liver function by stimulating bile production, which is essential for detoxification and fat metabolism. A simple way to incorporate dandelion root is by preparing a decoction. Add 1 to 2 teaspoons of dried root to 8 ounces of water in a small saucepan. Bring to a boil, then simmer gently for 15 to 20 minutes. Strain and drink the tea up to three times daily. For those who prefer convenience, dandelion root is also available in tincture form; use 1 to 2 ml three times daily.

Turmeric (Curcuma longa) contains curcumin, a compound that enhances the liver's ability to detoxify chemicals. To incorporate turmeric into your diet, you can add the powdered root to foods or take a supplement. When choosing a supplement, select one that contains piperine (black pepper extract) to enhance absorption. The recommended dosage is 400 to 600 mg of standardized curcumin extract three times daily.

Artichoke Leaf (Cynara scolymus) has been shown to stimulate bile production, which helps to remove toxins from the body and aid in fat digestion. Artichoke leaf extract can be taken in capsule form, with a typical dosage of 300 to 600 mg daily. Look for products standardized to contain 5% cynarin for consistency in potency.

Burdock Root (Arctium lappa) is another herb that supports detoxification through its diuretic properties, helping to eliminate toxins through increased urine production. Additionally, it contains inulin, a prebiotic that promotes healthy gut flora. To prepare a burdock root tea, steep 1 teaspoon of the dried root in 8 ounces of boiling water for 10 to 15 minutes. Drink this tea up to three times a day. Alternatively, burdock root can be consumed as a tincture, with a general recommendation of 2 to 4 ml three times daily.

When incorporating these herbs into your regimen, it's important to start with lower doses and gradually increase to the recommended dosage to assess your body's response. Always consult with a healthcare provider before beginning any new supplement, especially if you have existing health conditions or are taking medications, to ensure there are no contraindications or potential interactions.

Dandelion Root Detox Tea

Beneficial effects

Dandelion Root Detox Tea is a natural and effective way to support liver and gallbladder health. Dandelion root has been traditionally used for its diuretic properties, helping to flush toxins from the liver and gallbladder. It also supports digestion and can help reduce inflammation. This tea is a gentle way to aid the body's natural detoxification processes, promoting overall wellness.

Portions

Serves 2

Preparation time

10 minutes

Cooking time

5 minutes

Ingredients

- 2 tablespoons of dried dandelion root
- 4 cups of water
- Honey or lemon to taste (optional)

Instructions

1. Measure 4 cups of water into a medium-sized saucepan and bring to a boil over high heat.
2. Once the water is boiling, add 2 tablespoons of dried dandelion root to the saucepan.
3. Reduce the heat to low and let the dandelion root simmer for about 5 minutes. This allows the water to become infused with the dandelion root's beneficial properties.
4. After simmering, remove the saucepan from the heat and let the tea steep for an additional 5 minutes. This extra time helps to extract more of the dandelion root's flavors and therapeutic compounds.
5. Strain the tea through a fine mesh sieve into a large pitcher or directly into serving cups, discarding the used dandelion root.
6. If desired, add honey or a squeeze of lemon to each cup for additional flavor. Honey can provide a soothing sweetness, while lemon adds a refreshing tang and can enhance the detoxifying effects.
7. Serve the tea warm, or allow it to cool and serve over ice for a refreshing detox beverage.

Variations

- For an extra detox boost, add a slice of fresh ginger to the saucepan along with the dandelion root. Ginger has its own detoxifying properties and can add a warming, spicy flavor to the tea.
- Combine with milk thistle tea for additional liver support. Milk thistle is another herb known for its beneficial effects on liver health.
- For a sweeter, more complex flavor, add a cinnamon stick during the simmering process.

Storage tips

Any leftover tea can be stored in a sealed container in the refrigerator for up to 3 days. Reheat gently on the stove or enjoy cold for a refreshing detox drink.

Tips for allergens

For those with allergies or sensitivities to honey, stevia or maple syrup can serve as sweetener alternatives. Ensure any additional herbs or spices used are free from allergens specific to the individual's needs.

Scientific references

- "The Diuretic Effect in Human Subjects of an Extract of Taraxacum officinale Folium over a Single Day" published in the Journal of Alternative and Complementary Medicine, which discusses the diuretic properties of dandelion.
- "Taraxacum officinale and related species—An ethnopharmacological review and its potential as a commercial medicinal plant" published in the Journal of Ethnopharmacology, highlighting the various medicinal benefits of dandelion, including liver support.

Mucilage-Rich Herbs for Digestive Health

Mucilage-rich herbs have emerged as a cornerstone in the natural management of digestive disorders such as Irritable Bowel Syndrome (IBS) and Leaky Gut Syndrome. These herbs contain a polysaccharide substance known as mucilage, which becomes a slick gel when mixed with water. This gelatinous material coats and soothes the mucous membranes of the gastrointestinal tract, providing a protective barrier against acidity and irritation, which can be particularly beneficial for those suffering from IBS and Leaky Gut.

Marshmallow root (Althaea officinalis) is a prime example of a mucilage-rich herb with a long history of use in digestive health. To harness its benefits, one can prepare a cold infusion by soaking 1 to 2 tablespoons of dried marshmallow root in about 4 cups of cold water overnight. This method allows for the extraction of mucilage without the heat that can destroy its soothing properties. The next day, strain the mixture and drink it on an empty stomach to maximize absorption and effectiveness. This preparation helps in reducing inflammation and soothing the lining of the digestive tract.

Slippery elm (Ulmus rubra) is another herb known for its high mucilage content. A simple way to incorporate slippery elm into your diet is by preparing a gruel. Mix 1 tablespoon of slippery elm powder with 2 cups of hot water. Stir well until the mixture thickens. If desired, you can add natural sweeteners like honey or maple syrup for taste. Consuming this gruel can aid in healing the gut lining by providing a protective layer and reducing inflammation.

Licorice root (Glycyrrhiza glabra), beyond its mucilage content, contains glycyrrhizin, which has anti-inflammatory and immune-boosting properties. To make a licorice root tea, add 1 teaspoon of dried licorice root to a cup of boiling water and steep for about 10 minutes. It's important to note that licorice root can elevate blood pressure in some individuals, so it's advisable to use deglycyrrhizinated licorice (DGL), which has the glycyrrhizin removed, to avoid this side effect.

Plantain seeds (Plantago spp.), not to be confused with the banana-like fruit, also contain mucilage and can be used to soothe the digestive tract. A simple way to use plantain seeds is by adding them to smoothies or making a tea. To prepare the tea, steep 1 teaspoon of plantain seeds in a cup of hot water for 10 to 15 minutes. This tea can be consumed several times a day to help reduce gut inflammation and irritation.

Aloe vera, widely recognized for its healing properties on the skin, also contains mucilage and can be beneficial for digestive health when taken internally. The inner gel of the aloe vera leaf can be extracted and mixed with water or juice. Consuming 2 to 4 ounces of aloe vera gel daily can help soothe the lining of the digestive tract and promote healing. However, it's crucial to ensure that the aloe product is free from aloin, a compound found in the outer leaf that can be irritating to the digestive system.

When incorporating mucilage-rich herbs into your regimen for IBS and Leaky Gut, it's essential to start with small doses and gradually increase to the recommended amounts to monitor your body's response. Additionally, maintaining hydration is crucial when consuming mucilage-rich herbs, as they absorb water and can otherwise lead to dehydration. Always consult with a healthcare provider before beginning any new treatment, especially if you have existing health conditions or are taking medications, to ensure safety and appropriateness.

Marshmallow Root Gut-Soothing Powder

Beneficial effects

Marshmallow root powder is renowned for its high mucilage content, which provides a soothing protective layer on the digestive tract. This can be particularly beneficial for individuals suffering from conditions like irritable bowel syndrome (IBS), leaky gut syndrome, and other forms of digestive irritation or inflammation. The mucilage can help to reduce gut inflammation, ease digestion, and promote the healing of the mucous membranes. Additionally, marshmallow root has been shown to support healthy gut flora, further aiding in digestive health.

Ingredients
- 1/4 cup dried marshmallow root
- 1 cup filtered water for grinding (optional)
- A coffee grinder or mortar and pestle

Instructions

1. Begin by ensuring the dried marshmallow root is finely chopped or broken into small pieces. This will facilitate a more uniform grinding process.

2. If using a coffee grinder, place the dried marshmallow root inside and grind it to a fine powder. If a mortar and pestle is being used, grind the pieces with consistent pressure until a fine powder is achieved. The goal is to create a powder that is as fine as possible to maximize its surface area for better mucilage release.

3. (Optional) For those preferring a slightly moist powder for immediate use, gradually add filtered water, a teaspoon at a time, to the ground marshmallow root in a bowl. Stir continuously until a paste-like consistency is achieved. This can be directly mixed into teas or warm water.

4. Transfer the marshmallow root powder (dry or moist) into a small, airtight container for storage.

Variations

- To enhance the gut-soothing effects, you can mix the marshmallow root powder with other digestive-friendly herbs such as slippery elm or licorice root powder. Use equal parts of each herb for a balanced blend.
- For an added flavor and digestive boost, mix in a small amount of cinnamon or ginger powder.

Storage tips

Store the marshmallow root powder in an airtight container in a cool, dry place. If kept dry, the powder can last for several months without losing its potency. If you've prepared a moist version, it's best used within a week and kept refrigerated to maintain freshness.

Tips for allergens

For individuals with specific plant allergies, ensure that the marshmallow root has been sourced from a supplier that avoids cross-contamination with other herbs or plants. Always start with a small dose to test for any adverse reactions, especially when mixing with other herbs.

Scientific references

- "The effect of herbal medicines on the inflammation of mucous membranes" published in the Journal of Phytotherapy Research, which discusses the soothing properties of marshmallow root on the digestive tract.
- "Prebiotic potential of herbal medicines used in digestive health and disease" found in the Journal of Gastroenterology, highlights the support marshmallow root provides to healthy gut flora.

BOOK 6: RESPIRATORY HEALTH

CHAPTER 1: DECONGESTANTS AND MUCOLYTICS

Clear Airways Naturally

To effectively clear airways naturally, employing a combination of herbal remedies known for their decongestant and mucolytic properties can be highly beneficial. These herbs work by thinning mucus and facilitating its expulsion, thereby relieving congestion and improving respiratory function. Here is a detailed guide on how to utilize these herbs for respiratory health.

Eucalyptus (Eucalyptus globulus) is renowned for its potent decongestant capabilities. To harness its benefits, add 2 to 3 drops of eucalyptus essential oil to a bowl of hot water. Cover your head with a towel, lean over the bowl, and inhale the steam for 5 to 10 minutes. The steam inhalation process helps to loosen mucus, allowing for easier breathing. Ensure the water is not boiling at the moment of inhalation to avoid steam burns.

Thyme (Thymus vulgaris) possesses expectorant properties that can aid in clearing mucus from the airways. Prepare a thyme infusion by steeping 1 teaspoon of dried thyme leaves in 1 cup of boiling water for 10 minutes. Strain and drink this tea up to three times daily. Thyme's active compounds, such as thymol, help in thinning the mucus and facilitating its removal from the respiratory tract.

Peppermint (Mentha piperita) contains menthol, a compound that helps soothe sore throats and acts as a natural decongestant. To make a peppermint tea, steep 1 tablespoon of dried peppermint leaves in 1 cup of boiling water for 10 minutes. Strain and drink up to twice daily. Alternatively, you can add a few drops of peppermint essential oil to a diffuser to help clear nasal passages.

Mullein (Verbascum thapsus) is beneficial for its mucilage content and soothing properties, making it ideal for irritated respiratory tracts. Prepare a mullein leaf tea by adding 1 to 2 teaspoons of dried mullein leaves to 1 cup of boiling water. Let it steep for 10 to 15 minutes, then strain to remove any fine hairs. Drinking this tea can help in reducing respiratory congestion.

Licorice Root (Glycyrrhiza glabra) acts as an expectorant, helping to loosen and expel mucus, while also soothing the respiratory system. Brew a licorice root tea by steeping 1 teaspoon of dried licorice root in 1 cup of boiling water for 10 minutes. Strain and consume the tea once daily. Note that licorice root should be avoided by individuals with high blood pressure, pregnant women, or those on certain medications due to potential health risks and interactions.

For those looking to integrate these remedies into their daily routine, it's important to start with small doses to monitor the body's response. Gradually increasing to the recommended amounts can help ensure tolerance and effectiveness. Additionally, maintaining adequate hydration is crucial when using mucolytic herbs, as fluid intake can further aid in thinning mucus and facilitating its expulsion.

When selecting herbs, opt for high-quality, organic sources to ensure the absence of contaminants that could irritate the respiratory system. For essential oils, choose therapeutic-grade oils that are safe for inhalation and free from synthetic additives.

Incorporating these herbal remedies into your respiratory health regimen can offer natural and effective relief from congestion and mucus buildup. Remember, while these natural approaches can be highly beneficial, they should complement and not replace the advice of a healthcare professional, especially in cases of chronic respiratory conditions or acute infections.

Thyme and Eucalyptus Vapor Rub

Beneficial effects

Thyme and eucalyptus vapor rub harnesses the powerful antimicrobial and decongestant properties of both thyme and eucalyptus, making it an effective remedy for relieving symptoms of the common cold, such as congestion and coughing. Thyme contains thymol, an essential oil with strong antiseptic abilities, which can help reduce coughs by relaxing the muscles of the trachea. Eucalyptus oil, on the other hand, is widely recognized for its ability to clear nasal passages, ease breathing, and combat respiratory infections.

Ingredients

- ¼ cup coconut oil
- ¼ cup olive oil
- ¼ cup grated beeswax
- 20 drops eucalyptus essential oil

- 10 drops thyme essential oil
- 5 drops peppermint essential oil (optional for extra cooling effect)
- Small glass jar or metal tin for storage

Instructions

1. Begin by setting up a double boiler. Fill a medium saucepan with about 2 inches of water and place it on the stove over medium heat. Allow the water to reach a simmer.

2. In a heat-resistant bowl that fits snugly over the saucepan without touching the water, combine the coconut oil, olive oil, and grated beeswax. The gentle heat from the simmering water below will melt the mixture.

3. Stir the mixture occasionally with a heat-resistant spatula or spoon until the beeswax is completely melted and the oils have combined, forming a uniform liquid.

4. Once melted, carefully remove the bowl from the heat. Allow the mixture to cool for a few minutes but not solidify.

5. Add the eucalyptus, thyme, and optional peppermint essential oils to the slightly cooled mixture. Stir well to ensure the essential oils are evenly distributed throughout the mixture.

6. Pour the mixture into a small glass jar or metal tin. Allow it to cool and solidify completely at room temperature. This may take several hours.

7. Once solidified, seal the container with a lid to prevent the essential oils from evaporating.

Variations

- For sensitive skin, reduce the amount of essential oils by half to test for skin sensitivity.
- Add lavender essential oil for its soothing properties and a pleasant aroma.
- For a vegan version, replace beeswax with an equal amount of candelilla wax.

Storage tips

Store the vapor rub in a cool, dry place away from direct sunlight. The shelf life is approximately 1 year. If the rub changes in smell, color, or texture, it should be discarded.

Tips for allergens

Individuals with sensitivities to eucalyptus or thyme should perform a patch test before applying the rub extensively. For those allergic to coconut oil, an alternative carrier oil such as almond oil can be used. Always ensure that the essential oils used are 100% pure and free from additives that could cause allergic reactions.

CHAPTER 2: CHRONIC RESPIRATORY CONDITIONS

Chronic respiratory conditions, such as asthma, chronic obstructive pulmonary disease (COPD), and bronchitis, require a nuanced approach to management and treatment. Herbal remedies can play a supportive role in alleviating symptoms and improving lung health. It's crucial to understand the properties of each herb and how they can be used effectively to support respiratory health.

Mullein (Verbascum thapsus) is renowned for its expectorant properties, making it beneficial for expelling respiratory tract congestion. For individuals with chronic bronchitis or COPD, a daily tea made from mullein leaves can help reduce mucus buildup. To prepare, steep 1-2 teaspoons of dried mullein leaves in boiling water for 10-15 minutes. Strain and drink up to three times daily.

Licorice Root (Glycyrrhiza glabra) has anti-inflammatory and demulcent properties, offering soothing relief for irritated throat and bronchial tissues. It's particularly useful for those with dry, non-productive coughs. Create a licorice root decoction by simmering one teaspoon of the root in a cup of water for 10-15 minutes. It's recommended to consume this decoction once daily. Note: Licorice root is not recommended for individuals with high blood pressure, kidney disease, or those who are pregnant.

Ginger (Zingiber officinale), with its potent anti-inflammatory effects, can help reduce airway inflammation and inhibit airway contraction. A simple ginger tea, made by steeping fresh ginger slices in boiling water for several minutes, can be consumed throughout the day to harness these benefits.

Turmeric (Curcuma longa) contains curcumin, a compound with strong anti-inflammatory properties that can help reduce inflammation in the airways. Adding turmeric to meals or taking it as a supplement can be beneficial. For a therapeutic drink, mix 1 teaspoon of turmeric powder with a glass of warm milk or plant-based milk and drink once daily.

Peppermint (Mentha piperita) is another herb that can provide relief from respiratory symptoms due to its menthol content, which helps relax the muscles of the respiratory tract. Peppermint tea can be made by steeping dried peppermint leaves in boiling water for 10 minutes. Drinking this tea 2-3 times a day can help alleviate symptoms of congestion and promote easier breathing.

Eucalyptus (Eucalyptus globulus) is widely used for its decongestant properties. Eucalyptus oil can be added to a diffuser or a few drops placed in a bowl of hot water for steam inhalation. This method helps clear the airways and reduce congestion. However, eucalyptus oil should be used with caution, especially around young children and pets.

Thyme (Thymus vulgaris) has been traditionally used for respiratory conditions due to its antiseptic and expectorant properties. A thyme tea can be prepared by steeping dried thyme leaves in boiling water for 10 minutes. This tea can be consumed 2-3 times daily to help relieve cough and congestion.

When incorporating herbal remedies into a treatment plan for chronic respiratory conditions, it's important to consult with a healthcare provider, especially for those already taking prescribed medications. Herbs can interact with medications and may not be suitable for everyone. Additionally, managing chronic respiratory conditions often requires a comprehensive approach that includes medication, lifestyle changes, and possibly physical therapy. Herbal remedies can complement this approach by providing symptomatic relief and supporting overall lung health.

Mullein Lung-Healing Tea
Beneficial effects
Mullein tea is celebrated for its soothing properties on the respiratory system, making it an excellent choice for those dealing with chronic respiratory conditions such as bronchitis, asthma, and general lung discomfort. The active compounds in mullein, like saponins, flavonoids, and mucilage, contribute to its expectorant, anti-inflammatory, and demulcent actions. This means it can help in loosening mucus, reducing inflammation, and soothing irritated tissues in the respiratory tract.

Portions
Serves 2
Preparation time
5 minutes
Cooking time

15 minutes

Ingredients

- 2 tablespoons dried mullein leaves
- 4 cups of water
- 1 teaspoon honey (optional, for taste)
- 1 teaspoon lemon juice (optional, for added vitamin C and flavor)

Instructions

1. Begin by bringing 4 cups of water to a boil in a medium-sized pot.
2. While the water is heating, measure out 2 tablespoons of dried mullein leaves. Ensure the leaves are crumbled to increase the surface area for infusion, which maximizes the release of beneficial compounds.
3. Once the water reaches a rolling boil, reduce the heat to a simmer and add the mullein leaves to the pot. Cover the pot with a lid to prevent the escape of volatile compounds.
4. Allow the mullein leaves to simmer gently for about 10 to 15 minutes. This slow simmering process helps to extract the mucilage, flavonoids, and other therapeutic compounds from the leaves.
5. After simmering, remove the pot from the heat and let it sit, covered, for an additional 5 minutes to further steep.
6. Strain the tea through a fine mesh strainer or a piece of cheesecloth into a large pitcher or directly into tea cups. This step is crucial to remove the fine hairs found on mullein leaves, which can be irritating to the throat.
7. If desired, stir in a teaspoon of honey to sweeten the tea and add a teaspoon of lemon juice for a vitamin C boost and to enhance the flavor.

Variations

- For added respiratory support, include a pinch of dried ginger or turmeric in the tea while simmering. Both spices are known for their anti-inflammatory properties.
- Combine mullein with other respiratory-supportive herbs such as licorice root or marshmallow root for a more potent herbal remedy.

Storage tips

If you have leftover tea, it can be stored in a sealed container in the refrigerator for up to 2 days. Reheat gently on the stove or enjoy cold, though warm tea is more soothing for respiratory issues.

Tips for allergens

For those with allergies to honey, maple syrup or agave nectar make suitable substitutes. Always ensure that the mullein leaves are sourced from a reputable supplier to avoid contamination with allergens.

Scientific references

- "Pharmacological activity of Verbascum thapsus (Mullein): An anti-inflammatory and analgesic agent," published in the Phytotherapy Research journal, highlights the anti-inflammatory properties of mullein.

CHAPTER 3: SEASONAL ALLERGIES

Seasonal allergies, also known as hay fever or allergic rhinitis, affect millions of people and can significantly impact daily life. The primary culprits behind these allergies are pollen from trees, grasses, and weeds, as well as mold spores that are more prevalent during certain times of the year. Herbal remedies can offer a natural approach to managing the symptoms of seasonal allergies, which include sneezing, nasal congestion, itchy eyes, and throat irritation. Below are detailed descriptions of herbs known for their ability to support the body's response to allergens and how to utilize them effectively.

Nettles (Urtica dioica) have been traditionally used for their natural antihistamine properties. To harness nettles' full potential, it's recommended to start consuming nettle tea or capsules several weeks before allergy season begins. For tea, steep 1-2 teaspoons of dried nettle leaves in boiling water for 10-15 minutes. Drinking 2-3 cups daily can help manage allergy symptoms.

Goldenrod (Solidago virgaurea) is often mistakenly blamed for causing hay fever because it blooms simultaneously with ragweed, a common allergen. However, goldenrod can actually be beneficial for those with seasonal allergies due to its anti-inflammatory and antiseptic properties. A tea made from goldenrod can be prepared by steeping 1 teaspoon of dried flowers in a cup of boiling water for about 15 minutes. Drinking this tea once or twice a day during allergy season can help alleviate symptoms.

Butterbur (Petasites hybridus) is another herb with promising antihistamine effects. Studies suggest that butterbur may be as effective as some over-the-counter antihistamines. When choosing a butterbur supplement, it's crucial to select a product that is labeled PA-free (pyrrolizidine alkaloids-free), as PAs can be harmful to the liver. The recommended dose can vary, so follow the manufacturer's instructions or consult with a healthcare provider.

Quercetin is a natural compound found in many plants and foods, such as onions, apples, and berries. It has been shown to stabilize mast cells, reducing the release of histamine, which is a key factor in allergic reactions. While not an herb, quercetin supplements can be an integral part of a natural allergy relief regimen. For best results, start taking quercetin 6-8 weeks before allergy season at a dose of 500 mg twice daily.

Local Honey contains trace amounts of pollen from local plants, which may help desensitize the body to these allergens over time. Incorporating 1-2 tablespoons of local honey into your daily diet year-round can potentially reduce the severity of seasonal allergy symptoms. It's important to note that because the pollen types in honey are not the same ones that typically cause hay fever, results can vary from person to person.

Bromelain, an enzyme found in pineapple, can reduce nasal swelling and thin mucus, making it easier to breathe. Bromelain supplements are another adjunct to consider for managing seasonal allergies. The recommended dosage is typically 500-1000 mg daily, taken in divided doses, but it's advisable to consult with a healthcare provider for personalized advice.

Spirulina, a type of blue-green algae, has been studied for its potential to improve symptoms of allergic rhinitis, thanks to its anti-inflammatory and immune-modulating effects. Taking 1-2 grams of spirulina daily during allergy season may help reduce symptoms such as nasal discharge, sneezing, nasal congestion, and itching.

Incorporating these herbs and supplements into your routine can offer a holistic approach to managing seasonal allergies. However, it's essential to consult with a healthcare provider before starting any new herbal remedy, especially if you are pregnant, nursing, or taking other medications, to ensure they are appropriate for your individual health needs. Additionally, while herbal remedies can provide relief, they are most effective when combined with other strategies, such as avoiding known allergens, using air purifiers, and maintaining a healthy diet and lifestyle to support overall immune function.

Nettles and Goldenrod for Histamine Reduction

Nettles (Urtica dioica) and Goldenrod (Solidago virgaurea) are two powerful herbs that have garnered attention for their ability to naturally reduce histamine levels in the body, offering relief from the symptoms of seasonal allergies. Histamine is a compound released by cells in response to injury and in allergic and inflammatory reactions, causing contraction of smooth muscle and dilation of capillaries. The mechanism through which nettles and goldenrod exert their effects involves several pathways, including the inhibition of histamine release from mast cells, which are immune cells involved in allergic reactions.

Nettles contain compounds such as quercetin, a natural flavonoid that stabilizes mast cells, preventing them from releasing histamine. Quercetin is known for its antioxidant, anti-inflammatory, and antihistamine properties. To utilize nettles for histamine reduction, it's recommended to use the dried leaves to prepare a tea. Steep 1 to 2 teaspoons of dried nettle leaves in boiling water for 10 to 15 minutes. This tea can be consumed 2 to 3 times a day during allergy season to help manage symptoms. For those who prefer a more convenient approach, nettle capsules are available and can be taken according to the manufacturer's instructions, typically starting several weeks before the onset of allergy season.

Goldenrod, on the other hand, works by reducing inflammation and possibly inhibiting enzymes involved in the allergic response, thereby mitigating the symptoms associated with high histamine levels. Despite common misconceptions, goldenrod is not a significant allergen as its pollen is too heavy to be airborne. Instead, its flowers can be used to make a soothing tea that supports the body's response to seasonal allergies. To prepare goldenrod tea, steep 1 teaspoon of dried goldenrod flowers in a cup of boiling water for about 15 minutes. Drinking this tea once or twice a day can help alleviate allergy symptoms.

It's important to source nettles and goldenrod from reputable suppliers to ensure purity and potency. When harvesting goldenrod, ensure correct identification as it can be easily confused with other plants. Both nettles and goldenrod should be dried properly to preserve their medicinal qualities. For drying, spread the herbs in a single layer on a clean surface in a well-ventilated, dark, and dry place. Once dried, store the herbs in airtight containers away from light and moisture to maintain their efficacy.

While nettles and goldenrod offer a natural way to manage histamine-related symptoms, individuals should consult with a healthcare provider before starting any new herbal regimen, especially those who are pregnant, nursing, or on medication, as herbs can interact with medications. Additionally, starting with small doses and gradually increasing allows one to monitor the body's response to these herbs.

Incorporating nettles and goldenrod into a holistic approach to managing seasonal allergies can significantly improve quality of life during allergy season. Alongside these herbs, maintaining a healthy diet rich in anti-inflammatory foods, staying hydrated, and using air purifiers can further enhance the body's ability to cope with allergens.

Nettles and Lemon Allergy Relief Tea

Beneficial effects

Nettles and Lemon Allergy Relief Tea leverages the natural antihistamine properties of nettles and the immune-boosting power of lemon to provide relief from seasonal allergies. Nettles have been shown to naturally block the body's ability to produce histamine, which can reduce symptoms like sneezing, nasal congestion, and itching. Lemon, rich in Vitamin C, supports the immune system and acts as a detoxifying agent, which can further alleviate allergy symptoms. This herbal tea blend offers a gentle, natural approach to managing seasonal allergies, promoting respiratory health and overall wellness.

Portions

Serves 2

Preparation time

5 minutes

Cooking time

10 minutes

Ingredients

- 2 tablespoons dried nettle leaves
- 1/2 lemon, freshly squeezed
- 2 cups of water
- Honey (optional, to taste)

Instructions

1. Begin by bringing 2 cups of water to a boil in a medium-sized saucepan.

2. Once the water is boiling, add 2 tablespoons of dried nettle leaves to the saucepan.

3. Reduce the heat to low and allow the nettles to simmer for about 10 minutes. This slow simmering process helps to extract the beneficial compounds from the nettles without destroying their antihistamine properties.

4. After simmering, remove the saucepan from the heat and let the tea steep for an additional 5 minutes, allowing the flavors and therapeutic compounds to further infuse into the water.

5. Strain the tea through a fine mesh sieve into a teapot or directly into serving cups, discarding the nettle leaves.

6. Stir in the juice of half a lemon into the tea. The lemon not only adds a refreshing flavor but also contributes Vitamin C, enhancing the tea's allergy-relief benefits.

7. If desired, add honey to taste. Honey can sweeten the tea and may also offer additional soothing effects for the throat.

8. Serve the tea warm for immediate relief from allergy symptoms.

Variations

- For a cold beverage option, allow the tea to cool to room temperature, then refrigerate until chilled. Serve over ice for a refreshing allergy relief drink.
- Add a slice of fresh ginger while simmering the nettles for an extra anti-inflammatory boost and a warming flavor.
- Combine with peppermint leaves during the steeping process for added flavor and to enhance the decongestant properties of the tea.

Storage tips

If there is leftover tea, it can be stored in a sealed container in the refrigerator for up to 2 days. Enjoy it cold, or gently reheat on the stove or in a microwave for a warm, soothing drink.

Tips for allergens

For those with allergies or sensitivities to honey, consider using maple syrup or agave nectar as sweetener alternatives. Ensure that the nettles are sourced from a reputable supplier to avoid contamination with other allergens.

Scientific references

- "The effect of Urtica dioica (Stinging Nettle) on the severity of allergic rhinitis: a randomized, double-blind, placebo-controlled trial" published in Phytotherapy Research, which discusses the benefits of nettles in reducing allergy symptoms.
- "Vitamin C in the treatment and/or prevention of obesity, hypertension, cardiovascular disease and cancer: an update" from the International Journal of Medical Sciences, highlighting the immune-boosting properties of lemon.

BOOK 7: CARDIOVASCULAR HEALTH

CHAPTER 1: HERBS FOR BLOOD PRESSURE

Hawthorn (Crataegus spp.) is widely recognized for its cardiovascular benefits, particularly in regulating blood pressure. The berries, leaves, and flowers of the hawthorn plant contain potent antioxidants that help dilate blood vessels, improve blood flow, and protect against blood vessel damage. For those looking to incorporate hawthorn into their regimen, a standardized extract of 300 to 600 mg daily, divided into two or three doses, is often recommended. Alternatively, hawthorn tea can be made by steeping 1-2 teaspoons of dried hawthorn berries, leaves, or flowers in boiling water for at least 10 minutes. Drinking this tea 2-3 times a day can support cardiovascular health.

Garlic (Allium sativum) has been shown to have a significant impact on reducing blood pressure in individuals with hypertension. Garlic supplements are available in various forms, including aged garlic extract, garlic oil, and garlic powder. The recommended dose for blood pressure management is approximately 600-900 mg daily, divided into multiple doses. These supplements should contain about 1.2% allicin, the active component in garlic responsible for its health benefits. For those preferring to use fresh garlic, incorporating one to two cloves into your diet daily can also confer cardiovascular benefits.

Olive Leaf (Olea europaea) extract is another powerful herb for managing hypertension. Olive leaf works by relaxing the arteries, lowering systemic blood pressure, and improving arterial health. The recommended dosage for olive leaf extract is 500 mg twice daily, standardized to contain 6-15% oleuropein, the active compound. Olive leaf can also be consumed as a tea; steep 1 teaspoon of dried leaves in hot water for 8-10 minutes and drink 1-2 cups daily.

Beetroot (Beta vulgaris) is not traditionally an herb but is included for its high nitrate content, which the body converts into nitric oxide, a molecule that helps dilate blood vessels and lower blood pressure. Beetroot juice or powder is the most effective form for blood pressure management. Drinking 250-500 ml of beetroot juice daily or taking 3-5 grams of beetroot powder can offer cardiovascular benefits.

Celery Seed (Apium graveolens) has been used traditionally for centuries to treat hypertension. Celery seed can be taken as a supplement, with a recommended dose of 600-900 mg daily, or used in cooking. Additionally, celery seed tea can be a beneficial drink; simmer 1 teaspoon of the seeds in water for 15-20 minutes and consume daily.

Dandelion (Taraxacum officinale) leaf is a diuretic that can help lower blood pressure by reducing blood volume. Dandelion leaf tea can be made by steeping 1-2 teaspoons of dried leaves in boiling water for 10 minutes. Drinking 1-2 cups of dandelion leaf tea daily can support blood pressure regulation. However, it's important to monitor blood pressure closely when using diuretic herbs, especially for those on blood pressure medications, as it may lead to hypotension.

When incorporating these herbs into your health regimen for blood pressure management, it's crucial to consult with a healthcare provider, especially if you are already taking prescribed medications for hypertension. Herbs can interact with medications, and it's essential to ensure that any herbal supplements or teas are used safely and effectively. Additionally, lifestyle factors such as diet, exercise, and stress management play a significant role in managing blood pressure and should be considered alongside herbal remedies for optimal cardiovascular health.

Balancing Blood Pressure with Herbs

Hawthorn and garlic stand out in the realm of natural remedies for their cardiovascular benefits, especially in the management and regulation of blood pressure. Hawthorn, scientifically known as Crataegus species, is a plant whose berries, leaves, and flowers are rich in flavonoids and oligomeric proanthocyanidins, compounds known for their potent antioxidant properties. These components play a crucial role in dilating blood vessels, enhancing blood flow, and protecting against blood vessel damage, which can help in the normalization of blood pressure. To effectively incorporate hawthorn into a daily regimen for blood pressure management, one can utilize a standardized extract, which is often recommended at a dosage of 300 to 600 mg daily, divided into two or three doses. This ensures a consistent intake of the active compounds. Alternatively, preparing a tea from 1-2 teaspoons of dried hawthorn berries, leaves, or flowers steeped in boiling water for at least 10 minutes and consumed 2-3 times a day can also support cardiovascular health. It's essential to source hawthorn from reputable suppliers to ensure the quality and potency of the herb.

Garlic, known scientifically as Allium sativum, has been extensively studied for its cardiovascular health benefits, including its ability to lower high blood pressure. Garlic's active component, allicin, is responsible for its health benefits. However, allicin is only formed when garlic is crushed or chopped and is highly volatile. For those looking to benefit from garlic's blood pressure-lowering effects, incorporating one to two fresh garlic cloves into the diet daily is beneficial. The cloves should be crushed or chopped and allowed to sit for a few minutes before consumption to maximize the formation of allicin. For individuals who prefer not to consume fresh garlic, garlic supplements are an alternative, with a recommended dose of 600-900 mg daily, divided into multiple doses. These supplements should specify their allicin potential to ensure they provide therapeutic benefits.

When considering the use of hawthorn and garlic for managing blood pressure, it's crucial to understand the importance of consistency and patience. The cardiovascular benefits of these herbs build over time, and their full effects on blood pressure may not be immediately apparent. Regular monitoring of blood pressure is advisable to gauge the effectiveness of these remedies and adjust dosages as necessary. Additionally, while hawthorn and garlic can be powerful allies in cardiovascular health, they should be part of a broader approach that includes a healthy diet, regular physical activity, and stress management techniques.

It's also important to consult with a healthcare provider before starting any new supplement, especially for individuals already taking prescribed medications for hypertension, as herbs can interact with medications. A healthcare provider can offer guidance on appropriate dosages and ensure that hawthorn and garlic supplements are used safely and effectively alongside conventional treatments.

Incorporating hawthorn and garlic into a holistic approach to blood pressure management can offer significant benefits. However, their use should be viewed as part of a comprehensive strategy for cardiovascular health that emphasizes a balanced diet, physical activity, and regular healthcare consultations.

Hawthorn Berry Tea for Heart Health

Hawthorn Berry Tea is a revered herbal remedy known for its cardiovascular benefits, particularly its ability to help regulate blood pressure and support heart health. To prepare Hawthorn Berry Tea, you will need the following:

Ingredients:
- 1-2 teaspoons of dried **hawthorn berries**
- 8 ounces (about 1 cup) of water
- Optional: honey or lemon to taste

Tools:
- Teapot or saucepan
- Strainer or tea infuser
- Measuring spoons
- Kettle or another method to boil water
- Cup for serving

Preparation Steps:
1. **Boil Water:** Begin by boiling 8 ounces of water. Using a kettle will allow for more precise control of the water temperature. The ideal temperature for extracting the beneficial compounds from hawthorn berries without destroying them is just below boiling, around 200°F.
2. **Measure Hawthorn Berries:** While the water is heating, measure out 1-2 teaspoons of dried hawthorn berries. The amount can be adjusted based on personal preference for strength. More berries will result in a stronger tea.
3. **Prepare the Berries:** If using a teapot, place the dried hawthorn berries directly into the pot. For those using a saucepan, the berries can be added directly to the water once it's heated. If you prefer to use a tea infuser, place the berries inside the infuser and then place it in your cup.
4. **Steep the Tea:** Once the water has reached the correct temperature, pour it over the hawthorn berries. Allow the tea to steep for 10-15 minutes. Steeping for at least 10 minutes is crucial to ensure the maximum extraction of the hawthorn berries' beneficial compounds, such as flavonoids and oligomeric proanthocyanidins, which are known for their antioxidant properties.
5. **Strain and Serve:** After steeping, strain the tea to remove the berries. If you used a tea infuser, simply remove it from the cup. At this point, you can add honey or lemon to taste, although it's recommended to try the tea plain first to truly appreciate its unique flavor.

6. **Enjoy:** Drink the hawthorn berry tea while it's warm to enjoy its full benefits. Consuming this tea 2-3 times a day can support cardiovascular health, but it's important to start with one cup a day to monitor how your body responds.

Additional Tips:

- Always source your hawthorn berries from reputable suppliers to ensure they are free from contaminants and have been properly dried and stored.
- Hawthorn Berry Tea can be part of a holistic approach to cardiovascular health, which includes a balanced diet, regular exercise, and stress management practices.
- Consult with a healthcare provider before incorporating Hawthorn Berry Tea into your regimen, especially if you are currently taking medication for heart conditions or blood pressure, as hawthorn can interact with some medications.

By following these detailed steps, you can prepare a therapeutic cup of Hawthorn Berry Tea to support your cardiovascular health.

CHAPTER 2: CHOLESTEROL MANAGEMENT WITH HERBS

Managing cholesterol levels is crucial for cardiovascular health, and herbal remedies offer a natural approach to complement traditional treatments. **Fenugreek** seeds, known for their soluble fiber content, can aid in reducing low-density lipoprotein (LDL) or "bad" cholesterol. Incorporating **fenugreek** into your diet can be as simple as adding powdered seeds to warm water or blending them into smoothies. For a daily dose, aim for about 5-10 grams of powdered **fenugreek** seeds.

Cinnamon, another potent herb, has been shown to lower total cholesterol levels when consumed regularly. Sprinkling half a teaspoon of **cinnamon** on your morning oatmeal or incorporating it into your coffee can make a significant difference over time. It's not just for flavor; **cinnamon**'s active compounds work to reduce cholesterol absorption in the intestines.

Garlic has long been celebrated for its health benefits, including its ability to manage cholesterol. Allicin, the active component in **garlic**, helps prevent LDL oxidation, thus reducing plaque formation in arteries. For effective cholesterol management, consuming one to two fresh **garlic** cloves daily or taking aged **garlic** supplements as directed can offer cardiovascular benefits.

Red yeast rice is another powerful tool in the cholesterol-lowering arsenal. It contains monacolin K, the same active ingredient found in certain prescription cholesterol-lowering medications. However, due to its potency, it's essential to consult with a healthcare provider before adding **red yeast rice** supplements to your regimen, especially if you're already taking cholesterol medication.

Plant sterols and stanols, found in fortified foods and supplements, mimic cholesterol's structure, helping block its absorption in the digestive tract. Incorporating products enriched with plant sterols or taking supplements as advised can significantly lower LDL cholesterol levels.

For those seeking to manage their cholesterol through diet and lifestyle changes, incorporating these herbs and supplements can offer a complementary approach. However, it's crucial to consult with a healthcare provider before starting any new supplement, especially if you have existing health conditions or are taking medications. Regular monitoring of cholesterol levels will help gauge the effectiveness of these herbal remedies and ensure your cardiovascular health remains on track.

Herbs to Lower LDL Naturally

Incorporating specific herbs into one's diet can play a significant role in managing and reducing LDL cholesterol levels, a key factor in cardiovascular health. Among these, artichoke leaf extract stands out for its ability to inhibit cholesterol synthesis. The active compound in artichoke, cynarin, not only enhances bile production but also facilitates the removal of cholesterol from the body. To harness these benefits, one might consider taking artichoke supplements, available in capsule form, with a recommended dosage of 300-600 mg daily. It's important to look for supplements that specify the content of cynarin to ensure efficacy.

Another noteworthy herb is Guggul, a resin derived from the Mukul myrrh tree, which has been used in Ayurvedic medicine for centuries to improve lipid profiles. Guggulsterones, the active compounds, are believed to increase the liver's metabolism of LDL cholesterol. For those considering Guggul supplements, a typical dosage ranges from 500-1000 mg, taken in divided doses. However, due to its potent nature, one should monitor liver function and lipid levels regularly when using Guggul, especially in conjunction with other cholesterol-lowering medications.

Psyllium husk, widely recognized for its fiber content, also plays a pivotal role in lowering LDL cholesterol. By forming a gel-like substance in the intestines, it binds to cholesterol, preventing its absorption. Incorporating psyllium into one's diet can be as simple as adding a teaspoon of psyllium husk powder to a glass of water or a smoothie, ideally taken before meals to maximize its cholesterol-binding effects. Aim for a daily intake of 10-15 grams, but start with a lower dose to assess tolerance.

Green tea, rich in catechins and polyphenols, offers antioxidant properties that can aid in lowering LDL cholesterol levels. Regular consumption of green tea, aiming for 3-4 cups daily, can contribute to a healthier lipid profile. For those who prefer a more concentrated form, green tea extract supplements are an alternative, with recommended dosages typically around 250-500 mg per day. It's crucial to ensure that the extract is standardized for EGCG, the most active catechin, to optimize health benefits.

Lastly, red clover, containing isoflavones, has been shown to have a mild effect on reducing LDL cholesterol. These phytoestrogens can mimic the effects of estrogen, potentially influencing lipid metabolism.

Incorporating red clover can be through teas or supplements, with a suggested intake of one to two cups of tea daily or a supplement dose as advised by a healthcare provider. As with any supplement, it's essential to consult with a healthcare professional before starting, particularly for those with hormone-sensitive conditions.

When considering these herbs for cholesterol management, it's imperative to integrate them into a balanced diet and healthy lifestyle for optimal results. Regular exercise, maintaining a healthy weight, and avoiding foods high in saturated fats are foundational steps in managing cholesterol levels. Additionally, monitoring cholesterol levels through regular check-ups will provide insights into the effectiveness of these herbal interventions and whether adjustments are needed.

Fenugreek and Cinnamon Cholesterol-Balancing Tonic

Beneficial effects

Fenugreek and cinnamon are both renowned for their health-promoting properties, particularly in the context of cardiovascular health. Fenugreek seeds contain soluble fiber, which can help in reducing cholesterol levels by inhibiting the absorption of cholesterol in the intestines. Cinnamon, on the other hand, has been shown to improve insulin sensitivity and lower blood sugar levels, which can indirectly support cholesterol management. Together, this tonic is designed to aid in balancing cholesterol levels, supporting overall heart health.

Portions

Serves 2

Preparation time

5 minutes

Cooking time

10 minutes

Ingredients

- 1 teaspoon of fenugreek seeds
- 1 cinnamon stick (or 1/2 teaspoon ground cinnamon)
- 2 cups of water
- Honey or stevia to taste (optional)

Instructions

1. Begin by lightly crushing the fenugreek seeds using a mortar and pestle to release their flavor and beneficial oils. If you don't have a mortar and pestle, a rolling pin or the back of a spoon against a hard surface works as well.
2. In a small saucepan, bring 2 cups of water to a boil. Once boiling, add the crushed fenugreek seeds and the cinnamon stick to the water.
3. Reduce the heat to a simmer and allow the mixture to cook for 10 minutes. This slow simmering process helps to extract the active compounds from the fenugreek seeds and cinnamon, infusing the water with their beneficial properties.
4. After 10 minutes, remove the saucepan from the heat. Let the tonic steep for an additional 5 minutes with the lid on to further concentrate the flavors and healthful components.
5. Strain the tonic through a fine mesh sieve into two cups, removing the fenugreek seeds and cinnamon stick. If you used ground cinnamon, there's no need to strain.
6. If desired, sweeten the tonic with honey or stevia to taste. Stir well to ensure the sweetener is fully dissolved.
7. Serve the tonic warm for maximum benefits.

Variations

- For a refreshing twist, add a slice of fresh ginger or a few mint leaves while simmering the tonic.
- Incorporate a slice of lemon or orange for a vitamin C boost and a tangy flavor.
- For those who prefer a cold beverage, allow the tonic to cool to room temperature, then refrigerate and serve chilled.

Storage tips

This tonic is best enjoyed fresh, but if you have leftovers, they can be stored in a sealed container in the refrigerator for up to 2 days. Reheat gently on the stove or enjoy cold.

Tips for allergens

For individuals with allergies to honey, stevia serves as a great alternative sweetener. Always ensure that the fenugreek seeds and cinnamon are sourced from reputable suppliers to avoid cross-contamination with allergens.

Scientific references

- "The effect of fenugreek on lipid profile: A meta-analysis of randomized controlled trials" published in the Journal of Ethnopharmacology, which discusses the cholesterol-lowering effects of fenugreek.
- "Cinnamon: Potential Role in the Prevention of Insulin Resistance, Metabolic Syndrome, and Type 2 Diabetes" published in the Journal of Diabetes Science and Technology, highlighting the beneficial impact of cinnamon on insulin sensitivity and blood sugar levels.

BOOK 8: IMMUNE-BOOSTING HERBAL MEDICINE

CHAPTER 1: HERBS FOR IMMUNE RESPONSE

Elderberry (Sambucus nigra) is renowned for its potent antiviral properties, making it a frontline defense in boosting the immune system rapidly. To harness elderberry's benefits, consider creating an Elderberry Immune Syrup. Start with 1 cup of dried elderberries and 4 cups of water. Bring to a boil, then simmer until the liquid is reduced by half. Strain the mixture, pressing the berries to extract maximum juice. While still warm, mix in 1 cup of honey for its antibacterial properties. For adults, take 1 tablespoon daily during cold and flu season or every 3-4 hours if symptoms arise.

Echinacea (Echinacea purpurea) is another herb that stimulates the immune system by increasing the production of white blood cells, which fight infections. A simple Echinacea tea can be made by steeping 1-2 teaspoons of dried echinacea root or leaves in boiling water for 15 minutes. Drink 2-3 cups daily at the first sign of cold or flu symptoms to enhance immune response.

Vitamin C-rich herbs like Rosehips (Rosa canina) are crucial for immune function. To make a Rosehip tea, use 1-2 teaspoons of dried rosehips per cup of boiling water, steep for 10-15 minutes, and drink 2-3 times daily. This tea is not only high in vitamin C but also provides antioxidants that support overall health.

Astragalus (Astragalus membranaceus) is a powerful adaptogen that boosts the body's defense mechanism. Incorporate Astragalus into your diet by adding a few slices of the root to soups or stews, allowing it to simmer and infuse its properties into the dish. It's particularly beneficial when consumed during the colder months for preventive health care.

Garlic (Allium sativum), with its natural antibiotic and antiviral properties, is effective in fighting infections and enhancing immune function. Incorporate fresh garlic into your meals, aiming for 1-2 cloves per day. For a more potent intake, finely mince a clove of garlic, let it sit for 15 minutes to activate its allicin compound, then swallow with water or mix it into a teaspoon of honey.

Ginger (Zingiber officinale) is well-known for its anti-inflammatory and antioxidative properties. For an immune-boosting drink, add 1 inch of fresh ginger root to boiling water, simmer for 20 minutes, and drink warm. You can enhance the flavor and benefits by adding lemon juice and honey to taste.

Turmeric (Curcuma longa), with its active compound curcumin, offers significant anti-inflammatory benefits. Create a turmeric latte by warming 1 cup of milk (dairy or plant-based), stirring in 1 teaspoon of turmeric powder, a pinch of black pepper (to enhance absorption), and honey to taste. Drink this daily to support immune health.

For those seeking to fortify their immune system, incorporating these herbs into your daily regimen can offer a natural and effective way to enhance your body's defenses. Remember, consistency is key in herbal supplementation for immune support. Additionally, always consult with a healthcare provider before starting any new herbal regimen, especially if you have existing health conditions or are taking medications.

Elderberry and Echinacea for Infections

Elderberry (Sambucus nigra) and Echinacea (Echinacea purpurea) stand out in the realm of immune-boosting herbs due to their extensive history of use and the backing of modern scientific research. These plants offer a dynamic approach to enhancing the body's defense mechanisms against infections. To leverage the full potential of these herbs, it's crucial to understand their unique properties, optimal preparation methods, and recommended dosages.

Elderberry is celebrated for its rich content of flavonoids, specifically anthocyanins, which possess potent antioxidant and antiviral properties. These compounds are believed to inhibit the replication of viruses, thereby shortening the duration and severity of cold and flu symptoms. To prepare an elderberry syrup, start with high-quality, organic dried elderberries. Combine 1 cup of dried elderberries with 4 cups of water in a saucepan. Bring the mixture to a boil, then reduce the heat and simmer for about 45 minutes to an hour, until the liquid has reduced by almost half. Strain the liquid, pressing the berries to extract as much juice as possible. While the liquid is still warm, stir in 1 cup of raw, local honey. This not only adds sweetness but also enhances the syrup's antibacterial properties. The recommended dosage for adults is 1 tablespoon of syrup daily for immune support during cold and flu season, and every 3-4 hours when experiencing acute symptoms.

Echinacea, on the other hand, boosts the immune system by increasing the production of white blood cells, which play a crucial role in fighting infections. It also enhances the activity of the phagocytes, cells that engulf and digest pathogens. For an effective Echinacea preparation, use the root or aerial parts of Echinacea purpurea or Echinacea angustifolia. To make a simple tea, steep 1-2 teaspoons of dried Echinacea in a cup of boiling water for 15 minutes. This tea can be consumed 2-3 times daily at the onset of cold or flu symptoms. For a more concentrated dose, Echinacea tinctures are available. The typical dosage is 1-2 ml, taken three times daily during active infections.

When combining elderberry and Echinacea, you create a powerful synergistic effect that can significantly bolster the immune system's ability to combat viral infections. A combined regimen might include taking the elderberry syrup daily for preventive care during peak cold and flu seasons and introducing Echinacea tea or tincture at the first sign of illness, continuing its use for the duration of symptoms.

It's important to source these herbs from reputable suppliers to ensure they are of high quality and free from contaminants. Organic sources are preferable to minimize exposure to pesticides and other harmful chemicals. Additionally, while these herbs are generally considered safe for most people, individuals with autoimmune diseases, pregnant women, and those on immunosuppressive medications should consult with a healthcare provider before use due to the immune-stimulating effects of Echinacea.

Incorporating elderberry and Echinacea into your wellness routine represents a proactive approach to enhancing immune function and protecting against infections. By understanding the specific benefits, preparation methods, and dosages of these herbs, individuals can effectively harness their natural healing powers.

Elderberry Immune Syrup Recipe

To create an effective **Elderberry Immune Syrup**, gather the following ingredients:
- **1 cup of dried elderberries**: Ensure they are organic to avoid pesticides and other chemicals.
- **4 cups of water**: Use filtered water to ensure purity and enhance the natural flavors of the ingredients.
- **1 cup of raw, local honey**: Local honey not only sweetens the syrup but also introduces local pollen, which can help with seasonal allergies.
- **A fine mesh strainer or cheesecloth**: This is essential for separating the elderberries from the liquid after boiling.
- **A large saucepan**: Choose a saucepan that can comfortably hold the liquid volume, allowing for evaporation.
- **A storage container**: Preferably glass, such as a mason jar, for storing the syrup. Ensure it's sterilized to keep the syrup preserved.

Preparation Steps:
1. **Combine the elderberries and water** in the large saucepan. Bring the mixture to a boil over high heat, then reduce to a simmer. Allow the mixture to simmer for about 45 minutes to an hour. The goal is to reduce the liquid by about half, concentrating the mixture to intensify the flavors and benefits.
2. **Strain the mixture** using the fine mesh strainer or cheesecloth over a bowl. Press the berries to extract as much liquid as possible. Compost or discard the elderberries after straining.
3. **While the liquid is still warm** (not hot, to preserve the beneficial enzymes in the honey), add the raw, local honey. Stir thoroughly until the honey is completely dissolved. The warmth of the liquid will help to incorporate the honey smoothly.
4. **Transfer the syrup** to the sterilized glass container. If using a mason jar, use a canning funnel to avoid spills. Seal the container tightly.
5. **Storage**: Store the elderberry syrup in the refrigerator. The cold environment will help preserve the syrup's potency and extend its shelf life. Typically, the syrup can be stored for up to two months when refrigerated.

Usage Guidelines:
- For **daily immune support** during cold and flu season, adults can take 1 tablespoon of elderberry syrup daily. Children over the age of one can take 1 teaspoon daily.
- During **acute illness**, the dosage can be increased to every 3-4 hours, but consult with a healthcare provider before doing so, especially for children.

Important Notes:
- **Do not give honey** to children under one year of age due to the risk of botulism.
- **Consult with a healthcare provider** before using elderberry syrup if you are pregnant, nursing, have any medical conditions, or are taking medications.

- **Elderberries must be cooked** before consumption to eliminate any potentially harmful toxins present in the raw berries.

This **Elderberry Immune Syrup** recipe combines the antiviral and immune-boosting properties of elderberries with the antibacterial benefits of honey, creating a powerful natural remedy for enhancing immune health.

CHAPTER 2: LONG-TERM IMMUNE STRENGTHENING

Astragalus (Astragalus membranaceus) is a cornerstone herb for long-term immune strengthening, known for its adaptogenic properties that help the body resist stressors of all kinds, whether physical, chemical, or biological. The root of the Astragalus plant is used in herbal medicine, typically available in forms such as dried slices, powders, tinctures, and capsules. For incorporating Astragalus into your diet, consider adding a few slices of the root to soups or stews. This method allows the Astragalus to simmer and infuse its properties into the dish without overwhelming the flavor profile. It's particularly beneficial when consumed during the colder months for preventive health care. The recommended daily dosage for dried root is 9-15 grams, but it's advisable to start with a lower dose to assess tolerance.

Reishi Mushroom (Ganoderma lucidum), another powerful adaptogen, supports immune function and helps combat stress. Reishi can be consumed in various forms, including teas, powders, and capsules. To make a Reishi tea, simmer about 5 grams of dried Reishi mushroom in 4 cups of water for 2 hours, strain, and drink the tea throughout the day. The bitter taste of Reishi might be off-putting to some, so combining it with other herbs or a bit of honey can improve its palatability. Regular consumption can significantly enhance the immune system's resilience over time.

Vitamin D is crucial for immune function, and while not an herb, it's an essential component of long-term immune health. The best source of Vitamin D is sunlight, but supplements can be beneficial, especially in areas with limited sun exposure. The recommended daily allowance (RDA) for Vitamin D is 600-800 IU, but many experts suggest higher doses, up to 2000 IU, for optimal immune function. Always check with a healthcare provider before starting any new supplement regimen.

Probiotics, found in fermented foods like yogurt, kefir, sauerkraut, and supplements, play a vital role in maintaining gut health, which is directly linked to the immune system. A healthy gut flora supports the immune system by enhancing the gut barrier and producing antimicrobial compounds. Aim for a variety of fermented foods in your diet or consider a probiotic supplement with at least 1 billion colony-forming units (CFUs) and multiple strains of bacteria.

Zinc is a mineral essential for immune cell function and signaling. A deficiency in zinc can lead to a weakened immune response. Foods rich in zinc include beef, oysters, pumpkin seeds, and lentils. For those considering supplementation, the recommended daily intake of zinc is 8 mg for women and 11 mg for men, but doses up to 40 mg can be used for short-term immune support under a healthcare provider's guidance.

Elderberry (Sambucus nigra) has been mentioned for its immediate immune-boosting properties, but it also plays a role in long-term immune health. Elderberry's high antioxidant content helps protect cells from damage and supports the body's natural defense mechanisms. For daily support, elderberry syrup can be taken in doses of 1 tablespoon per day for adults and 1 teaspoon per day for children over one year old.

Incorporating these herbs and nutrients into your daily regimen can significantly contribute to a robust and resilient immune system over the long term. Remember, consistency is key, and it's essential to combine these strategies with a healthy lifestyle, including adequate sleep, regular exercise, stress management, and a balanced diet. Always consult with a healthcare provider before starting any new supplement, especially if you have existing health conditions or are taking medications.

Adaptogenic Support: Astragalus & Reishi

Adaptogenic herbs like **Astragalus** and **Reishi** play a pivotal role in bolstering the body's immune system over the long term. These herbs are renowned for their ability to modulate the immune response, enhancing the body's ability to fend off and recover from illness. Here, we delve into how to incorporate Astragalus and Reishi into your wellness regimen for immune support.

Astragalus (Astragalus membranaceus), a staple in traditional Chinese medicine, is celebrated for its immune-boosting and antiviral properties. To harness these benefits, consider adding Astragalus root to your daily routine. Start with dried Astragalus root, available at health food stores or online. A simple method is to prepare a decoction: measure out 1 to 2 tablespoons of the dried root, add it to 4 cups of water, and simmer for approximately 30 minutes. Strain and consume the liquid, drinking 1 to 2 cups daily. This decoction can be stored in the refrigerator for up to three days. For convenience, Astragalus is also available in capsule or tincture form; follow the manufacturer's dosage recommendations.

Reishi mushroom (Ganoderma lucidum), often called the "mushroom of immortality," supports immune health and helps combat stress. To incorporate Reishi into your diet, begin with dried Reishi mushrooms. These can be steeped in hot water to make a tea. Take 1 to 2 grams of dried Reishi slices, add to a pot with 4 cups of water, and simmer for about 2 hours. The resulting tea will have a bitter taste, which can be softened with honey or mixed with other herbal teas for flavor. Drinking 1 cup of Reishi tea daily is a good start. Reishi is also available in powder, capsule, or tincture form, offering a more straightforward approach for daily intake. Again, adhere to the dosage instructions provided by the product manufacturer.

When using **Astragalus and Reishi** together, it's important to note that these herbs work synergistically to enhance each other's effects on the immune system. A balanced approach could involve alternating between Astragalus and Reishi tea each day or combining the two in a single brew. For those preferring supplements, look for formulas that include both herbs to simplify your regimen.

Remember, while Astragalus is generally considered safe for most people, it should be used with caution by those with autoimmune diseases or those taking immunosuppressive drugs, as it could potentially enhance immune function. Similarly, Reishi can interact with certain medications, including anticoagulants and immunosuppressants, and may not be suitable for individuals with specific health conditions. Always consult with a healthcare provider before adding these or any new supplements to your routine, especially if you have existing health concerns or are on medication.

Incorporating **Astragalus and Reishi** for adaptogenic support is a proactive step towards long-term immune strengthening. By understanding the specific preparation and consumption methods for these powerful herbs, individuals can effectively enhance their body's resilience against illness and stress, contributing to overall health and well-being.

Astragalus and Reishi Immune Tonic

Beneficial effects
Astragalus and Reishi mushrooms are two powerful adaptogens that work synergistically to enhance the immune system. Astragalus is known for its ability to increase the production of white blood cells, which are crucial for fighting off infections. Reishi, often referred to as the "mushroom of immortality," supports immune health by modulating the immune response and reducing inflammation. Together, this tonic can help to build long-term immune resilience, making it an excellent choice for those looking to support their immune system naturally.

Ingredients
- 1/4 cup dried Astragalus root slices
- 1/4 cup dried Reishi mushroom slices
- 4 cups of water
- 1 tablespoon honey (optional, for sweetness)
- 1 slice of ginger (optional, for additional immune support and flavor)

Instructions
1. Combine the dried Astragalus root slices and dried Reishi mushroom slices in a medium-sized pot.
2. Add 4 cups of water to the pot, ensuring that the herbs are fully submerged.
3. Bring the mixture to a boil over high heat, then reduce the heat to a simmer.
4. Allow the mixture to simmer gently for 1 to 2 hours, or until the liquid has reduced by half. This slow simmering process helps to extract the beneficial compounds from the Astragalus and Reishi, creating a potent tonic.
5. If using, add a slice of ginger to the pot during the last 30 minutes of simmering for additional flavor and immune support.
6. After simmering, remove the pot from the heat and let it cool slightly.
7. Strain the tonic through a fine mesh strainer or cheesecloth into a large bowl or pitcher, discarding the solid herb remnants.
8. Stir in honey to taste, if desired, until it dissolves completely.
9. Serve the tonic warm, or allow it to cool completely and then transfer it to a glass jar or bottle for storage.

Variations
- For a citrus twist, add a few slices of lemon or orange during the last 10 minutes of simmering. This adds a refreshing flavor and vitamin C, which further supports the immune system.
- Incorporate a cinnamon stick during simmering for added warmth and blood sugar regulation benefits.

- Blend the strained tonic with a small amount of fresh juice, such as apple or pomegranate, for added antioxidants and flavor.

Storage tips

Store the cooled tonic in an airtight glass jar or bottle in the refrigerator for up to one week. Gently reheat on the stove or enjoy cold, shaking well before use.

Tips for allergens

For those with allergies or sensitivities to honey, substitute it with maple syrup or simply omit it for a less sweet tonic. Ensure that the Astragalus and Reishi mushrooms are sourced from reputable suppliers to avoid contamination with allergens.

Scientific references

- "Astragalus membranaceus: A Review of its Protection Against Inflammation and Gastrointestinal Cancers" published in the American Journal of Chinese Medicine, which discusses Astragalus's immune-boosting properties.
- "Ganoderma lucidum (Reishi mushroom) for cancer treatment," found in the Cochrane Database of Systematic Reviews, highlights the immune-modulating effects of Reishi mushrooms.

CHAPTER 3: SEASONAL HERBAL BLENDS

As the seasons change, so do the needs of our bodies, particularly our immune system. To address these shifting requirements, incorporating seasonal herbal blends into your wellness routine can offer targeted support for immune health. Each season brings its own set of challenges and opportunities for strengthening the body's defenses, and by aligning our herbal practices with these cycles, we can enhance our resilience and vitality.

Spring: A time of renewal, spring is ideal for cleansing and revitalizing the body after the winter months. A blend focusing on detoxification and immune system awakening can be beneficial. Herbs like **dandelion root**, known for its liver-supportive properties, and **nettle leaf**, rich in nutrients and a natural antihistamine, make a perfect combination. To prepare a spring tonic, simmer 1 tablespoon each of dried dandelion root and nettle leaf in 4 cups of water for 15 minutes. Strain and drink 1 cup in the morning to stimulate detoxification and boost immunity.

Summer: With the abundance of warmth and outdoor activities, summer calls for cooling and hydrating herbs to prevent overheating and maintain hydration. **Hibiscus** and **peppermint** serve as excellent choices for a summer blend, offering cooling effects and aiding in digestion. For a refreshing iced tea, steep 2 tablespoons of dried hibiscus flowers and 1 tablespoon of peppermint leaves in 4 cups of boiling water. Cool and serve over ice for a thirst-quenching drink that also supports immune health.

Fall: As temperatures begin to drop, preparing the body for the colder months is key. Immune-boosting herbs that also provide warmth, such as **ginger** and **elderberry**, are ideal. Ginger, with its warming and anti-inflammatory properties, and elderberry, known for its antiviral benefits, can be combined to create a potent immune-supporting syrup. Simmer 1/2 cup of dried elderberries and 2 tablespoons of freshly grated ginger in 3 cups of water until reduced by half. Strain, add honey to taste, and take 1 tablespoon daily to enhance immune function.

Winter: This season is all about sustaining the immune system and warding off colds and flu. Herbs like **echinacea**, which can enhance the body's natural defense mechanism, and **thyme**, with its antimicrobial properties, are perfect for a winter tea blend. To make, steep 1 tablespoon of dried echinacea and 1 teaspoon of thyme leaves in 4 cups of boiling water for 10 minutes. Drinking this tea 2-3 times a day can help maintain immune strength during the winter months.

For each of these seasonal blends, it's important to source high-quality, organic herbs to ensure the maximum benefit and reduce exposure to pesticides. Additionally, while these herbs are generally safe for most people, individual reactions can vary. It's advisable to start with small doses to see how your body responds and consult with a healthcare provider, especially if you have existing health conditions or are taking medications. By aligning herbal practices with the seasons, we can proactively support our body's immune system and overall well-being throughout the year. These seasonal blends offer a natural and holistic approach to health that can be easily incorporated into daily routines, providing a foundation for a vibrant and healthy life.

Preparing for Cold and Flu Season

As cold and flu season approaches, fortifying your immune system becomes paramount. A strategic approach involves the use of specific herbs known for their immune-enhancing properties. To effectively prepare for this season, incorporating a daily regimen of herbal teas and supplements can provide a natural defense mechanism against common viral infections.

Elderberry (Sambucus nigra) is widely recognized for its antiviral effects, particularly against the flu virus. To utilize elderberry, consider making an elderberry syrup by combining 1 cup of dried elderberry with 4 cups of water. Boil the mixture until it is reduced by half, then strain and mix with 1 cup of honey. Adults can take 1 tablespoon of this syrup daily for immune support, and half a tablespoon for children. This syrup can be stored in a refrigerator for up to two weeks.

Echinacea (Echinacea purpurea) is another herb that boosts the immune system by increasing the production of white blood cells. A simple way to incorporate echinacea is by preparing a tea. Add 1 teaspoon of dried echinacea root to 1 cup of boiling water and steep for 10-15 minutes. Drinking 1-2 cups of echinacea tea daily can help enhance immune function.

Astragalus (Astragalus membranaceus), a root used in Traditional Chinese Medicine, is known for its deep immune-system-boosting effects. To incorporate astragalus into your routine, add slices of the dried root to soups or stews. The root slices are virtually tasteless and can be removed before serving. Alternatively, astragalus can be taken as a tincture; follow the manufacturer's instructions for dosage.

Vitamin C-rich herbs such as **rose hips (Rosa canina)** and **camu camu (Myrciaria dubia)** can also support the immune system. Rose hips can be steeped in hot water to make a vitamin C-rich tea, which can be consumed daily. Camu camu powder can be added to smoothies or yogurt, providing a potent dose of vitamin C with antiviral properties.

Garlic (Allium sativum), with its natural antibiotic and immune-boosting properties, can be easily integrated into daily meals. Consuming 1-2 cloves of raw garlic daily, either minced in salad dressings or as a supplement, can offer protective benefits during flu season.

For those seeking to combine these herbs for a comprehensive approach, consider creating a **Cold and Flu Season Herbal Blend**. Mix equal parts dried elderberry, echinacea, and rose hips, adding a quarter part of astragalus root. To make a tea, use 1 tablespoon of this blend per cup of boiling water, steeping for 15-20 minutes. This tea can be consumed 2-3 times daily, with the option to sweeten with honey, which also possesses antimicrobial properties.

When selecting herbs, ensure they are of high quality and organically sourced to avoid the intake of pesticides. Begin integrating these herbs into your regimen at the onset of cold and flu season, or even a few weeks prior, to build up your immune defenses.

It's important to note that while these herbs are generally safe for most individuals, those with autoimmune diseases, pregnant women, or those on certain medications should consult with a healthcare provider before starting any new herbal regimen. This precaution ensures the avoidance of any potential interactions or side effects.

By proactively incorporating these immune-boosting herbs into your daily routine, you can enhance your body's natural defenses, potentially reducing the severity and duration of cold and flu symptoms.

Cold Season Herbal Tea Blend

Beneficial effects

This Cold Season Herbal Tea Blend combines the immune-boosting and respiratory-supportive properties of elderberry, echinacea, and peppermint. Elderberry is renowned for its antiviral effects, helping to prevent or shorten the duration of colds and flu. Echinacea enhances the body's immune response, while peppermint offers relief from coughs and congestion. Together, these herbs create a powerful ally during the cold season, supporting overall respiratory health and immune function.

Portions

Serves 4

Preparation time

5 minutes

Cooking time

15 minutes

Ingredients

- 1/4 cup dried elderberries
- 2 tablespoons dried echinacea leaves
- 2 tablespoons dried peppermint leaves
- 4 cups of water
- Honey or lemon (optional, for taste)

Instructions

1. In a medium saucepan, bring 4 cups of water to a boil.
2. Once boiling, add the dried elderberries to the saucepan. Reduce the heat to a simmer.
3. Allow the elderberries to simmer for 10 minutes. This process extracts their antiviral properties and deep, rich flavor.
4. Add the dried echinacea leaves to the saucepan, simmering for an additional 3 minutes. Echinacea is added later in the process to preserve its immune-boosting compounds.
5. Finally, turn off the heat and add the dried peppermint leaves. Cover the saucepan with a lid and let the mixture steep for 5 minutes. Peppermint is added last to maintain its menthol flavor and soothing properties.
6. Strain the tea through a fine mesh sieve into a large pitcher or directly into tea cups, pressing on the solids to extract as much liquid as possible.

7. If desired, sweeten with honey or add a squeeze of lemon to enhance the tea's flavor and add a vitamin C boost.

8. Serve the tea warm to enjoy its maximum benefits.

Variations

- For a spicier kick, add a slice of fresh ginger or a cinnamon stick during the simmering process.
- Combine with licorice root for additional soothing throat support.
- For a caffeine boost, add a bag of green tea during the last 3 minutes of steeping.

Storage tips

Cool any leftover tea and store it in a sealed container in the refrigerator for up to 3 days. Reheat gently on the stove or enjoy chilled.

Tips for allergens

For those with allergies or sensitivities to honey, maple syrup or agave nectar are suitable sweeteners. Ensure that the herbs are sourced from reputable suppliers to avoid cross-contamination with allergens.

Scientific references

- "Elderberry Supplementation Reduces Cold Duration and Symptoms in Air-Travellers: A Randomized, Double-Blind Placebo-Controlled Clinical Trial" published in the journal Nutrients, which discusses the benefits of elderberry on cold and flu symptoms.
- "Echinacea purpurea: Pharmacology, phytochemistry and analysis methods" published in the Pharmacognosy Reviews, highlighting the immune-boosting properties of echinacea.
- "Peppermint Oil in the Acute Treatment of Tension-Type Headache" from the journal Schmerz, detailing the soothing effects of peppermint on headaches and respiratory conditions.

BOOK 9: HERBAL REMEDIES FOR EMOTIONAL WELLBEING

CHAPTER 1: NERVINES FOR STRESS AND ANXIETY

Nervines are a class of herbal remedies specifically beneficial for the nervous system, offering relief from stress and anxiety. These herbs work by directly impacting the central nervous system to calm, soothe, and support nerve function. Incorporating nervines into your daily routine can be a gentle yet effective way to manage everyday stressors, improve sleep quality, and enhance overall emotional wellbeing. Here, we detail how to use some of the most effective nervines, including **chamomile**, **valerian root**, **lemon balm**, and **lavender**, providing specific recommendations for preparation and consumption.

Chamomile (Matricaria recutita) is widely recognized for its calming properties. To harness these benefits, prepare chamomile tea by steeping 1-2 teaspoons of dried chamomile flowers in 8 ounces of boiling water for 5-10 minutes. This tea can be consumed 2-3 times daily, especially in the evening to promote restful sleep. For those who prefer, chamomile is also available in capsule form or as a liquid extract. Follow the manufacturer's instructions for dosage.

Valerian Root (Valeriana officinalis) is another powerful nervine known for its sedative qualities, making it particularly useful for those with sleep disturbances. To prepare valerian root tea, steep 1 teaspoon of the dried root in 1 cup of hot water for 10 minutes. It's recommended to drink valerian tea 30 minutes to 2 hours before bedtime. Valerian is also available in tincture and capsule forms; however, it's important to start with a lower dose to assess tolerance, as some individuals may experience grogginess.

Lemon Balm (Melissa officinalis), with its mild sedative effects, can help reduce anxiety and promote a sense of calm. For a soothing lemon balm tea, use 1-2 tablespoons of dried lemon balm leaves per cup of boiling water, steeping for 10 minutes. Drinking lemon balm tea 2-3 times a day can help alleviate stress and ease nervous tension. Lemon balm can also be taken as a tincture or in capsules according to the dosage on the product label.

Lavender (Lavandula angustifolia) is renowned not only for its pleasant aroma but also for its ability to decrease anxiety and improve sleep quality. To enjoy lavender's benefits, add a few drops of lavender essential oil to a diffuser before bedtime or dilute with a carrier oil and apply topically to the temples and wrists. Additionally, brewing a tea with 1 teaspoon of dried lavender flowers in 8 ounces of boiling water for 5 minutes can be a delightful way to wind down in the evening. Note that lavender essential oil should not be ingested unless the product is specifically labeled for such use.

When incorporating these nervines into your regimen, it's crucial to consider any potential interactions with medications or underlying health conditions. Always consult with a healthcare provider before starting any new herbal treatment, especially if you are pregnant, nursing, or have a medical condition. Remember, while nervines can significantly aid in managing stress and anxiety, they should be part of a comprehensive approach to emotional wellbeing, including a balanced diet, regular exercise, and adequate sleep.

Calming Herbs: Chamomile and Valerian

Chamomile and valerian root are two of the most revered herbs in the realm of natural remedies for their calming and sedative properties. These plants have been utilized for centuries to alleviate stress and anxiety, promote relaxation, and support restful sleep. Here, we delve into the specifics of how to effectively use chamomile and valerian root to harness their benefits.

Chamomile (Matricaria recutita), with its delicate, apple-like aroma, is not only a pleasure to the senses but also a potent herb for calming the nervous system. To prepare a chamomile infusion, you'll need:
- 1-2 teaspoons of dried chamomile flowers
- 8 ounces of boiling water

Place the chamomile flowers in a teapot or cup and pour the boiling water over them. Cover and steep for 5-10 minutes to allow the therapeutic properties to be released. Strain the tea and enjoy it warm. For those experiencing stress or difficulty sleeping, drinking chamomile tea 2-3 times a day, especially before bedtime, can be particularly beneficial. Chamomile is also available in pre-packaged tea bags for convenience, but ensure they are of high quality and organic, if possible, to maximize benefits.

Valerian Root (Valeriana officinalis) is another powerhouse herb known for its ability to improve sleep quality and reduce the time it takes to fall asleep. Unlike chamomile, valerian root has a very strong, earthy odor, which some may find off-putting, but its effectiveness is unparalleled. For valerian root tea:
- 1 teaspoon of dried valerian root

- 1 cup of hot water

Add the valerian root to the hot water and let it steep for 10 minutes. Due to its potent flavor, you may wish to add honey or mix it with another herbal tea to improve the taste. Drinking a cup of valerian root tea about 30 minutes to 2 hours before bedtime can significantly enhance sleep quality. Valerian is also available in capsules and tinctures for those who prefer not to drink the tea due to its strong flavor.

When using **chamomile and valerian root** together, they can offer a synergistic effect that is particularly effective for those with severe stress, anxiety, or sleep disorders. A combination tea can be made by mixing 1 teaspoon of dried chamomile flowers with 1 teaspoon of dried valerian root in 8 ounces of boiling water. Steep for 10 minutes, strain, and drink before bedtime.

It's important to note that while both chamomile and valerian root are generally considered safe for most people, they can interact with certain medications and conditions. For example, chamomile should be used with caution by those who are pregnant or have a history of severe allergies, especially to plants in the daisy family. Valerian root, while safe for short-term use, should not be taken with alcohol or sedative medications, and its long-term safety remains unclear.

Always consult with a healthcare provider before starting any new herbal regimen, particularly if you are pregnant, nursing, or have existing health conditions or concerns. With proper use, chamomile and valerian root can be powerful tools in your natural wellness toolkit for combating stress and promoting a peaceful, restful state of being.

Chamomile and Lavender Relaxation Tea

Beneficial effects

Chamomile and Lavender Relaxation Tea combines the calming properties of chamomile with the soothing effects of lavender, making it an ideal beverage for stress relief and promoting relaxation before bedtime. Chamomile is widely recognized for its ability to ease anxiety and induce sleep, while lavender contributes to reducing stress levels and improving sleep quality. This herbal blend can help soothe the nervous system, making it perfect for unwinding after a long day.

Portions

Serves 2

Preparation time

5 minutes

Cooking time

10 minutes

Ingredients

- 2 tablespoons dried chamomile flowers
- 1 tablespoon dried lavender buds
- 3 cups of water
- Honey or lemon (optional, for taste)

Instructions

1. Begin by bringing 3 cups of water to a boil in a medium-sized saucepan.
2. Once the water reaches a rolling boil, remove the saucepan from the heat.
3. Add 2 tablespoons of dried chamomile flowers and 1 tablespoon of dried lavender buds to the hot water. If you have a tea infuser or a tea ball, you can use it to contain the herbs for easier removal later.
4. Cover the saucepan with a lid to prevent the escape of essential oils and allow the herbs to steep for 8 to 10 minutes. The longer you steep, the stronger the flavor and therapeutic benefits.
5. After steeping, strain the tea through a fine mesh sieve into teacups or a teapot, pressing on the herbs to extract as much liquid as possible. Discard the used herbs.
6. If desired, sweeten the tea with honey or add a squeeze of lemon to enhance the flavor. Stir well to ensure any added sweeteners are fully dissolved.
7. Serve the tea warm to enjoy its maximum calming effects.

Variations

- For a cooler, refreshing version, allow the tea to cool to room temperature, then refrigerate and serve over ice.
- Add a cinnamon stick or a few slices of fresh ginger to the water before boiling for a warming, spicy twist.
- Combine with a small amount of peppermint leaves during steeping for a refreshing minty flavor.

Storage tips

If you have leftover tea, it can be stored in a sealed container in the refrigerator for up to 2 days. Enjoy it cold, or gently reheat on the stove or in a microwave for a warm, soothing drink.

Tips for allergens

For those with allergies or sensitivities to honey, maple syrup or agave nectar make suitable sweetener alternatives. Always ensure that the chamomile and lavender are sourced from reputable suppliers to avoid contamination with allergens.

Scientific references

- "Chamomile: A herbal medicine of the past with a bright future" published in Molecular Medicine Reports, which discusses the anxiolytic (anxiety-reducing) and sedative effects of chamomile.
- "Lavender and the Nervous System" found in Evidence-Based Complementary and Alternative Medicine, highlighting lavender's efficacy in alleviating stress and improving sleep quality.

CHAPTER 2: UPLIFTING HERBS FOR DEPRESSION

Depression, a common but serious mood disorder, affects millions globally. It's characterized by persistent sadness, lack of interest in activities, and a range of physical and emotional problems, significantly impacting daily functioning. While conventional treatment typically involves medication and psychotherapy, herbal remedies offer a complementary approach that can support emotional wellbeing. This section delves into uplifting herbs known for their potential to alleviate symptoms of depression, focusing on **St. John's Wort**, **Lemon Balm**, and **Saffron**.

St. John's Wort (Hypericum perforatum) has been extensively studied for its antidepressant properties. It's believed to work by increasing the levels of neurotransmitters in the brain, such as serotonin, dopamine, and norepinephrine, which play an essential role in regulating mood. For those considering St. John's Wort, it's available in various forms, including capsules, teas, and tinctures. A standard dose is 300 mg of an extract, taken three times daily, which should be standardized to contain 0.3% hypericin. It's crucial to note that St. John's Wort can interact with a wide range of medications, including antidepressants, birth control pills, and blood thinners, so consulting with a healthcare provider before starting is essential.

Lemon Balm (Melissa officinalis), a member of the mint family, is renowned for its calming effects on the nervous system, making it beneficial for those experiencing depression with anxiety. Lemon Balm can be consumed as a tea by steeping 1-2 teaspoons of dried herb in boiling water for 10 minutes. It's also available in capsules and tinctures for those preferring a more concentrated form. The recommended dose for capsules is 300-500 mg, taken up to three times daily. Lemon Balm should be used with caution in combination with sedative medications due to its calming effects.

Saffron (Crocus sativus), often referred to as the "sunshine spice," has shown promise in clinical studies for its ability to improve symptoms of depression, possibly due to its influence on serotonin metabolism. Saffron can be incorporated into the diet by adding it to dishes or taken as a supplement. The recommended dose for depression is 30 mg of saffron extract daily, divided into two 15 mg doses. Given its high cost as a spice, ensuring the authenticity of saffron supplements is crucial when selecting a product.

When incorporating these herbs into a regimen for depression, it's important to maintain realistic expectations and understand that herbal remedies can complement but not replace conventional treatments prescribed by healthcare professionals. Additionally, lifestyle factors such as diet, exercise, and sleep play a critical role in managing depression. Therefore, a holistic approach that includes these elements, alongside herbal remedies, can offer the best support for emotional wellbeing.

Finally, while these herbs have been associated with positive outcomes in some individuals, responses can vary. Starting with lower doses and gradually adjusting based on personal tolerance and effectiveness, under the guidance of a healthcare provider, is advisable. Monitoring for any side effects or interactions with other medications is also essential to ensure safety and efficacy in the management of depression.

St. John's Wort & Lemon Balm for Mood

St. John's Wort (Hypericum perforatum) and Lemon Balm (Melissa officinalis) are two potent herbs renowned for their mood-enhancing properties, offering a natural approach to mitigating symptoms of depression and elevating emotional wellbeing. When considering the use of these herbs, it's essential to understand their active components, optimal dosages, and preparation methods to maximize their therapeutic benefits.

St. John's Wort operates primarily through its active compounds, hypericin and hyperforin, which are believed to contribute to its antidepressant and anti-anxiety effects. These compounds work by influencing neurotransmitter activity in the brain, including serotonin, dopamine, and norepinephrine, which play pivotal roles in regulating mood. For those seeking to incorporate St. John's Wort into their regimen, it's advisable to start with a standardized extract of 300 mg, taken three times daily. This dosage ensures a consistent intake of its active ingredients, aiming for a cumulative effect over time, typically observed after 4-6 weeks of consistent use. It's crucial to source St. John's Wort from reputable suppliers to ensure the extract's potency and purity. Additionally, individuals should be aware of St. John's Wort's potential interactions with pharmaceutical medications, including antidepressants, birth control pills, and blood thinners, necessitating a consultation with a healthcare provider before commencing its use.

Lemon Balm, on the other hand, is cherished for its calming and mood-stabilizing effects, attributed to its rich content of rosmarinic acid and terpenes. These compounds have been shown to enhance cognitive function, alleviate stress, and promote relaxation without sedation. To harness Lemon Balm's mood-enhancing benefits, a daily intake of 300-600 mg of its extract is recommended, preferably in the form of capsules or a standardized extract for consistency. Alternatively, Lemon Balm tea, prepared by steeping 1-2 teaspoons of dried herb in hot water for 10-15 minutes, offers a soothing and therapeutic beverage that can be enjoyed up to three times daily. When selecting Lemon Balm, opting for organically grown herbs or extracts can ensure the absence of pesticides and maximize the therapeutic constituents.

Combining St. John's Wort and Lemon Balm presents a synergistic approach to mood enhancement, where St. John's Wort's antidepressant action complements Lemon Balm's stress-relieving properties. A holistic regimen might include the standardized doses of St. John's Wort alongside Lemon Balm tea or extract, adjusted according to individual responses and under the guidance of a healthcare professional. This combination should be approached with caution, especially when other medications are involved, to avoid potential herb-drug interactions.

In preparing these herbs, precision and consistency in dosing are paramount. For St. John's Wort, utilizing a standardized extract ensures accurate dosing, while for Lemon Balm, both dried herb for tea and extracts offer flexibility in preparation methods. The quality of herbs significantly influences their efficacy; thus, sourcing from certified organic producers and reputable suppliers becomes crucial. Storage also plays a vital role in preserving the herbs' potency, where they should be kept in a cool, dark, and dry place to maintain their therapeutic properties.

Incorporating St. John's Wort and Lemon Balm into one's wellness routine for mood enhancement requires an informed approach, emphasizing the importance of understanding each herb's characteristics, optimal dosages, and potential interactions. By adhering to recommended guidelines and consulting healthcare professionals, individuals can safely explore the mood-enhancing benefits of these time-honored herbs, contributing to an overall strategy for emotional wellbeing and depression management.

Lemon Balm Uplifting Infusion

Beneficial effects

Lemon Balm Uplifting Infusion is a soothing beverage designed to elevate mood and alleviate symptoms of stress and anxiety. Lemon balm, a member of the mint family, has been used for centuries to improve mood and cognitive function, thanks to its natural calming effects. This herbal infusion harnesses the aromatic and therapeutic properties of lemon balm to provide a gentle, natural way to enhance emotional wellbeing.

Portions

Serves 2

Preparation time

5 minutes

Cooking time

10 minutes

Ingredients

- 2 tablespoons of dried lemon balm leaves
- 2 cups of boiling water
- Honey or stevia to taste (optional)
- A few slices of fresh lemon for garnish (optional)

Instructions

1. Boil 2 cups of water in a kettle or a pot. Once boiling, remove from heat.
2. Place 2 tablespoons of dried lemon balm leaves in a tea infuser or directly into a teapot.
3. Pour the hot water over the lemon balm leaves, ensuring they are fully submerged.
4. Cover the teapot or cup and let the lemon balm steep for 10 minutes. This allows the water to become infused with the lemon balm's essential oils and therapeutic properties.
5. After steeping, remove the tea infuser or strain the infusion to remove the lemon balm leaves.
6. If desired, sweeten the infusion with honey or stevia according to taste.
7. Serve the infusion in cups, and for an added touch of freshness, garnish with a slice of fresh lemon in each cup.

Variations
- For a cooling summer drink, let the infusion cool to room temperature, then refrigerate until cold. Serve over ice.
- Add a sprig of fresh mint or a few leaves of fresh lemon balm to the infusion for an extra burst of flavor and freshness.
- Combine with chamomile in the evening for a relaxing blend that can help promote a restful night's sleep.

Storage tips
If you have leftover lemon balm infusion, it can be stored in a sealed container in the refrigerator for up to 2 days. Enjoy it chilled or gently reheat on the stove or in a microwave.

Tips for allergens
For those with allergies or sensitivities to honey, stevia is a suitable sweetener alternative that does not trigger common allergies. Always ensure that the lemon balm and any other herbs used are sourced from reputable suppliers to avoid contamination with allergens.

Scientific references
- "Melissa officinalis L. – A review of its traditional uses, phytochemistry and pharmacology" published in the Journal of Ethnopharmacology, which discusses the mood-enhancing and cognitive-improving effects of lemon balm.
- "Anxiolytic effects of a combination of Melissa officinalis and Valeriana officinalis during laboratory induced stress" found in Phytotherapy Research, highlighting the stress-relieving properties of lemon balm when used in herbal blends.

BOOK 10: HERBAL FIRST AID ESSENTIALS

CHAPTER 1: EMERGENCY HERBAL REMEDIES

In the realm of emergency herbal remedies, **Calendula and Yarrow Healing Salve** stands out as a versatile and potent solution for treating cuts, burns, and bruises. This salve harnesses the anti-inflammatory and healing properties of both calendula and yarrow, making it an essential component of any herbal first aid kit. Here's a detailed breakdown of how to prepare this healing salve:

Ingredients:
- 1 cup of calendula-infused oil (To prepare, fill a jar with dried calendula flowers, cover with a carrier oil such as olive or almond oil, seal the jar, and place in a sunny spot for 4-6 weeks, shaking daily. Strain the oil through cheesecloth before use.)
- 1/4 cup of yarrow-infused oil (Follow the same process as for the calendula-infused oil, using dried yarrow flowers.)
- 1/4 cup of beeswax pellets (Ensure they are pure and free from impurities for the best healing properties.)
- Optional: 10-15 drops of lavender essential oil for its soothing and antimicrobial benefits.

Tools:
- Double boiler (If you don't have one, place a heat-safe bowl over a pot of simmering water.)
- Glass jar or metal tin for storage
- Cheesecloth or fine mesh strainer
- Stirring utensil (A wooden spoon or spatula is ideal.)

Preparation Steps:
1. Combine the calendula and yarrow-infused oils in the top part of the double boiler or heat-safe bowl. Heat gently over simmering water until the oils are warm but not boiling.
2. Add the beeswax pellets to the warmed oil mixture, stirring continuously until the beeswax is completely melted and the mixture is well combined.
3. Remove from heat. If using, add the lavender essential oil to the mixture at this point and stir well to ensure even distribution.
4. Carefully pour the liquid salve into your chosen storage container. Allow it to cool and solidify at room temperature. This may take several hours.
5. Once solidified, seal the container with a lid to prevent contamination and store in a cool, dark place.

Application:
- To use, clean the affected area with mild soap and water and pat dry.
- Apply a small amount of the salve directly to cuts, burns, or bruises.
- Cover with a clean bandage or gauze if necessary.
- Reapply 2-3 times daily until the wound begins to heal.

Safety Precautions:
- Always patch test a small area of skin before widespread use to ensure there is no allergic reaction.
- Do not apply to open or weeping wounds.
- Consult a healthcare professional if symptoms persist or if there is any concern about the wound's healing process.

This **Calendula and Yarrow Healing Salve** recipe is designed to be simple yet effective, suitable for those with varying levels of herbal knowledge and accessible to individuals with different educational backgrounds. The detailed steps ensure precision in preparation, while the specific recommendations for materials, tools, and techniques aim to provide clarity and enhance the overall effectiveness of the remedy.

Treating Cuts, Burns, and Bruises

Calendula and yarrow, two potent herbs renowned for their healing properties, offer a natural and effective way to treat cuts, burns, and bruises. These plants have been used for centuries in traditional medicine, thanks to their anti-inflammatory, antimicrobial, and astringent qualities. When combined in a salve, they create a powerful remedy that can accelerate the healing process, reduce the risk of infection, and alleviate pain and inflammation.

To prepare a Calendula and Yarrow Healing Salve, you will need the following ingredients and tools:

Ingredients:

- 1/2 cup of dried calendula petals, known for their ability to speed up wound healing and reduce inflammation.
- 1/2 cup of dried yarrow leaves and flowers, which are valued for their antimicrobial and pain-relieving properties.
- 1 cup of carrier oil, such as olive oil or coconut oil, to infuse with the herbs. These oils are chosen for their skin-soothing benefits and ability to carry the medicinal properties of the herbs into the skin.
- 1/4 cup of beeswax, to solidify the oil into a salve form. Beeswax also adds a protective layer over wounds, which helps keep them clean and moisturized.
- Optional: A few drops of lavender essential oil for additional antimicrobial and soothing effects.

Tools:
- A double boiler or a makeshift one using a glass bowl over a pot of simmering water. This is used to gently heat the oil and beeswax without burning them.
- A fine mesh strainer or cheesecloth for filtering the herb-infused oil.
- A clean, dry jar or tin for storing the salve.

Preparation Steps:
1. Begin by infusing the carrier oil with calendula and yarrow. Combine the dried herbs and the carrier oil in a double boiler, and let them gently simmer over low heat for 2-3 hours. This slow process allows the oil to extract the healing compounds from the herbs.
2. After the infusion is complete, carefully strain the oil through a fine mesh strainer or cheesecloth into a clean bowl, making sure to squeeze out as much oil as possible from the herbs.
3. Return the strained oil to the double boiler, and add the beeswax. Heat the mixture gently, stirring frequently, until the beeswax is completely melted and incorporated into the oil.
4. Remove the mixture from the heat, and if desired, stir in a few drops of lavender essential oil for its soothing scent and additional healing properties.
5. Quickly pour the liquid salve into your prepared jar or tin before it begins to solidify. Allow it to cool and harden at room temperature.

Application:
To use the Calendula and Yarrow Healing Salve, first clean the affected area with mild soap and water. Pat the area dry with a clean towel. With clean hands or a spatula, apply a small amount of the salve directly to the cut, burn, or bruise. If necessary, cover with a bandage or clean cloth. The salve can be applied 2-3 times daily until the wound heals. It's important to monitor the area for signs of infection or allergic reaction, especially if it's the first time using the salve.

Safety Precautions:
While calendula and yarrow are generally safe for topical use, it's crucial to perform a patch test before applying the salve extensively, especially if you have sensitive skin or allergies to plants in the Asteraceae family. Discontinue use if irritation or allergic reaction occurs. For serious burns or deep cuts, seek professional medical advice before applying any home remedies.

This detailed guide to creating and using a Calendula and Yarrow Healing Salve is designed to be accessible to individuals with varied levels of herbal knowledge and from different educational backgrounds. The step-by-step instructions ensure clarity and precision in preparation, while the inclusion of specific recommendations for materials, tools, and techniques enhances the overall effectiveness and safety of the remedy.

Calendula and Yarrow Healing Salve
Beneficial effects
Calendula and yarrow are both renowned for their healing properties, particularly when it comes to skin care. Calendula is celebrated for its anti-inflammatory, antimicrobial, and astringent qualities, making it an excellent choice for soothing and repairing damaged skin. Yarrow, on the other hand, is known for its ability to stop bleeding, heal wounds, and reduce inflammation. Together, these herbs create a powerful salve that can be used to treat cuts, scrapes, burns, and other skin irritations, promoting faster healing and reducing the risk of infection.

Portions
Makes approximately 8 ounces of salve
Preparation time
15 minutes

Cooking time
2 hours (includes infusion and cooling time)
Ingredients
- 1 cup of calendula petals, freshly picked and dried
- 1 cup of yarrow flowers and leaves, freshly picked and dried
- 1.5 cups of olive oil or coconut oil
- 1/4 cup of beeswax pellets
- Optional: 10-15 drops of lavender essential oil for added antimicrobial and soothing properties
Instructions
1. Begin by sterilizing a glass jar and a metal spoon in boiling water for 5 minutes. Dry thoroughly.
2. Place the dried calendula petals and yarrow flowers and leaves into the sterilized glass jar.
3. Pour the olive oil or coconut oil over the herbs, ensuring they are completely submerged. Seal the jar tightly.
4. Use a double boiler method to infuse the oil: Fill a saucepan with a few inches of water and place the sealed jar in the saucepan. Heat the water to a gentle simmer and let the jar sit in the simmering water for 2 hours. This process slowly infuses the oil with the healing properties of the herbs.
5. After 2 hours, carefully remove the jar from the water and let it cool slightly.
6. Strain the infused oil through a cheesecloth or fine mesh strainer into a clean bowl, squeezing or pressing the herbs to extract as much oil as possible. Discard the herbs.
7. Add the beeswax pellets to the infused oil. If the oil has cooled and solidified, gently reheat it until the beeswax melts, stirring constantly with the sterilized metal spoon.
8. Once the beeswax is fully melted and combined with the oil, remove from heat. If using, stir in the lavender essential oil.
9. Pour the mixture into small tins or glass jars for storage. Let the salve cool and solidify at room temperature.
10. Once solidified, seal the containers. Label them with the contents and date.
Variations
- For vegan salve, substitute beeswax with an equal amount of candelilla wax.
- Add vitamin E oil as a natural preservative and to boost skin healing.
- Incorporate other healing herbs such as plantain or comfrey for additional therapeutic benefits.
Storage tips
Store the salve in a cool, dark place. It should last for up to 1 year. If the salve smells rancid or changes color, discard it.
Tips for allergens
For those with sensitivities to beeswax or any of the essential oils, ensure to perform a patch test before applying the salve extensively. Substitute beeswax with candelilla wax for a bee product-free version.
Scientific references
- "Anti-inflammatory and wound healing activity of a growth substance in Aloe vera," published in the Journal of the American Podiatric Medical Association, highlights the healing properties of herbal ingredients similar to those in calendula.
- "Yarrow (Achillea millefolium L.): A neglected panacea? A review of its pharmacology, therapeutic potential and mechanisms of action," in the Journal of Ethnopharmacology, discusses yarrow's healing effects.

CHAPTER 2: COUGHS & RESPIRATORY EMERGENCIES

In the face of coughs and respiratory emergencies, having a well-prepared herbal remedy can be a game-changer. This section delves into the preparation of a **Marshmallow Root Cough Syrup**, a soothing solution for coughs and throat irritation. Marshmallow root (Althaea officinalis) is renowned for its mucilaginous properties, offering a protective layer over the throat and reducing irritation that leads to coughing.

Ingredients:
- 2 tablespoons of dried marshmallow root
- 1 quart of filtered water
- 1 cup of raw, local honey
- Optional: 2 tablespoons of lemon juice for added vitamin C and flavor

Tools:
- Medium saucepan
- Strainer or cheesecloth
- Measuring cups and spoons
- Sterilized glass jar with lid

Preparation Steps:
1. **Infuse Marshmallow Root:** Combine the marshmallow root with the filtered water in a medium saucepan. Bring the mixture to a boil, then reduce the heat and simmer gently for 20 minutes. This slow simmering process allows the water to become infused with the mucilaginous compounds of the marshmallow root.
2. **Strain:** After simmering, remove the saucepan from the heat. Strain the liquid through a strainer or cheesecloth into a large bowl, pressing the marshmallow root to extract as much liquid as possible. Discard the spent herbs.
3. **Add Honey:** While the liquid is still warm (but not hot), add the raw honey to the marshmallow infusion. Stir thoroughly until the honey is completely dissolved. The honey acts as a natural cough suppressant and also gives the syrup a pleasant taste. If you choose to add lemon juice, do so at this stage.
4. **Bottle:** Pour the finished syrup into a sterilized glass jar. Secure the lid tightly. Label the jar with the contents and date.

Usage:
- For adults, take 1 tablespoon of the syrup up to 4 times a day. For children over the age of one, administer 1 teaspoon up to 4 times a day. Due to the honey content, this syrup is not recommended for children under one year of age.

Storage:
- Store the cough syrup in the refrigerator. It will keep for up to 2 months. Always check the syrup before use; if it shows any signs of spoilage, discard it.

Safety Precautions:
- While marshmallow root is generally considered safe, it's important to consult with a healthcare provider before using this remedy, especially for individuals with diabetes (due to the honey content), pregnant or nursing women, and parents considering it for children.

Additional Tips:
- For an extra immune boost, consider adding a teaspoon of dried echinacea to the marshmallow root during the simmering process. Echinacea can enhance the body's immune response, making it a valuable addition during cold and flu season.
- Ensure the honey is added to warm, not hot, liquid to preserve its natural enzymes and benefits.

This detailed guide to creating a Marshmallow Root Cough Syrup is designed to be accessible and straightforward, allowing individuals of varying levels of herbal knowledge and from different educational backgrounds to prepare an effective remedy for coughs and respiratory discomfort. The emphasis on specific ingredients, precise measurements, and clear instructions ensures that the preparation process is both simple and successful, providing a natural and soothing solution for those seeking relief from coughs and throat irritation.

Herbal Solutions for Respiratory Distress

In addressing acute respiratory distress, a condition characterized by sudden and severe difficulty in breathing, herbal remedies can serve as adjunctive treatments to conventional care. The focus here is on herbs known for their expectorant, anti-inflammatory, and soothing properties that can help alleviate symptoms associated with this condition. It's crucial to understand the properties of each herb, how to prepare them, and the appropriate dosages to ensure safety and effectiveness.

Mullein (Verbascum thapsus) is a key herb for respiratory health, particularly due to its expectorant and soothing qualities. To prepare a mullein leaf tea, which can help loosen congestion and ease breathing, you'll need:
- 1 to 2 teaspoons of dried mullein leaves
- 1 cup of boiling water
- A strainer or tea ball

Steep the mullein leaves in boiling water for 10 to 15 minutes, ensuring a prolonged infusion time to extract the active compounds effectively. Strain the tea to remove the leaves, as they can be irritating if ingested. Drinking this tea 2 to 3 times a day can provide relief.

Licorice root (Glycyrrhiza glabra) is another beneficial herb, acting as an anti-inflammatory and demulcent, soothing irritated mucous membranes. For a licorice root decoction:
- 1 teaspoon of dried licorice root
- 1 cup of water

Combine the licorice root with water in a small saucepan and bring to a boil. Reduce the heat and simmer for 10 to 15 minutes to allow the licorice to release its therapeutic properties. Strain and drink up to two cups a day. Note: Licorice root is contraindicated in cases of high blood pressure, heart disease, and during pregnancy.

Thyme (Thymus vulgaris) is renowned for its antimicrobial and expectorant properties, making it excellent for respiratory infections that can accompany or exacerbate respiratory distress. To make a thyme infusion:
- 1 teaspoon of dried thyme
- 1 cup of boiling water

Steep the thyme in boiling water for 5 to 10 minutes, then strain. Thyme tea can be consumed 2 to 3 times daily. Adding honey, which has antimicrobial and soothing effects, can enhance the therapeutic benefits and taste.

Eucalyptus (Eucalyptus globulus) is effective for its decongestant properties. Eucalyptus should not be ingested but can be used in a steam inhalation:
- 2 to 3 drops of eucalyptus essential oil
- A bowl of boiling water

Add the eucalyptus oil to the boiling water, drape a towel over your head, and inhale the steam for 5 to 10 minutes. This method helps to open up the airways and ease breathing. Ensure the room is well-ventilated and avoid direct contact with the eyes.

Peppermint (Mentha piperita) also serves as a decongestant due to its high menthol content. Peppermint tea can be made by:
- 1 teaspoon of dried peppermint leaves
- 1 cup of boiling water

Steep the peppermint leaves in boiling water for 10 minutes, strain, and drink. Alternatively, peppermint essential oil can be used in steam inhalation, similar to eucalyptus, but should not be ingested or applied undiluted to the skin.

It's imperative to source high-quality, organic herbs to ensure the absence of contaminants and to use precise measurements for both the herbs and water to maintain the efficacy of the remedies. Always consult with a healthcare provider before incorporating new herbal treatments, especially for serious conditions like acute respiratory distress, to avoid contraindications and ensure they complement existing treatments. While these herbal remedies can provide symptomatic relief, they are not substitutes for professional medical intervention in emergencies.

Marshmallow Root Cough Syrup
Beneficial effects

Marshmallow root has been traditionally used for its soothing properties on the throat and digestive system. Its mucilaginous content provides a protective layer on the mucous membranes, offering relief from coughing and irritation caused by colds or allergies. This cough syrup combines marshmallow root with honey and lemon, both known for their antimicrobial and soothing effects, to create a natural remedy for coughs and sore throats.

Portions
Makes about 16 ounces

Preparation time
10 minutes

Cooking time
20 minutes

Ingredients
- 1/2 cup dried marshmallow root
- 4 cups filtered water
- 1 cup honey (preferably raw and local)
- 1/4 cup lemon juice (freshly squeezed)

Instructions
1. In a medium saucepan, combine the dried marshmallow root with the filtered water. Place the saucepan on the stove and bring the mixture to a boil over high heat.
2. Once boiling, reduce the heat to low and let the mixture simmer for about 20 minutes. This slow simmering process allows the water to become infused with the mucilaginous properties of the marshmallow root.
3. After simmering, remove the saucepan from the heat. Strain the liquid through a fine mesh sieve or cheesecloth into a large bowl, pressing on the marshmallow root to extract as much liquid as possible. Discard the marshmallow root after straining.
4. While the liquid is still warm (but not hot), add the honey to the marshmallow infusion. Stir continuously until the honey is completely dissolved. The warmth of the liquid will help to incorporate the honey smoothly without destroying its beneficial enzymes.
5. Stir in the lemon juice, mixing thoroughly. The lemon juice adds a refreshing flavor and vitamin C, which can help to boost the immune system.
6. Allow the mixture to cool to room temperature. Once cooled, transfer the cough syrup into a clean glass bottle or jar with a tight-fitting lid.
7. Label the bottle or jar with the contents and date.

Variations
- For added antimicrobial properties, include 1 tablespoon of ginger root (freshly grated) during the simmering process.
- If honey is not suitable, substitute it with maple syrup or vegetable glycerin, adjusting the amount to taste.
- Add a few cloves or a cinnamon stick during simmering for additional flavor and soothing properties.

Storage tips
Store the cough syrup in the refrigerator for up to 3 months. Shake well before each use as natural separation may occur.

Tips for allergens
For those with allergies to honey, maple syrup or vegetable glycerin are suitable alternatives that do not compromise the syrup's soothing effects. Always ensure that the marshmallow root is sourced from reputable suppliers to avoid contamination with allergens.

Scientific references
- "The effect of marshmallow root extract on cough reflex sensitivity" published in the Journal of Alternative and Complementary Medicine, which discusses the soothing properties of marshmallow root on the throat and its potential in treating coughs.

BOOK 11: HERBAL REMEDIES FOR CHILDREN

CHAPTER 1: GENTLE HERBS FOR COMMON AILMENTS

In addressing common ailments in children, gentle herbs stand out for their efficacy and safety. When selecting herbs for children, it's crucial to opt for those with a long history of safe use, both in traditional practices and confirmed by modern research. Here, we delve into specific herbs and their applications for common pediatric concerns, ensuring that parents and caregivers can confidently administer these natural remedies.

Chamomile (Matricaria recutita) is renowned for its calming effects, making it an excellent choice for soothing teething discomfort and promoting restful sleep. Prepare a mild chamomile tea by steeping 1 teaspoon of dried flowers in 1 cup of boiling water for 5-10 minutes. Strain and allow the tea to cool to a safe temperature before offering it to the child. For teething, a clean cloth dipped in chamomile tea and then frozen can provide chewable relief.

Catnip (Nepeta cataria), beyond its well-known effects on felines, possesses mild sedative properties beneficial for children experiencing restlessness or digestive upset. A tea made from 1 teaspoon of dried catnip leaves steeped in 1 cup of boiling water for 10 minutes can help ease minor tummy troubles and facilitate relaxation. Always ensure the tea is cooled sufficiently before serving.

Fennel (Foeniculum vulgare) is effective against gas and colic in infants. To prepare fennel tea, crush 1 teaspoon of fennel seeds and steep in 1 cup of boiling water for 10 minutes. Strain and cool the tea to a suitable temperature. Fennel tea can be given in small doses throughout the day to alleviate gas pains.

Ginger (Zingiber officinale) is a go-to remedy for nausea and digestive issues. For children, a mild ginger tea can be made by steeping a small slice of fresh ginger (about the size of a nickel) in 1 cup of boiling water for 5 minutes. Strain and cool the tea before offering it in small sips to help settle the stomach.

Peppermint (Mentha piperita) offers relief from headaches and minor aches due to its natural analgesic properties. A peppermint tea, prepared by steeping 1 teaspoon of dried peppermint leaves in 1 cup of boiling water for 5-10 minutes, can be given to children over the age of 5. Ensure the tea is cooled to a safe temperature before consumption.

When introducing any new herb to a child's regimen, start with small amounts to monitor for any adverse reactions. It's also paramount to consult with a healthcare provider before administering herbal remedies to children, especially in the case of ongoing medical conditions or the use of prescription medications. The recommended dosages provided here are for children aged 2-12 years. For infants under 2, professional guidance is strongly advised to ensure safety and appropriateness of the herbal remedy.

Soothing Teething Pain with Chamomile

Chamomile, scientifically known as Matricaria recutita, and Catnip, known as Nepeta cataria, are two herbs celebrated for their gentle soothing properties, making them ideal for addressing the discomfort associated with teething in children. When a child is teething, they may experience a range of symptoms including irritability, trouble sleeping, and a tendency to chew on objects. The calming effects of Chamomile, coupled with the mild sedative properties of Catnip, can provide natural relief during this challenging period.

To prepare a Chamomile and Catnip blend for teething pain, begin by sourcing high-quality, organic dried Chamomile flowers and Catnip leaves. The importance of using organic herbs cannot be overstated, as it ensures the absence of pesticides and chemicals, safeguarding your child's health. For the preparation, you will need:

- 1 teaspoon of dried Chamomile flowers
- 1 teaspoon of dried Catnip leaves
- 1 cup of boiling water

Start by boiling water in a clean, stainless steel pot. Once the water reaches a rolling boil, remove it from the heat. In a teapot or heat-safe container, combine the Chamomile flowers and Catnip leaves. Pour the hot water over the herbs, ensuring they are fully submerged. Cover the teapot or container with a lid to prevent the escape of essential oils and aromas. Let the herbs steep for about 10 minutes. This duration is crucial as it allows the therapeutic properties of the herbs to infuse into the water, creating a potent herbal remedy.

After steeping, strain the tea through a fine mesh sieve or a cheesecloth to remove the herb particles, ensuring a smooth tea that is safe for your child. Allow the tea to cool to room temperature to avoid any risk of burning.

For infants and young children, it is essential to test the temperature of the tea before administration to ensure it is comfortably warm but not hot.

For teething relief, the Chamomile and Catnip tea can be offered to the child to sip. Alternatively, for younger children or those who might not readily drink the tea, soaking a clean, small washcloth in the tea and then chilling it in the refrigerator creates a soothing teether. The child can chew on the cool, damp cloth, benefiting from the analgesic properties of the herbs while the coldness helps to numb the gums and reduce inflammation.

It is recommended to administer this herbal remedy sparingly, starting with small amounts to observe how the child reacts. While Chamomile and Catnip are generally safe for children, every child is unique, and it's prudent to monitor for any adverse reactions. Consulting with a pediatrician or a professional herbalist before introducing any new herbal remedy to your child's regimen is always advised, especially if the child is under two years of age or has specific health conditions.

Remember, the goal is to provide gentle relief to your teething child, utilizing the natural, time-tested properties of Chamomile and Catnip. By preparing this herbal remedy with care and attention to detail, you can offer your child a safe and effective option for teething discomfort, harnessing the power of nature's own medicine cabinet.

Chamomile Teething Relief Tea

Beneficial effects
Chamomile Teething Relief Tea provides a gentle, natural remedy for soothing the discomfort associated with teething in babies. Chamomile is renowned for its calming and anti-inflammatory properties, making it an ideal choice to ease gum irritation, reduce inflammation, and help babies relax, potentially leading to better sleep during this challenging period.

Portions
Makes about 2 cups

Preparation time
5 minutes

Cooking time
10 minutes

Ingredients
- 2 tablespoons dried chamomile flowers
- 2 cups of water
- Optional: 1 teaspoon of honey (for babies over 1 year old) or a pinch of cinnamon for flavor

Instructions
1. In a small saucepan, bring 2 cups of water to a gentle boil.
2. Remove the saucepan from the heat and add 2 tablespoons of dried chamomile flowers to the hot water.
3. Cover the saucepan with a lid to prevent the escape of essential oils and allow the chamomile to steep for 8 to 10 minutes. The longer steeping time ensures a stronger infusion, maximizing the soothing effects of the chamomile.
4. After steeping, strain the tea through a fine mesh sieve into a clean container, pressing on the chamomile flowers to extract as much liquid as possible. Discard the used chamomile flowers.
5. Allow the tea to cool to room temperature before serving to ensure it is safe for baby's consumption. If desired, you can refrigerate the tea to cool it down more quickly.
6. For babies over 1 year old, you may sweeten the tea with a teaspoon of honey to enhance the flavor. Alternatively, a pinch of cinnamon can be added for babies of any age, but always ensure the tea is completely cooled to the appropriate temperature before serving.

Variations
- For additional calming effects, a small amount of lavender can be added to the chamomile during the steeping process. However, use lavender sparingly due to its strong flavor.
- To create a larger batch, simply double or triple the recipe. Adjust the amount of chamomile proportionally to ensure the tea maintains its intended therapeutic benefits.

Storage tips
Store any leftover tea in a sealed container in the refrigerator for up to 48 hours. Warm the tea gently to room temperature before serving again, but do not reheat in the microwave as hot spots could form and burn the baby's mouth.

Tips for allergens

For babies with sensitivities or allergies, ensure that the chamomile used is pure and not mixed with other herbs that could potentially cause a reaction. Always introduce new ingredients to babies individually and watch for any signs of allergic reactions.

Scientific references

- "Chamomile: A herbal medicine of the past with bright future" published in Molecular Medicine Reports, which discusses the anti-inflammatory and sedative effects of chamomile, supporting its use in relieving teething discomfort.

- "Safety and efficacy of herbal remedies in obstetrics—review and clinical implications" in Midwifery, highlighting the safe use of chamomile in children for various ailments, including teething discomfort.

CHAPTER 2: IMMUNE SUPPORT FOR KIDS

Building immunity in children is a critical aspect of their development, ensuring they can resist infections and maintain optimal health. A robust immune system is the foundation of a healthy body, and certain herbs have been recognized for their ability to support and enhance the immune response in children. When considering herbal remedies for immune support, it's essential to focus on herbs known for their safety and efficacy in pediatric populations. Here, we delve into specific herbs and their applications for bolstering immune health in children, alongside preparation methods that are both child-friendly and effective.

Elderberry (Sambucus nigra) is celebrated for its antiviral properties, making it a cornerstone in pediatric immune support. Rich in antioxidants and vitamins that can help fight off viruses, elderberry is particularly beneficial during cold and flu season. For children, elderberry syrup is a palatable way to administer this herb. To prepare, simmer dried elderberries in water for about 45 minutes. Strain the mixture and add honey to taste once cooled. The recommended dosage is 1 teaspoon for children aged 2-12, taken daily during peak cold and flu season.

Echinacea (Echinacea purpurea) has been shown to enhance the immune system by increasing white blood cell production, a key component in the body's defense against illness. A simple echinacea tea can be made by steeping the dried root or flowers in boiling water for 10-15 minutes. Given its slightly bitter taste, mixing echinacea tea with a bit of honey or blending it with more palatable herbal teas like peppermint or chamomile can make it more appealing to children. The tea can be served once or twice a day, especially at the onset of cold symptoms.

Vitamin C-rich herbs such as rose hips (Rosa canina) and camu camu (Myrciaria dubia) offer immune-boosting benefits and can be easily incorporated into a child's diet. Rose hips, for instance, can be brewed into a tea or added to smoothies in powdered form. Camu camu, being one of the most potent sources of Vitamin C, can be purchased in powder form and added to juices or smoothies. A quarter teaspoon of camu camu powder or a single cup of rose hip tea daily is sufficient for enhancing immune function in children.

Garlic (Allium sativum), with its potent antibiotic and immune-boosting properties, can be included in children's meals to support their immune system. Incorporating finely minced garlic into pasta sauces, soups, or spreads can make it more acceptable to young palates. For optimal immune support, adding garlic towards the end of the cooking process preserves its medicinal properties.

When introducing herbal remedies for immune support, it's crucial to start with small doses to monitor for any adverse reactions. Additionally, consulting with a healthcare provider before beginning any new herbal regimen is paramount, especially for children with existing health conditions or those taking prescription medications. The herbs mentioned here are generally considered safe for children, but individual sensitivities can vary.

It's also important to note that while these herbs can support the immune system, they should not replace standard care practices such as vaccinations and other preventive measures recommended by healthcare professionals. Instead, they should be used as part of a holistic approach to health, complementing a balanced diet, regular physical activity, and adequate sleep, all of which are essential for maintaining a strong immune system in children.

By carefully selecting and preparing these herbs, parents and caregivers can provide natural, effective immune support for children, helping them to thrive and stay healthy throughout the year.

Building Immunity with Elderberry & Echinacea

Elderberry and Echinacea stand out as two potent herbs that play a significant role in enhancing the immune system, especially in children. Their efficacy in fighting off infections and boosting overall health is backed by both traditional use and scientific research. When it comes to preparing these herbs in a way that's both safe and appealing to children, specific methods and considerations are essential to ensure the remedies are effective and enjoyable.

Starting with Elderberry (Sambucus nigra), this herb is renowned for its antiviral properties and its ability to support the immune system. To harness these benefits for children, creating a homemade elderberry syrup is an effective approach. Begin by sourcing high-quality, dried elderberries. It's crucial to use dried berries from a reputable source to ensure they are free from pesticides and contaminants. For the preparation, you will need about half a cup of dried elderberries, two cups of water, and a natural sweetener, preferably honey, for its additional antimicrobial properties. However, remember that honey is not recommended for children under one year of age due to the risk of botulism, so consider alternatives like maple syrup for younger children.

Combine the elderberries and water in a saucepan and bring the mixture to a boil. Reduce the heat and allow it to simmer for about 45 minutes to an hour, reducing the liquid by almost half. This slow simmering process extracts the active compounds from the elderberries. After simmering, mash the berries to release any remaining juice and then strain the mixture through a fine mesh sieve or cheesecloth, pressing to get all the liquid out. Once the mixture has cooled to room temperature, stir in your sweetener of choice. The ratio of sweetener can vary, but a general guideline is to add one cup of honey per cup of liquid, adjusting based on your preference and considerations for the child's age. Store the syrup in a clean, airtight glass bottle in the refrigerator. The recommended dosage for immune support is a teaspoon a day for children aged 2-12, increasing to a tablespoon for older children and adults.

Echinacea (Echinacea purpurea), on the other hand, is known for its ability to stimulate the immune system by increasing white blood cell production. Preparing an Echinacea tincture or tea can be an effective way to incorporate this herb into a child's routine for immune support. For a tincture, fill a jar with dried Echinacea root or leaves, then cover it with a high-proof alcohol like vodka, which will extract the active compounds over time. Seal the jar and store it in a cool, dark place, shaking it daily for about four to six weeks. After this period, strain the liquid through cheesecloth, and it's ready to use. Given the alcohol content, use the tincture sparingly for children, diluting a few drops in water or juice. The exact dosage can vary, but a general guideline is 1-2 drops per 4 pounds of body weight, not exceeding three times a day.

For those preferring a non-alcoholic preparation, Echinacea tea is a suitable alternative. Steep one teaspoon of dried Echinacea in a cup of boiling water for 10-15 minutes. The tea can have a slightly bitter taste, so consider blending it with more palatable herbs or adding a natural sweetener to make it more appealing to children. Serving the tea warm, especially during cold months, can provide soothing immune support.

When introducing these herbal remedies, it's vital to monitor for any allergic reactions or side effects, as individual sensitivities can vary. Always consult with a healthcare provider before adding new herbal supplements to a child's regimen, particularly if the child is under medical care or taking prescription medications. While Elderberry and Echinacea are generally considered safe, their use should complement a holistic approach to health, including a balanced diet, adequate hydration, and proper sleep, to support a robust immune system in children.

Elderberry Gummies for Kids

Beneficial effects

Elderberry gummies for kids harness the natural immune-boosting properties of elderberries, making them an excellent choice for supporting your child's immune system. Elderberries are rich in vitamins and antioxidants, which can help to fight off colds and flu. These gummies offer a fun and tasty way for kids to enjoy the benefits of elderberries, making them more likely to take their daily dose without fuss.

Portions

Makes approximately 50 gummies

Preparation time

10 minutes

Cooking time

5 minutes

Ingredients

- 3/4 cup elderberry syrup (homemade or store-bought)
- 1/4 cup water
- 1/2 cup unflavored gelatin powder
- 2 tablespoons honey (optional, adjust based on the sweetness of the elderberry syrup)
- Silicone molds or a glass dish for setting the gummies

Instructions

1. In a small saucepan, combine the elderberry syrup and water. Warm the mixture over low heat, but do not boil.

2. Gradually sprinkle the gelatin powder over the liquid, whisking constantly to prevent any lumps from forming. Continue to whisk until the gelatin is completely dissolved, about 2-3 minutes.

3. Remove the saucepan from the heat. If using honey, stir it into the mixture now until well combined. The warmth of the mixture will help dissolve the honey evenly.

4. Carefully pour the mixture into silicone molds. If you don't have silicone molds, you can pour the mixture into a glass dish and cut it into bite-sized pieces once set.

5. Place the molds or glass dish in the refrigerator for at least 2 hours, or until the gummies are firm to the touch.

6. Once the gummies have set, gently pop them out of the molds or cut them into pieces if using a glass dish.

7. Store the gummies in an airtight container in the refrigerator.

Variations

- For an added vitamin C boost, mix in a teaspoon of vitamin C powder with the elderberry syrup before heating.
- Incorporate other immune-supportive ingredients like echinacea or vitamin D drops for additional benefits. Adjust the amount of water accordingly if liquid additives are used.
- To make vegan elderberry gummies, substitute agar powder for gelatin at a ratio of 1:1. Note that the setting times and textures may vary.

Storage tips

Keep the elderberry gummies in an airtight container in the refrigerator for up to two weeks. For longer storage, they can be frozen and thawed as needed.

Tips for allergens

For children with allergies to honey, substitute it with maple syrup or omit it altogether if the elderberry syrup is already sweetened. Always ensure that the gelatin or agar powder used does not contain any additives that could cause allergic reactions.

Scientific references

- "Elderberry Supplementation Reduces Cold Duration and Symptoms in Air-Travellers: A Randomized, Double-Blind Placebo-Controlled Clinical Trial" published in the journal Nutrients, which supports the immune-boosting effects of elderberry.

CHAPTER 3: TUMMY TROUBLES IN CHILDREN

Tummy troubles in children, ranging from mild indigestion to more persistent conditions like colic and constipation, can often be alleviated with carefully selected herbal remedies. These natural solutions offer gentle yet effective relief, emphasizing the importance of using herbs that are safe and well-tolerated by young bodies. Here, we detail the preparation and application of several herbal remedies tailored for children's digestive issues, ensuring parents and caregivers can confidently address these common ailments.

Slippery Elm (Ulmus rubra) is a remarkable herb known for its mucilaginous properties, which can soothe the digestive tract and relieve irritation. To prepare a Slippery Elm porridge for digestive discomfort, mix 1 teaspoon of Slippery Elm powder with 2 teaspoons of cold water to form a paste. Gradually add 1 cup of boiling water, stirring constantly to prevent lumps. Cook the mixture on low heat for 2-3 minutes until it thickens. Once cooled to a safe temperature, it can be given to the child; the bland taste is usually well accepted, but a small amount of natural sweetener like maple syrup can be added if necessary. This remedy is particularly suitable for children experiencing gastritis or mild stomach ulcers, providing a protective layer to the stomach lining.

Licorice Root (Glycyrrhiza glabra), with its natural sweetness, is often more readily accepted by children. It acts as a demulcent, soothing the digestive system, and as an anti-inflammatory, reducing intestinal inflammation. To prepare a Licorice Root tea, add 1 teaspoon of dried Licorice Root to 1 cup of boiling water. Steep for 10 minutes, then strain. Ensure the tea is cooled to a safe temperature before offering it to the child. Due to its potent properties, Licorice Root tea should be used with caution and only for short periods, as excessive use can lead to adverse effects like elevated blood pressure. It is not recommended for children under 2 years of age or those with health conditions that could be exacerbated by Licorice Root.

Chamomile (Matricaria recutita) is widely recognized for its calming effects on the digestive system, making it an excellent choice for treating colic, gas, and indigestion in children. To make Chamomile tea, steep 1 teaspoon of Chamomile flowers in 1 cup of boiling water for 5-10 minutes. Strain and cool the tea to a suitable drinking temperature. Chamomile tea can be given to children in small, frequent sips throughout the day. Its gentle sedative properties also make it beneficial for children experiencing restlessness or difficulty sleeping due to digestive discomfort.

Ginger (Zingiber officinale) is effective in treating nausea and improving digestion. A mild Ginger tea can be made by steeping a small piece of fresh Ginger (no larger than 1 inch) in 1 cup of boiling water for 5 minutes. Strain and allow the tea to cool before giving it to the child. Ginger should be used sparingly in young children; a few sips of the tea throughout the day is sufficient. Due to its warming properties, Ginger is particularly useful in cases of cold stomach, where digestion is sluggish.

Peppermint (Mentha piperita) is another herb that can relieve symptoms of indigestion and gas. However, Peppermint tea should be used with caution in very young children or those with reflux, as it can sometimes exacerbate these conditions. To prepare Peppermint tea, steep 1 teaspoon of dried Peppermint leaves in 1 cup of boiling water for 10 minutes. Strain and cool the tea to a safe temperature before offering it to children over 5 years of age. Peppermint tea can be particularly refreshing and soothing for upset stomachs, promoting relaxation of the digestive tract muscles.

When introducing herbal remedies for tummy troubles in children, it's crucial to observe the child's response closely. Start with small doses to ensure there are no adverse reactions. Always consult with a healthcare provider before beginning any new treatment, especially for ongoing conditions or if the child is taking other medications. Remember, the goal is to provide gentle, natural support to the child's digestive system, enhancing their overall comfort and well-being.

Relieving Colic with Fennel

Fennel (**Foeniculum vulgare**) is a potent herb known for its carminative properties, making it an excellent choice for relieving colic and upset stomachs in children. The active compounds in fennel, such as anethole, fenchone, and estragole, contribute to its antispasmodic and gas-relieving effects. Here is a detailed guide on how to prepare and use fennel tea for this purpose.

Ingredients:
- 1 teaspoon of crushed fennel seeds
- 1 cup (8 ounces) of boiling water

Tools:
- Mortar and pestle or a spice grinder
- Kettle for boiling water
- Strainer or fine mesh sieve
- Measuring teaspoon
- Heat-resistant cup or teapot

Preparation Steps:

1. **Crush the Fennel Seeds**: Begin by using a mortar and pestle or a spice grinder to lightly crush 1 teaspoon of fennel seeds. This process helps to release the essential oils and active compounds from the seeds, enhancing the tea's effectiveness.

2. **Boil Water**: Heat 1 cup (8 ounces) of water in a kettle until it reaches a rolling boil. The high temperature of the water is crucial for extracting the beneficial properties of the fennel seeds effectively.

3. **Steep the Fennel Seeds**: Place the crushed fennel seeds into a heat-resistant cup or teapot. Pour the boiling water over the seeds, ensuring they are fully submerged. Cover the cup or teapot with a lid or a small plate to prevent the escape of the essential oils during the steeping process.

4. **Allow the Tea to Steep**: Let the fennel seeds steep in the boiling water for 10 minutes. This duration is optimal for creating a potent infusion. Steeping for less time may result in a weaker tea that might not provide the desired relief for colic and upset stomachs.

5. **Strain the Tea**: After steeping, use a strainer or fine mesh sieve to strain the tea into another cup, removing the fennel seeds. This step ensures a smooth tea that is pleasant to drink.

6. **Cool the Tea to a Safe Temperature**: Before offering the tea to a child, it is essential to let it cool down to a safe, warm temperature. Testing the tea's temperature before administration can prevent accidental burns.

Dosage and Administration:
- For children aged 2-4 years, offer 1-2 teaspoons of the cooled fennel tea up to three times a day.
- For children aged 5-12 years, the dosage can be increased to 2-4 tablespoons of tea up to three times a day.

Important Considerations:
- Always start with a small dose to monitor the child's response to the herb.
- Consult with a pediatrician before introducing fennel tea, especially if the child is under two years old, has a medical condition, or is taking medication.
- Ensure the child is not allergic to fennel or related plants in the Apiaceae family, such as carrots or celery.

Fennel tea can be a gentle and natural way to alleviate colic and upset stomachs in children, offering relief from discomfort and promoting digestive health. By following these detailed preparation and administration guidelines, caregivers can safely use this herbal remedy to support their child's well-being.

Fennel and Peppermint Tummy Tea

Beneficial effects

Fennel and peppermint tea combines the soothing properties of fennel seeds with the calming effects of peppermint leaves, making it an excellent natural remedy for easing tummy troubles in children. Fennel is known for its ability to relieve gas and bloating, while peppermint can help relax the muscles of the digestive tract, reducing cramps and nausea. This gentle herbal tea is ideal for soothing digestive discomfort and promoting a healthy digestive system in children.

Portions

Serves 2

Preparation time

5 minutes

Cooking time

10 minutes

Ingredients
- 1 tablespoon dried fennel seeds
- 1 tablespoon dried peppermint leaves
- 2 cups boiling water
- Honey or maple syrup to taste (optional, for children over 1 year old)

Instructions

1. Begin by boiling 2 cups of water in a kettle or a saucepan.

2. While the water is boiling, measure out 1 tablespoon of dried fennel seeds and 1 tablespoon of dried peppermint leaves.

3. Place the fennel seeds and peppermint leaves into a tea infuser or directly into a teapot.

4. Once the water has reached a rolling boil, pour it over the fennel seeds and peppermint leaves in the teapot.

5. Cover the teapot with a lid to prevent the escape of essential oils and allow the tea to steep for 10 minutes. This steeping time allows the water to become infused with the medicinal properties of the herbs.

6. After steeping, remove the tea infuser or strain the tea to remove the loose herbs. Ensure all plant material is removed to avoid any choking hazard for children.

7. If desired, sweeten the tea with a small amount of honey or maple syrup, but only for children over 1 year old. Stir well to ensure the sweetener is fully dissolved.

8. Allow the tea to cool to a safe, warm drinking temperature before serving to a child.

Variations

- For a stronger digestive aid, add a slice of fresh ginger to the tea while it steeps.
- To make a cold remedy version, include a small piece of cinnamon stick during the steeping process for its warming properties.
- For children who prefer a cooler beverage, allow the tea to cool completely and serve it over ice for a refreshing herbal drink.

Storage tips

Any leftover tea can be stored in a sealed container in the refrigerator for up to 24 hours. Reheat gently or serve cold, but always check the temperature before giving it to a child.

Tips for allergens

For children with sensitivities, ensure that the fennel and peppermint are pure and not mixed with other herbs that could potentially cause a reaction. Always introduce new ingredients to children individually and watch for any signs of allergic reactions.

Scientific references

- "Effect of Foeniculum vulgare Mill. (fennel) on pain and menstrual duration in primary dysmenorrhea" published in the Journal of Pediatric and Adolescent Gynecology, which discusses the antispasmodic properties of fennel.
- "Peppermint Oil in the Acute Treatment of Tension-Type Headache" from Schmerz, highlighting peppermint's muscle-relaxing and pain-relieving effects.

BOOK 12: HERBS FOR WOMEN'S HEALTH

CHAPTER 1: HORMONAL BALANCE WITH HERBS

Hormonal imbalances can significantly impact women's health, manifesting through various symptoms such as mood swings, irregular menstrual cycles, and fatigue. Herbal remedies offer a natural path to restoring balance and enhancing well-being. When selecting herbs for hormonal regulation, it's crucial to understand their properties, how they interact with the body, and the most effective ways to use them.

Vitex (Vitex agnus-castus), also known as Chaste Tree Berry, is renowned for its ability to regulate menstrual cycles and improve symptoms of premenstrual syndrome (PMS). For optimal results, Vitex should be taken consistently over a period of several months. A standard dose can range from 160 to 240 mg of extract daily. It's important to note that Vitex may interact with hormonal medications, so consulting with a healthcare provider before starting is advisable.

Black Cohosh (Actaea racemosa) has been traditionally used to ease menopause symptoms, including hot flashes and sleep disturbances. The recommended dosage is typically 20 to 40 mg of the standardized extract twice daily. However, due to its estrogenic effects, women with a history of breast cancer or those on hormone replacement therapy should use Black Cohosh under the guidance of a healthcare professional.

Maca (Lepidium meyenii) is a root vegetable native to Peru, often used to enhance libido and energy levels. Maca works by supporting the endocrine system to balance hormone levels. It can be consumed in powder form, with a general recommendation of 1 to 3 teaspoons per day mixed into smoothies or food. Given its energizing properties, it's best taken in the morning.

Red Raspberry Leaf (Rubus idaeus) is beneficial for menstrual health, known for toning the uterine muscles and easing menstrual cramps. It can be consumed as a tea, with 1 to 2 teaspoons of dried leaves steeped in hot water for 10 minutes. Drinking 1 to 3 cups daily is a common practice, especially in the week leading up to menstruation.

Dong Quai (Angelica sinensis), often referred to as "female ginseng," is used for menstrual regularity and to alleviate menopausal symptoms. The typical dosage is 3 to 15 grams of the root in decoction. However, Dong Quai should be avoided during menstruation as it can increase bleeding. Additionally, it may interact with blood thinners and other medications.

Incorporating these herbs into your wellness routine requires patience and consistency. Start with one herb to monitor its effects on your body before introducing another. Always source high-quality, organic herbs to ensure purity and efficacy. Remember, while herbal remedies can offer significant benefits for hormonal balance, they should complement a holistic approach to health that includes a balanced diet, regular exercise, and adequate sleep. Consulting with a healthcare provider, particularly one experienced in herbal medicine, is essential to tailor a regimen that best suits your individual needs and conditions.

Vitex for Menstrual Cycle Regulation

Vitex, scientifically known as Vitex agnus-castus, plays a pivotal role in the natural regulation of menstrual cycles and the alleviation of symptoms associated with premenstrual syndrome (PMS) and other menstrual disorders. This herb, often referred to as Chaste Tree Berry, exerts its effects by modulating the pituitary gland, which in turn regulates the balance of female hormones, primarily progesterone and estrogen. The efficacy of Vitex in menstrual cycle regulation is attributed to its active compounds, such as flavonoids, iridoid glycosides, and essential oils, which collectively contribute to its therapeutic properties.

For individuals seeking to incorporate Vitex into their wellness regimen for menstrual cycle regulation, it is recommended to opt for a standardized extract of Vitex agnus-castus, ensuring a consistent dosage of its active components. The typical dosage range for Vitex extract is between 160 to 240 mg per day, taken in the morning to align with the body's natural hormonal rhythm. It is crucial to maintain a consistent daily intake, as the benefits of Vitex are cumulative and may take several cycles (usually 3 to 6 months) to manifest fully.

When selecting a Vitex supplement, look for products that specify the concentration of agnuside or casticin, as these are among the herb's primary active compounds. A product labeled as containing 0.5% agnuside or casticin, for instance, provides a quantifiable measure of potency. Additionally, opting for supplements that have undergone third-party testing for purity and potency can further ensure the quality of the product.

Incorporating Vitex into one's daily routine requires minimal preparation. The extract is typically available in capsule or liquid tincture form. For capsules, simply follow the manufacturer's recommended dosage, usually one capsule taken with water in the morning. If using a liquid tincture, the recommended approach is to dilute the specified amount (often 20-30 drops) in a small amount of water or juice, also taken in the morning. It's important to read and adhere to the product's specific instructions, as concentrations and formulations can vary.

While Vitex is generally well-tolerated, it's essential to be aware of potential interactions, especially for those on hormonal medications, including birth control pills or hormone replacement therapy. Consulting with a healthcare provider before starting Vitex is advisable to ensure it is appropriate for your individual health profile and to avoid any adverse interactions with existing medications.

To monitor the effects of Vitex on menstrual cycle regulation, keeping a menstrual diary can be beneficial. Record the start and end dates of your period, any symptoms experienced throughout the cycle, and any changes in the flow or duration of your period. This record can help identify patterns or improvements over time and can be a valuable tool for discussions with healthcare providers regarding the effectiveness of Vitex for your specific situation.

In summary, Vitex agnus-castus is a well-established herbal remedy for those seeking a natural approach to menstrual cycle regulation and the relief of PMS symptoms. By understanding the appropriate dosage, selection criteria for supplements, and method of intake, individuals can effectively incorporate Vitex into their wellness routine, potentially experiencing improved hormonal balance and menstrual health over time.

Vitex Hormonal Balance Tincture
Beneficial effects
Vitex, also known as Chaste Tree Berry, has been traditionally used to help balance hormones, particularly in women. It can alleviate symptoms of PMS, menopause, and may support fertility. Vitex works by affecting the hypothalamus and pituitary glands, helping to increase progesterone levels and reduce prolactin, which can lead to hormonal balance.

Portions
Makes about 1 pint (16 ounces)

Preparation time
10 minutes

Cooking time
24 hours for maceration

Ingredients
- 1 cup dried Vitex berries
- 2 cups high-proof alcohol (vodka or brandy, at least 80 proof)
- Glass jar with a tight-fitting lid

Instructions
1. Begin by measuring 1 cup of dried Vitex berries. If the berries are whole, lightly crush them with a mortar and pestle to increase their surface area, which will help to extract more of their beneficial properties.
2. Transfer the crushed Vitex berries into a clean, dry glass jar.
3. Pour 2 cups of high-proof alcohol over the berries, ensuring they are completely submerged. The alcohol should be at least 80 proof to effectively preserve the tincture and extract the active compounds from the Vitex berries.
4. Secure the lid tightly on the jar to prevent evaporation and contamination. Shake the jar gently to mix the berries with the alcohol.
5. Label the jar with the contents and the date you started the maceration.
6. Store the jar in a cool, dark place for at least 4 weeks. This is the maceration period, during which time the alcohol will extract the active compounds from the Vitex berries. Shake the jar gently every day to help the process.
7. After 4 weeks, strain the mixture through a fine mesh sieve or cheesecloth into another clean, dry glass jar or bottle. Press or squeeze the berries to extract as much liquid as possible.
8. Discard the solid berry remnants. The liquid that remains is your Vitex hormonal balance tincture.
9. Label the container with the contents and the date of completion.

Variations
- For a non-alcoholic version, replace the alcohol with apple cider vinegar or vegetable glycerin, though the extraction process may differ slightly and the shelf life will be shorter.
- Add other hormone-balancing herbs such as red raspberry leaf or black cohosh to the tincture for added benefits. Adjust the proportions based on your preferences and needs.

Storage tips
Store the tincture in a cool, dark place. It should remain potent for up to 5 years if stored properly. Ensure the lid is always tightly secured to prevent evaporation.

Tips for allergens
For those with allergies or sensitivities to alcohol, consider the non-alcoholic version mentioned in the variations. Always ensure you are not allergic to Vitex or any other herbs you may add to your tincture.

Scientific references
- "Effect of Vitex agnus-castus on premenstrual syndrome: A meta-analysis and systematic review," published in the Journal of Ethnopharmacology, highlights the efficacy of Vitex in reducing PMS symptoms.
- "Vitex agnus-castus in the treatment of menopausal symptoms: a systematic review," in the Journal of Alternative and Complementary Medicine, discusses the potential benefits of Vitex for menopausal symptom relief.

CHAPTER 2: HERBS FOR PREGNANCY AND POSTPARTUM

Pregnancy and postpartum periods are transformative times in a woman's life, where the body undergoes significant changes requiring support for both physical and emotional well-being. Herbal remedies can offer gentle, natural support during these times, focusing on nutrients and balance without the harsh effects of pharmaceuticals. It's crucial, however, to approach herbal use with caution, prioritizing safety for both mother and baby. Here, we delve into specific herbs known for their efficacy in supporting pregnancy and postpartum health, alongside detailed instructions for their safe use.

Red Raspberry Leaf (Rubus idaeus) is widely recognized for its benefits during pregnancy. Rich in vitamins and minerals, it is particularly noted for its high magnesium, potassium, iron, and B-vitamins content, which are essential for pregnancy health. Red Raspberry Leaf works to strengthen the uterine walls and may decrease labor time. For use, steep 1-2 teaspoons of dried leaves in hot water for 10 minutes. Drinking 1-3 cups of this tea daily, starting in the second trimester, is recommended.

Ginger (Zingiber officinale) is effective in managing nausea and vomiting, common in the first trimester of pregnancy. To prepare ginger tea, slice fresh ginger root and steep in boiling water for 10-15 minutes. Limit intake to 2-3 cups daily to avoid potential side effects. Ginger can also be consumed in small amounts in food.

Peppermint (Mentha piperita) offers relief from digestive discomforts like gas and bloating, which are frequent during pregnancy. Peppermint tea can be made by steeping 1 teaspoon of dried peppermint leaves in a cup of hot water for 5-10 minutes. Stick to 1-2 cups per day to prevent exacerbating heartburn, a common pregnancy issue.

Dandelion (Taraxacum officinale) leaves and root support liver function and help manage fluid retention. Dandelion tea, made from the root or leaves, can be consumed once daily. Use 1 teaspoon of dried root or leaves per cup of hot water, steeping for about 10 minutes.

Nettle (Urtica dioica) is a nutritional powerhouse, high in vitamins A, C, K, calcium, potassium, and iron, making it an excellent tonic during pregnancy. Nettle tea can be prepared by steeping 1 tablespoon of dried nettle leaves in a cup of hot water for 10-15 minutes. Due to its diuretic properties, limit consumption to 1 cup daily.

For postpartum recovery, the following herbs are beneficial:

Fenugreek (Trigonella foenum-graecum) is traditionally used to enhance milk production in breastfeeding mothers. Fenugreek can be taken as a tea or in capsule form. If choosing tea, steep 1 teaspoon of seeds in a cup of hot water for 10-15 minutes and drink 1-2 cups daily.

Chamomile (Matricaria recutita) aids in relaxation and sleep, which is crucial for postpartum recovery. Chamomile tea can be safely consumed 1-2 times daily. Steep 1-2 teaspoons of dried chamomile flowers in hot water for 5-10 minutes.

Motherwort (Leonurus cardiaca), known for its ability to reduce anxiety and promote heart health, can be particularly helpful for new mothers facing postpartum stress. Motherwort should not be used during pregnancy but can be introduced postpartum in tincture form, typically 15-30 drops in water, up to 3 times daily.

When incorporating herbs into your pregnancy and postpartum care, always prioritize organic sources to avoid pesticides and contaminants. It's also essential to consult with a healthcare provider before starting any new herbal regimen, especially during these sensitive times. While herbs offer a holistic approach to wellness, their interactions with the body are complex and require careful consideration to ensure they complement your overall health plan without causing harm.

Red Raspberry Leaf for Uterine Health

Red Raspberry Leaf (Rubus idaeus) stands out as a quintessential herb for women, particularly during the pregnancy and postpartum periods, due to its remarkable uterine toning capabilities. This herb is rich in vitamins and minerals, including magnesium, potassium, iron, and B-vitamins, which are crucial for maintaining pregnancy health. Its primary function is to strengthen the uterine walls, potentially making labor more efficient and possibly reducing labor time. The preparation and consumption of Red Raspberry Leaf tea are straightforward yet require attention to detail to ensure maximum efficacy and safety.

To prepare Red Raspberry Leaf tea, start by sourcing high-quality, organic dried leaves. The organic certification ensures that the herb is free from pesticides and other contaminants, which is especially important during pregnancy. Measure 1-2 teaspoons of the dried Red Raspberry Leaf and place it in a tea infuser or teapot. Boil water and then allow it to cool slightly before pouring over the leaves to avoid destroying the delicate vitamins and minerals. Steep the leaves in hot water for about 10 minutes. This duration extracts the beneficial components effectively without leading to excessive tannin release, which can make the tea overly astringent.

The recommended intake is 1-3 cups of tea daily, starting from the second trimester of pregnancy. Beginning the consumption of Red Raspberry Leaf tea in the first trimester is generally discouraged due to the theoretical risk of stimulating the uterus before pregnancy is well established. However, from the second trimester onwards, the tea can be consumed safely, offering support to the uterine muscles and preparing the body for labor.

It's important to note that while Red Raspberry Leaf is widely regarded as safe during the latter stages of pregnancy, individual responses can vary. Some women may experience Braxton Hicks contractions more frequently after consuming the tea, which, although usually harmless, can cause discomfort or concern. Therefore, it's advisable to start with a lower quantity of tea—such as one cup per day—and gradually increase to gauge personal tolerance.

Furthermore, integrating Red Raspberry Leaf tea into a daily routine can be a comforting ritual, providing a moment of relaxation and reflection. The tea has a mild, pleasant taste, which can be enhanced with a spoonful of honey or a slice of lemon if desired. For those who may not favor the taste of herbal teas, Red Raspberry Leaf can also be taken in capsule form, with the dosage and frequency following the manufacturer's recommendations. However, the tea form allows for better absorption of the herb's beneficial properties and offers the added hydration necessary during pregnancy.

In addition to its uterine toning benefits, Red Raspberry Leaf tea supports overall pregnancy wellness by supplying essential nutrients and antioxidants. Its iron content is particularly beneficial in preventing anemia, a common concern during pregnancy. The magnesium in the leaves can help alleviate leg cramps, while the potassium supports overall cardiovascular health.

While Red Raspberry Leaf is a powerful ally for pregnant and postpartum women, it's crucial to consult with a healthcare provider before incorporating it or any new herb into your wellness regimen. This ensures that it complements your individual health profile and any other treatments or supplements being used. Pregnant women with a history of cesarean sections, labor induction, or those carrying multiples should exercise particular caution and seek professional advice due to the potential for increased uterine activity.

Incorporating Red Raspberry Leaf into the pregnancy journey offers a natural, gentle way to support the body's preparation for childbirth. Its historical use and modern appreciation underscore its value in women's herbal medicine, making it a staple for those seeking holistic health and wellness during this transformative time.

Red Raspberry and Nettle Pregnancy Tea
Beneficial effects
Red Raspberry Leaf is celebrated for its potential to tone the uterus and ease labor pains, making it a favorite among pregnant women. Nettle, rich in vitamins and minerals, supports overall health and increases energy levels. Together, this tea blend offers a nourishing tonic that can support the body throughout pregnancy.
Portions
Serves 4
Preparation time
5 minutes
Cooking time
10 minutes
Ingredients
- 2 tablespoons dried Red Raspberry Leaf
- 2 tablespoons dried Nettle Leaf
- 4 cups of water
- Optional: Honey or lemon to taste
Instructions
1. Bring 4 cups of water to a boil in a medium-sized pot.
2. Once the water reaches a rolling boil, reduce the heat to low and add 2 tablespoons of dried Red Raspberry Leaf and 2 tablespoons of dried Nettle Leaf to the pot.

3. Cover the pot with a lid and let the herbs simmer on low heat for 10 minutes. This slow simmering allows the water to become infused with the nutrients and flavors of the herbs.

4. After 10 minutes, remove the pot from the heat. Let the tea steep, covered, for an additional 5 minutes to enhance the infusion.

5. Strain the tea through a fine mesh sieve or cheesecloth into a teapot or directly into cups, ensuring to catch any loose herb particles.

6. If desired, add honey or a squeeze of lemon to each cup for added flavor. Stir well to ensure any added sweeteners are fully dissolved.

7. Serve the tea warm. For a refreshing alternative, allow it to cool and serve over ice.

Variations

- For a more complex flavor, add a cinnamon stick or a few slices of fresh ginger to the pot during the simmering process.
- Incorporate a tablespoon of dried peppermint leaves for a refreshing twist and additional digestive benefits.
- To make a larger batch, simply double the ingredients. Adjust the steeping time slightly longer to maintain the strength of the infusion.

Storage tips

Store any leftover tea in a glass jar or pitcher in the refrigerator for up to 3 days. Reheat gently on the stove or enjoy cold.

Tips for allergens

For those with sensitivities, ensure the Red Raspberry Leaf and Nettle Leaf are sourced from reputable suppliers to avoid cross-contamination with allergens. If honey is not suitable, consider maple syrup or agave nectar as sweetener alternatives.

Scientific references

- "The effect of Red Raspberry Leaf tea consumption on labor outcomes" published in the Journal of Midwifery & Women's Health, which discusses the potential benefits of Red Raspberry Leaf in shortening labor.

CHAPTER 3: MENOPAUSE AND PERIMENOPAUSE SUPPORT

Sage (Salvia officinalis) is renowned for its ability to mitigate hot flashes and night sweats, common symptoms of menopause and perimenopause. The active components in sage, such as volatile oils and flavonoids, contribute to its estrogenic effects, providing a natural cooling sensation. To harness the benefits of sage, one can prepare sage tea by steeping 1 teaspoon of dried sage leaves in a cup of boiling water for about 5 to 10 minutes. It's advisable to limit consumption to 2-3 cups daily, as excessive intake may lead to adverse effects.

Soy Isoflavones (Glycine max) have been studied for their estrogen-like effects, which can be particularly beneficial during menopause. Isoflavones, a type of phytoestrogen found in soy, can help balance hormone levels and alleviate menopausal symptoms such as mood swings and hot flashes. Incorporating soy products like tofu, tempeh, and soy milk into the diet is an effective way to consume soy isoflavones. For those preferring supplementation, it's crucial to opt for products standardized to contain 40 to 80 mg of isoflavones and to consult with a healthcare provider for personalized advice.

Flaxseed (Linum usitatissimum), rich in lignans and omega-3 fatty acids, offers another phytoestrogen source that supports hormonal balance. Ground flaxseed can be easily added to smoothies, oatmeal, or yogurt, providing a daily dose of fiber and phytoestrogens. A general recommendation is to consume 1 to 2 tablespoons of ground flaxseed daily. It's important to start with a lower dose and gradually increase to avoid gastrointestinal discomfort.

Evening Primrose Oil (Oenothera biennis) is praised for its gamma-linolenic acid (GLA) content, an omega-6 fatty acid that can help manage menopausal symptoms such as hot flashes and mood disturbances. The typical dosage for evening primrose oil is 500 to 1000 mg, taken in capsule form up to three times daily. As with any supplement, it's advisable to discuss with a healthcare provider before beginning use, especially for those taking other medications.

Black Cohosh (Actaea racemosa) continues to be a cornerstone herb for menopause support, addressing symptoms like mood swings, sleep disturbances, and hot flashes. The recommended approach for black cohosh is a standardized extract, with a common dosage being 20 to 40 mg twice daily. Given its potent effects, black cohosh should be used under the guidance of a healthcare professional, particularly for women with a history of liver issues or those on hormone therapy.

When integrating these herbs into a menopause support regimen, it's essential to consider quality and sourcing. Opting for organic, non-GMO products ensures purity and potency. Additionally, understanding that the efficacy of these remedies can vary from person to person is crucial. Monitoring one's symptoms and adjusting dosages or combinations of herbs under professional supervision can lead to the most beneficial outcomes. It's also important to view herbal remedies as part of a comprehensive approach to wellness during menopause, which includes a balanced diet, regular physical activity, and stress management techniques.

Black Cohosh for Hot Flashes

Black Cohosh (Actaea racemosa), a perennial plant native to North America, has gained prominence for its effectiveness in managing menopausal symptoms, particularly hot flashes. This herb functions by mimicking the effects of estrogen in the body, which can significantly alleviate the frequency and intensity of hot flashes and other menopausal discomforts such as mood swings and sleep disturbances. The active compounds in Black Cohosh, including triterpene glycosides, have been identified as the primary contributors to its therapeutic effects. To harness these benefits, it is crucial to understand the appropriate preparation, dosage, and considerations for use.

For those looking to incorporate Black Cohosh into their wellness regimen, the standardized extract of the root is the most researched and recommended form. This ensures a consistent concentration of active compounds, enhancing both the efficacy and safety of the herb. The typical dosage for managing menopausal symptoms is 20 to 40 mg of the standardized extract, taken twice daily. This dosage can provide significant relief from hot flashes and improve overall quality of life during menopause. It is available in various forms, including capsules, tablets, and tinctures, allowing for flexibility in administration based on personal preference.

When selecting a Black Cohosh product, look for labels that specify the content of triterpene glycosides, measured as 27-deoxyactein, to ensure you are getting an effective dose. Products that have undergone third-party testing for purity and potency are also preferable, as this adds an extra layer of assurance regarding the quality of the supplement.

Incorporating Black Cohosh into your daily routine requires minimal preparation. If opting for capsules or tablets, simply take the supplement with water, ideally at the same times each day to maintain consistent levels of the herb in your system. For those who prefer tinctures, dilute the recommended amount in water or juice. It is important to adhere to the manufacturer's guidelines on dosage and administration to avoid potential side effects.

While Black Cohosh is generally well-tolerated, it is essential to be mindful of potential interactions and contraindications. Women with a history of hormone-sensitive conditions, such as breast cancer, should use Black Cohosh under the supervision of a healthcare provider. Additionally, because of its estrogenic effects, it is advisable to avoid combining Black Cohosh with hormone replacement therapy or birth control pills without professional guidance.

Monitoring your body's response to Black Cohosh is crucial for assessing its effectiveness and tolerability. Keeping a symptom diary can be helpful, noting the frequency and severity of hot flashes and other menopausal symptoms before and after starting the supplement. This record can provide valuable insights into the herb's impact and assist healthcare providers in making any necessary adjustments to your regimen. In summary, Black Cohosh offers a natural and effective option for managing hot flashes and other symptoms associated with menopause. By selecting a high-quality, standardized extract and adhering to recommended dosages, women can achieve significant relief while minimizing potential risks. As with any supplement, consultation with a healthcare provider is recommended to ensure Black Cohosh is appropriate for your individual health profile and to safely integrate it into your menopausal support strategy.

Black Cohosh and Sage Cooling Tea
Beneficial effects
Black Cohosh and Sage Cooling Tea is designed to naturally alleviate symptoms associated with menopause and perimenopause, such as hot flashes and night sweats. Black Cohosh has been traditionally used to support women's hormonal balance and reduce menopausal symptoms, while Sage is known for its natural cooling properties and ability to decrease excessive sweating. Together, these herbs create a soothing tea that can help manage the discomforts of menopause, promoting a sense of well-being and comfort.

Portions
Serves 2
Preparation time
5 minutes
Cooking time
15 minutes
Ingredients
- 1 teaspoon dried Black Cohosh root
- 1 teaspoon dried Sage leaves
- 2 cups of water
- Optional: Honey or lemon to taste
Instructions
1. Begin by bringing 2 cups of water to a boil in a small saucepan.
2. Once the water is boiling, add 1 teaspoon of dried Black Cohosh root and 1 teaspoon of dried Sage leaves to the saucepan.
3. Reduce the heat to low and let the herbs simmer gently for 15 minutes. This slow simmering process allows the water to become infused with the medicinal properties of the herbs.
4. After 15 minutes, remove the saucepan from the heat and let the tea steep for an additional 5 minutes. Steeping the tea off the heat allows the flavors and beneficial compounds to further infuse into the water without becoming bitter.
5. Strain the tea through a fine mesh sieve into a teapot or directly into cups, discarding the used herbs.
6. If desired, add honey or a squeeze of lemon to each cup for added flavor. Stir well to ensure any added sweeteners are fully dissolved.
7. Serve the tea warm to enjoy its full therapeutic benefits.
Variations

- For a stronger tea, increase the amount of Black Cohosh and Sage to 1.5 teaspoons each and steep for an additional 5 minutes.
- Add a cinnamon stick to the saucepan with the herbs for a warming, spicy note that complements the natural flavors of the tea.
- Incorporate a slice of fresh ginger during the simmering process for added digestive support and a zesty flavor profile.

Storage tips

This tea is best enjoyed fresh but can be stored in a sealed container in the refrigerator for up to 24 hours. Gently reheat on the stove or enjoy cold for a refreshing alternative.

Tips for allergens

For those with sensitivities to specific herbs, ensure that the Black Cohosh and Sage are sourced from reputable suppliers to avoid cross-contamination with allergens. If honey is not suitable, consider maple syrup or agave nectar as sweetener alternatives.

Scientific references

- "Efficacy of Black Cohosh-containing preparations on menopausal symptoms: a meta-analysis" published in Alternative Therapies in Health and Medicine, which discusses the benefits of Black Cohosh for menopausal symptom relief.
- "Salvia officinalis for hot flushes: towards determination of mechanism of activity and active principles" in Planta Medica, highlighting Sage's effectiveness in reducing menopausal hot flashes and night sweats.

BOOK 13: HERBS FOR MEN'S HEALTH

CHAPTER 1: ENHANCING ENERGY AND VITALITY

Ashwagandha, scientifically known as Withania somnifera, is a powerful adaptogen traditionally used in Ayurvedic medicine to enhance energy and vitality, particularly in men. This herb is renowned for its ability to increase stamina, reduce stress, and improve overall well-being. When incorporating ashwagandha into a daily wellness routine, it's essential to focus on quality, dosage, and consistency to achieve the best results.

Quality: Opt for organic ashwagandha root powder or extracts standardized to contain at least 5% withanolides, which are the active compounds believed to be responsible for the herb's health benefits. High-quality supplements are free from fillers, additives, and are non-GMO.

Dosage: The effective dosage of ashwagandha can vary depending on the form of the supplement. For root powder, a general recommendation is 1 to 2 teaspoons (3 to 6 grams) per day, mixed into a smoothie or milk. If using an extract, follow the manufacturer's instructions, but a common dosage is about 300 to 500 mg, twice daily. It's advisable to start with a lower dose to assess tolerance and gradually increase as needed.

Consistency: Like many herbal supplements, ashwagandha may take several weeks to exhibit its full benefits. Consistent daily use is key. Incorporate it into your morning or evening routine for best practices.

Preparation Method: Ashwagandha can be taken in various forms, including powders, capsules, and tinctures. For those using the powder form, a popular method is to mix it into a warm beverage, such as a turmeric latte or herbal tea. This not only makes the herb more palatable but also forms a comforting ritual that supports its stress-reducing properties.

Safety and Interactions: While ashwagandha is generally safe for most people, it's important to consult with a healthcare provider before starting any new supplement, especially for those with thyroid conditions, autoimmune diseases, or those taking medications for anxiety, depression, or insomnia. Pregnant or breastfeeding women should avoid ashwagandha.

Incorporating ashwagandha into your wellness routine can be a simple yet effective way to enhance energy and vitality. By focusing on quality, appropriate dosage, and consistency, and by considering the preparation method and safety guidelines, individuals can harness the full potential of this ancient herb to support their health and well-being.

Ashwagandha for Stress and Strength

Ashwagandha, scientifically known as Withania somnifera, stands out in the realm of herbal supplements for its adaptogenic properties, which are particularly beneficial for enhancing energy and vitality in men. This herb has been used for centuries in Ayurvedic medicine to combat stress and increase stamina, making it an invaluable asset for those looking to bolster their overall well-being. When considering the incorporation of ashwagandha into a daily wellness regimen, it is crucial to pay attention to the quality of the herb, the dosage, and the consistency of use to fully harness its potential benefits.

Selecting a high-quality ashwagandha product is the first step toward ensuring its efficacy. Look for organic ashwagandha root powder or extracts that are standardized to contain at least 5% withanolides, the active compounds that contribute to the herb's health-promoting effects. Products that are certified organic, non-GMO, and free from unnecessary fillers or additives are preferable, as they offer a purer form of the herb and minimize the risk of consuming contaminants.

The dosage of ashwagandha can vary depending on the form in which it is taken. For those opting for the root powder, a general guideline is to consume 1 to 2 teaspoons (3 to 6 grams) per day, which can be easily mixed into smoothies, milk, or warm beverages like herbal teas. This method not only facilitates consumption but also allows for the gradual absorption of the herb's active compounds. If using an extract, the recommended dosage typically ranges from 300 to 500 mg, taken twice daily. Starting with a lower dose and gradually increasing it allows the body to adapt to the herb and helps identify the most effective dosage for individual needs.

Consistency in taking ashwagandha is key to achieving its full benefits, which may take several weeks to become noticeable. Integrating the herb into a daily routine, whether in the morning to kickstart the day or in the evening to promote relaxation and recovery, can enhance its effectiveness in reducing stress and improving energy levels.

For those using ashwagandha powder, incorporating it into a warm beverage can enhance its palatability and increase its soothing effects. A popular preparation method involves blending the powder into a turmeric latte or mixing it with warm milk and honey to create a comforting drink that supports relaxation and stress reduction.

While ashwagandha is generally considered safe for most individuals, it is important to consult with a healthcare provider before adding it to your wellness routine, especially for those with pre-existing conditions such as thyroid disorders, autoimmune diseases, or those on medication for anxiety, depression, or insomnia. Pregnant or breastfeeding women are advised to avoid ashwagandha due to the lack of sufficient research on its safety in these populations.

By focusing on the quality of the ashwagandha, adhering to recommended dosages, maintaining consistency in its use, and considering the most suitable preparation method, individuals can effectively leverage the stress-reducing and energy-boosting properties of this powerful herb. This approach ensures that ashwagandha serves as a supportive element in enhancing men's health and vitality, contributing to a holistic wellness strategy that addresses both physical and mental well-being.

Ashwagandha Power Smoothie

Beneficial effects

Ashwagandha, known for its adaptogenic properties, helps the body manage stress and enhances energy levels without stimulating the heart. It also supports muscle strength and recovery, making it an ideal supplement for those looking to boost their vitality and performance. This smoothie combines ashwagandha with other nutrient-rich ingredients to create a powerful energy-boosting beverage.

Portions

Serves 1

Preparation time

5 minutes

Ingredients

- 1 cup almond milk (unsweetened)
- 1 banana (frozen for a creamier texture)
- 1 tablespoon ashwagandha powder
- 1 tablespoon peanut butter (unsweetened)
- 1 teaspoon honey (or to taste)
- 1/2 teaspoon cinnamon
- A pinch of sea salt
- Ice cubes (optional, for a colder smoothie)

Instructions

1. Start by gathering all your ingredients. Ensure the banana is peeled and frozen ahead of time for a smoother, creamier texture.
2. In a blender, add 1 cup of unsweetened almond milk as the liquid base. This will help in blending the ingredients smoothly and add a mild, nutty flavor to the smoothie.
3. Add the frozen banana into the blender. The banana not only adds sweetness but also contributes to the creamy consistency of the smoothie.
4. Incorporate 1 tablespoon of ashwagandha powder. This is the key ingredient for stress relief and energy boosting.
5. Add 1 tablespoon of unsweetened peanut butter for a dose of healthy fats and protein, enhancing the smoothie's satiety factor.
6. Drizzle 1 teaspoon of honey for a touch of natural sweetness. Adjust the quantity based on your preference.
7. Sprinkle 1/2 teaspoon of cinnamon for its warming flavor and blood sugar regulation benefits.
8. Add a pinch of sea salt to enhance the flavors and add trace minerals.
9. If you prefer a colder smoothie, add a few ice cubes to the blender.
10. Blend all the ingredients on high speed until smooth and creamy, ensuring there are no lumps and the ashwagandha powder is fully incorporated.
11. Taste the smoothie and adjust the sweetness if necessary by adding a bit more honey.
12. Pour the smoothie into a glass and enjoy immediately for the best flavor and nutrient intake.

Variations

- For a protein boost, add a scoop of your favorite protein powder.
- Substitute almond milk with coconut milk for a tropical twist.
- Add a handful of spinach for extra iron and greens without altering the taste significantly.

- For a nut-free version, use sunflower seed butter instead of peanut butter.

Storage tips

This smoothie is best enjoyed fresh. However, if needed, it can be stored in the refrigerator for up to 24 hours. Stir well before drinking as separation may occur.

Tips for allergens

For those with nut allergies, ensure to use a nut-free milk alternative and substitute peanut butter with a seed butter like sunflower seed butter. Always check the label on ashwagandha powder to ensure it's processed in a facility free of allergens you're sensitive to.

Scientific references

- "An Overview on Ashwagandha: A Rasayana (Rejuvenator) of Ayurveda" published in the African Journal of Traditional, Complementary and Alternative Medicines, which discusses the adaptogenic and health-promoting properties of ashwagandha.

CHAPTER 2: PROSTATE HEALTH WITH HERBS

Prostate health is a significant concern for many men, especially as they age. Herbal remedies can offer supportive care for prostate health, with several herbs standing out for their beneficial properties. **Saw Palmetto** (Serenoa repens) is widely recognized for its ability to support prostate health. It works by inhibiting the enzyme 5-alpha-reductase, which converts testosterone into dihydrotestosterone (DHT), a hormone that can contribute to prostate enlargement. For optimal results, look for standardized extracts of Saw Palmetto berries containing 85 to 95% fatty acids and sterols. The recommended dosage is 160 mg twice daily or 320 mg once daily.

Nettle Root (Urtica dioica) is another herb that supports prostate health, particularly in combination with Saw Palmetto. Nettle root helps by modulating sex hormone binding globulin (SHBG), which in turn can help reduce symptoms of benign prostatic hyperplasia (BPH). A typical dosage for nettle root extract is 300 to 600 mg daily. When selecting a nettle root supplement, ensure it is a root extract, as the leaves have different medicinal properties.

Pumpkin Seeds (Cucurbita pepo) are rich in zinc, a mineral essential for prostate health and function. They also contain phytosterols that may help reduce the size of the prostate. Consuming raw, unsalted pumpkin seeds daily or taking a pumpkin seed oil supplement can be beneficial. For oil, a dosage of 1 to 2 tablespoons daily is recommended.

Pygeum (Pygeum africanum) is derived from the bark of the African cherry tree and has been used for centuries in traditional medicine to treat urinary problems. It is believed to work by reducing inflammation and promoting the elimination of cholesterol that can build up in the prostate. Look for pygeum supplements standardized to contain 13% total sterols, with a recommended dosage of 100 to 200 mg daily.

Lycopene, a powerful antioxidant found in tomatoes, watermelons, and pink grapefruit, has been linked to a reduced risk of prostate cancer. While not an herb, lycopene supplementation can support prostate health. Aim for a dietary intake of lycopene from foods or consider a supplement providing at least 10 mg of lycopene daily.

Green Tea (Camellia sinensis) contains compounds called catechins, which have been shown to support prostate health and may protect against prostate cancer. Opt for a green tea extract standardized to contain at least 45% EGCG, the most active catechin, with a recommended dosage of 250 to 500 mg daily.

When incorporating these herbs into your wellness routine for prostate health, it's crucial to select high-quality supplements from reputable manufacturers. Always start with the lower end of the dosage range to assess tolerance and gradually increase as needed. Consistency is key, as the benefits of herbal supplements often take several weeks to manifest. Additionally, while these herbs can support prostate health, they should not replace conventional treatments or medications prescribed by a healthcare provider. Always consult with a healthcare professional before starting any new supplement, especially if you have pre-existing health conditions or are taking medications.

Saw Palmetto for Prostate Health

Saw Palmetto, scientifically known as Serenoa repens, has garnered attention for its potential benefits in supporting prostate health, particularly in the context of benign prostatic hyperplasia (BPH). This condition, characterized by the enlargement of the prostate gland, affects a significant number of men, especially as they age, leading to symptoms like increased urinary frequency, a weakened urine stream, and difficulty in starting urination. The active compounds in Saw Palmetto, primarily fatty acids and phytosterols, are believed to exert a therapeutic effect by inhibiting the enzyme 5-alpha-reductase. This enzyme is responsible for the conversion of testosterone into dihydrotestosterone (DHT), a hormone that plays a key role in the development of prostate enlargement.

For those considering the incorporation of Saw Palmetto into their wellness regimen for prostate health, it is crucial to select a supplement that ensures the highest quality and efficacy. Look for products that provide standardized extracts of Saw Palmetto berries, with a concentration of 85 to 95% fatty acids and sterols. This standardization is critical as it guarantees the presence of the bioactive constituents believed to be beneficial for prostate health. The recommended dosage for Saw Palmetto supplements typically ranges from 160 mg taken twice daily to 320 mg once daily. This dosage has been studied and is considered effective for the management of BPH symptoms.

When integrating Saw Palmetto into your daily routine, consistency is key. Herbal supplements often require time to manifest their full benefits, and Saw Palmetto is no exception. It may take several weeks or even months of consistent use before improvements in symptoms are noticed. Therefore, patience and adherence to the recommended dosage are essential. Furthermore, while Saw Palmetto is generally well-tolerated, it is important to be aware of potential side effects. Some individuals may experience mild gastrointestinal discomfort, headache, or dizziness. As with any supplement, it is advisable to start with the lower end of the recommended dosage to assess tolerance and gradually adjust as needed.

In addition to Saw Palmetto, maintaining overall prostate health should include a balanced diet rich in fruits, vegetables, and healthy fats, regular physical activity, and routine check-ups with a healthcare provider. It is also important to note that while Saw Palmetto can be a valuable part of a holistic approach to managing BPH symptoms, it should not be used as a substitute for medical treatment in cases of severe prostate conditions or cancer. Always consult with a healthcare professional before starting any new supplement, particularly if you are taking medications or have pre-existing health conditions.

Incorporating Saw Palmetto into a comprehensive approach to prostate health involves not only understanding the appropriate selection and dosage of the supplement but also integrating other lifestyle and dietary practices that support overall well-being. By doing so, individuals can work towards managing symptoms associated with BPH and enhancing their quality of life.

Saw Palmetto and Nettle Tea
Beneficial effects
Saw Palmetto and Nettle Tea combines the potent properties of saw palmetto, known for supporting prostate health, with the nutritional benefits of nettle, which aids in reducing inflammation and improving urinary flow. This herbal blend is particularly beneficial for men looking to naturally support their prostate health and urinary function.

Portions
Serves 2
Preparation time
5 minutes
Cooking time
15 minutes
Ingredients
- 1 tablespoon dried saw palmetto berries
- 1 tablespoon dried nettle leaves
- 2 cups of water
- Optional: Honey or lemon to taste

Instructions
1. Begin by bringing 2 cups of water to a boil in a medium-sized pot.
2. While the water is heating, measure out 1 tablespoon of dried saw palmetto berries. If the berries are whole, lightly crush them using a mortar and pestle to increase their surface area for a more effective infusion.
3. Measure out 1 tablespoon of dried nettle leaves, ensuring they are free from any debris or dust.
4. Once the water has reached a rolling boil, add both the saw palmetto berries and nettle leaves to the pot.
5. Reduce the heat to low, allowing the herbs to simmer gently for 15 minutes. This slow simmering process helps to extract the beneficial compounds from the herbs.
6. After 15 minutes, remove the pot from the heat. Cover the pot with a lid and allow the tea to steep for an additional 5 minutes. This steeping period enhances the strength and efficacy of the tea.
7. Strain the tea through a fine mesh sieve into a teapot or directly into cups, discarding the used herbs.
8. If desired, add honey or a squeeze of lemon to each cup for added flavor. Stir well to ensure any added sweeteners are fully dissolved.
9. Serve the tea warm to enjoy its full therapeutic benefits.

Variations
- For added flavor and health benefits, include a slice of fresh ginger or a cinnamon stick to the pot during the simmering process.
- Incorporate a teaspoon of dried peppermint leaves in the last 5 minutes of simmering for a refreshing twist.
- To make a stronger infusion, increase the amount of saw palmetto berries and nettle leaves to 1.5 tablespoons each and steep for up to 10 minutes longer.

Storage tips

This tea is best enjoyed fresh but can be stored in a sealed container in the refrigerator for up to 24 hours. Reheat gently on the stove or enjoy cold for a refreshing alternative.

Tips for allergens

For those with sensitivities, ensure the saw palmetto and nettle leaves are sourced from reputable suppliers to avoid cross-contamination with allergens. If honey is not suitable, consider maple syrup or agave nectar as sweetener alternatives.

Scientific references

- "Saw palmetto extract: its impact on prostate health" published in the Journal of Urology, which discusses the benefits of saw palmetto in supporting prostate health.
- "Nettle extract and its potential benefits in prostate and urinary health" found in the Phytotherapy Research journal, highlighting nettle's role in reducing inflammation and improving urinary flow in men.

BOOK 14: HERBS FOR DIGESTIVE HEALTH

CHAPTER 1: HERBAL CARMINATIVES FOR DIGESTION

Carminative herbs play a crucial role in digestive health by helping to relieve discomfort caused by gas and bloating. These herbs stimulate digestion, reduce intestinal gas, and soothe the digestive tract. Incorporating carminative herbs into your diet or wellness routine can be a simple, natural way to enhance digestive function and comfort. Here, we detail how to use some of the most effective carminative herbs, including **Peppermint**, **Fennel**, and **Ginger**, focusing on their preparation and application.

Peppermint (Mentha piperita) is renowned for its ability to soothe stomach issues and relieve symptoms of irritable bowel syndrome (IBS). To harness Peppermint's benefits, prepare a peppermint tea by steeping 1 to 2 teaspoons of dried peppermint leaves in boiling water for 10 minutes. Strain and enjoy the tea after meals to aid digestion. For those who prefer not to make tea, peppermint capsules are an alternative, with a recommended dose of 1-2 capsules taken 2-3 times daily, preferably before meals.

Fennel (Foeniculum vulgare) seeds are another excellent carminative that can be used to treat bloating, gas, and indigestion. Chew a half teaspoon of fennel seeds after meals, or brew a fennel tea by crushing the seeds slightly and steeping them in boiling water for 5-10 minutes. This not only aids in digestion but also freshens the breath. Fennel tea bags are also available for convenience, and the recommended consumption is one cup of tea, 2-3 times daily, especially after heavy meals.

Ginger (Zingiber officinale) is a powerful herb known for its anti-inflammatory and digestive properties. To make ginger tea, slice fresh ginger root and steep in boiling water for at least 10 minutes. Adding honey or lemon can enhance the flavor. Drinking ginger tea 20 minutes before meals can stimulate digestion and prevent discomfort. Ginger capsules are an alternative for those on the go, with a typical dosage being 1 gram daily, divided into two doses before meals.

For individuals looking to integrate these carminative herbs into their daily routine, consider the following tips:
- Start with small doses to see how your body reacts, gradually increasing as needed.
- Ensure herbs are of high quality, preferably organic, to avoid consuming pesticides and other chemicals.
- Consult with a healthcare provider, especially if you are pregnant, nursing, or have existing health conditions or are taking medications, as some herbs can interact with medications.

Remember, while carminative herbs are generally safe and effective for relieving digestive discomfort, they are part of a holistic approach to health. Maintaining a balanced diet, staying hydrated, and engaging in regular physical activity are also vital for optimal digestive health.

Peppermint and Fennel for Bloating

Peppermint and fennel are two of the most effective carminative herbs known for their ability to alleviate gas and bloating, making them invaluable in the realm of digestive health. These herbs work by relaxing the digestive tract muscles, which can help to release trapped gas and ease discomfort. To fully harness the benefits of peppermint and fennel for gas and bloating, it's essential to understand how to properly select, prepare, and use these herbs.

Starting with peppermint, or Mentha piperita, this herb is celebrated for its soothing menthol content, which provides a cooling effect on the digestive system. When selecting peppermint for digestive relief, opt for fresh leaves or high-quality dried leaves to ensure the potency of the essential oils. For preparation, peppermint tea is a popular and effective method. Use one tablespoon of fresh peppermint leaves or one teaspoon of dried leaves per cup of boiling water. Steep the leaves for 10 minutes before straining. This tea can be consumed 2-3 times daily, preferably between meals, to aid digestion and relieve bloating and gas. Peppermint oil capsules are another option, offering a convenient and concentrated way to obtain peppermint's benefits. It's recommended to follow the dosage instructions on the product label, as concentrations can vary.

Fennel, or Foeniculum vulgare, is another powerhouse herb with a long history of use in aiding digestion. Its seeds contain anethole, a compound that can help relax the digestive tract and reduce gas production. To utilize fennel seeds for digestive relief, you can chew on a half teaspoon of the seeds after meals. Alternatively, fennel tea is an excellent way to enjoy the benefits of this herb. Crush a teaspoon of fennel seeds and steep in a cup of boiling water for 5-10 minutes. Straining is optional, as consuming the seeds can increase the carminative effect. Fennel tea can be enjoyed 2-3 times daily, especially after meals, to help prevent or alleviate bloating and gas.

For those incorporating peppermint and fennel into their wellness routines, it's crucial to source these herbs from reputable suppliers to ensure they are free from contaminants and of the highest quality. Organic sources are preferable to minimize exposure to pesticides and other harmful chemicals. Additionally, while both peppermint and fennel are generally considered safe for most people, individuals with certain health conditions, such as gastroesophageal reflux disease (GERD) for peppermint or hormone-sensitive conditions for fennel, should consult with a healthcare provider before use. Pregnant or breastfeeding women should also seek medical advice prior to using these herbs.

Incorporating peppermint and fennel into your diet or wellness routine can be a simple yet effective way to manage digestive discomfort such as gas and bloating. Whether opting for teas, capsules, or chewing the seeds, these herbs offer a natural and accessible means to support digestive health. Remember, consistency in use and paying attention to how your body responds will help you determine the most effective way to incorporate these carminative herbs into your holistic health practices.

Peppermint and Fennel Tea for Bloating

Beneficial effects

Peppermint and Fennel Tea is a soothing, aromatic beverage known for its ability to alleviate bloating and digestive discomfort. Peppermint relaxes the digestive system and can relieve gas and spasms, while fennel seeds contain compounds that aid in digestion and reduce inflammation. Together, they create a powerful herbal remedy that can help soothe the stomach, reduce bloating, and promote overall digestive health.

Portions

Serves 2

Preparation time

5 minutes

Cooking time

10 minutes

Ingredients

- 1 tablespoon dried peppermint leaves
- 1 teaspoon fennel seeds
- 2 cups of water
- Optional: Honey or a slice of lemon for flavor

Instructions

1. Begin by bringing 2 cups of water to a boil in a small saucepan. While waiting for the water to boil, gather the peppermint leaves and fennel seeds.
2. Once the water reaches a rolling boil, add 1 tablespoon of dried peppermint leaves and 1 teaspoon of fennel seeds to the saucepan.
3. Reduce the heat to low, cover the saucepan with a lid, and let the mixture simmer gently for 10 minutes. This allows the water to become infused with the flavors and beneficial properties of the peppermint and fennel.
4. After 10 minutes, remove the saucepan from the heat. Let the tea steep, covered, for an additional 5 minutes to enhance the strength and efficacy of the infusion.
5. Strain the tea through a fine mesh sieve into teacups or a teapot, discarding the peppermint leaves and fennel seeds.
6. If desired, add honey or a slice of lemon to each cup for added flavor. Stir well to ensure any added sweeteners are fully dissolved.
7. Serve the tea warm to enjoy its digestive benefits.

Variations

- For a caffeine-free morning boost, add a slice of fresh ginger to the saucepan along with the peppermint and fennel for an extra digestive aid.
- Incorporate a cinnamon stick during the simmering process for a warming, spicy flavor that complements the cooling peppermint.
- To make a cold remedy, add a tablespoon of elderflower to the mix, which can help relieve cold symptoms in addition to soothing the digestive system.

Storage tips

This tea is best enjoyed fresh but can be stored in the refrigerator for up to 24 hours. Reheat gently on the stove or enjoy cold as a refreshing digestive aid.

Tips for allergens

For those with sensitivities, ensure the peppermint and fennel seeds are sourced from reputable suppliers to avoid cross-contamination with allergens. If honey is not suitable, consider maple syrup or agave nectar as sweetener alternatives.

Scientific references

- "Peppermint oil for the treatment of irritable bowel syndrome: a systematic review and meta-analysis" published in the Journal of Clinical Gastroenterology, which discusses the benefits of peppermint in relieving IBS symptoms.
- "Fennel and anise as estrogenic agents" published in the Journal of Ethnopharmacology, highlighting the anti-inflammatory and estrogen-like effects of fennel seeds, which can aid in digestion.

CHAPTER 2: GUT HEALING WITH DEMULCENTS

Herbal demulcents are a cornerstone in the natural treatment of digestive issues, particularly those involving irritation or inflammation of the gut lining. These herbs contain high levels of mucilage, a slippery, gel-like substance that, when mixed with water, forms a soothing film. This protective layer coats the mucous membranes of the digestive tract, offering relief from discomfort and aiding in the healing process of the gut lining. Understanding the specific herbs that fall into this category, their preparation, and application can significantly enhance digestive health.

Marshmallow Root (Althaea officinalis) is renowned for its high mucilage content. To harness its gut-soothing properties, a cold infusion is most effective. Combine one tablespoon of dried marshmallow root with one cup of cold water and let it steep overnight. Strain and drink on an empty stomach to maximize contact with the gut lining.

Slippery Elm (Ulmus rubra) shares similar demulcent properties. For a soothing drink, mix one teaspoon of slippery elm powder with a cup of hot water. The mixture will thicken as it cools, forming a gel-like consistency that coats the digestive tract, offering relief from irritation.

Licorice Root (Glycyrrhiza glabra), beyond its demulcent action, has additional healing properties that can be beneficial for gut health. Prepare a licorice root tea by simmering one teaspoon of the dried root in a cup of water for about 10 minutes. Strain and drink up to two cups a day. Note: Licorice root is not recommended for those with high blood pressure.

Flaxseed (Linum usitatissimum), while not a herb in the traditional sense, is a powerful demulcent. To create a flaxseed gel, soak one tablespoon of flaxseeds in three tablespoons of water for several hours or overnight. The resulting gel can be mixed into smoothies or oatmeal, providing a protective layer for the digestive tract.

For those dealing with chronic digestive issues such as irritable bowel syndrome (IBS) or leaky gut syndrome, incorporating these demulcent herbs into your daily routine can offer significant relief. It's important to remember that while these herbs are generally safe, they should be used in moderation and in consultation with a healthcare provider, especially if you are pregnant, nursing, or on medication.

Incorporating these herbs into your diet can be as simple as drinking the prepared teas or infusions daily, or adding the flaxseed gel to foods. Consistency is key to seeing improvements in digestive health. Additionally, combining the use of demulcent herbs with a diet rich in fiber and low in inflammatory foods can enhance the healing process of the gut lining.

Remember, the goal of using demulcent herbs is not only to relieve symptoms but to support the body's natural healing processes. With regular use and a holistic approach to health, these herbs can be a valuable part of a comprehensive plan for digestive wellness.

Marshmallow Root for IBS and Inflammation

Marshmallow root (**Althaea officinalis**) is a perennial herb that is highly valued for its soothing and protective properties, especially beneficial for individuals suffering from Irritable Bowel Syndrome (IBS) and inflammation of the digestive tract. The root contains a high percentage of mucilage, a gelatinous substance that swells upon contact with water, forming a protective layer on the lining of the digestive system. This action can provide relief from the discomfort associated with IBS and inflammatory conditions by reducing irritation and calming inflammation.

To prepare a **Marshmallow Root Cold Infusion**, which is the most effective method to extract its mucilaginous properties, follow these detailed steps:

1. **Selecting Marshmallow Root**: Opt for organic, dried marshmallow root to ensure the absence of pesticides and contaminants that can exacerbate digestive issues. The root should be light beige to white in color and have a fibrous texture.

2. **Preparation of the Infusion**: Measure one tablespoon of dried marshmallow root into a glass jar. Pour one cup (approximately 240 milliliters) of cold water over the herbs. Cold water is crucial as it extracts the mucilage without dissolving other substances that could irritate the gut.

3. **Steeping Time**: Seal the jar with a lid and let the mixture steep overnight, or for at least 8 to 12 hours. This long infusion period allows the cold water to slowly draw out the mucilage from the marshmallow root.

4. **Straining**: After steeping, strain the infusion using a fine mesh strainer or cheesecloth to remove the herb particles. The resulting liquid should be thick and slippery to the touch.

5. **Consumption**: Drink the marshmallow root infusion on an empty stomach to ensure that the mucilage can coat the digestive tract thoroughly. For best results, consume the infusion first thing in the morning before eating or drinking anything else.

6. **Dosage**: Individuals can start with one cup of marshmallow root infusion daily, monitoring their body's response. Depending on the severity of the symptoms and personal tolerance, the amount can be adjusted. It's advisable not to exceed three cups per day.

7. **Storage**: Any unused portion of the infusion should be refrigerated. Consume within 24 hours to ensure the potency of the mucilage.

Considerations and Cautions:

- While marshmallow root is generally safe for most people, those with diabetes should monitor their blood sugar levels closely as it may lower blood sugar.
- Pregnant or nursing women should consult with a healthcare provider before incorporating marshmallow root into their regimen due to limited research on its effects during pregnancy and lactation.
- Individuals taking prescription medications should discuss the use of marshmallow root with their healthcare provider to avoid potential interactions, as the mucilage can interfere with the absorption of oral medications.

Incorporating marshmallow root into your wellness routine can offer a natural and gentle option for managing IBS and digestive inflammation. Its ability to soothe the gut lining makes it a valuable herb in the holistic approach to digestive health.

Marshmallow Root Gut-Soothing Powder

Beneficial effects

Marshmallow Root Gut-Soothing Powder leverages the mucilaginous properties of marshmallow root, which forms a protective layer on the lining of the digestive tract. This soothing effect can help alleviate irritation and inflammation in the gut, making it beneficial for individuals experiencing symptoms of IBS, leaky gut syndrome, and other digestive issues. Marshmallow root is also known for its ability to hydrate and maintain moisture in the digestive system, promoting healthy bowel movements.

Portions

Makes approximately 1/2 cup of powder

Preparation time

15 minutes

Cooking time

N/A

Ingredients

- 1 cup dried marshmallow root
- Optional: 1/4 cup dried slippery elm bark for added digestive support

Instructions

1. Begin by sourcing high-quality, organic dried marshmallow root to ensure the purity and effectiveness of your gut-soothing powder. If including slippery elm bark, ensure it is also of high quality.

2. Using a clean coffee grinder or a high-powered blender, add the dried marshmallow root (and slippery elm bark if using) in small batches. Grinding in small amounts helps achieve a more uniform powder and prevents the machine from overheating.

3. Pulse the grinder or blender for 30 seconds to 1 minute, or until the marshmallow root (and slippery elm bark) is ground into a fine powder. The texture should be consistent, without any large pieces.

4. After each batch is ground to a fine powder, sift it through a fine mesh sieve into a mixing bowl. This step ensures that any unground pieces are removed, and you're left with only the finest powder for your digestive aid.

5. Once all the marshmallow root (and slippery elm bark) has been ground and sifted, gently stir the powder to ensure an even mix if you've used both herbs.

6. Transfer the gut-soothing powder into an airtight container. Glass jars with tight-fitting lids work well for storage and help maintain the powder's freshness.

Variations
- For added flavor and digestive benefits, consider mixing in a small amount of ground ginger or cinnamon powder to the marshmallow root powder.
- If you're addressing specific digestive issues, such as excessive gas, adding a small proportion of ground fennel or caraway seeds can offer additional relief.

Storage tips
Store your Marshmallow Root Gut-Soothing Powder in a cool, dry place away from direct sunlight. The powder can maintain its potency for up to 6 months when stored properly. Always use a dry spoon when measuring out the powder to prevent moisture from entering the container.

Tips for allergens
For individuals with sensitivities or allergies to specific herbs, ensure that the marshmallow root and any additional herbs used are processed in a facility that does not handle allergens. If you're allergic to any of the optional ingredients suggested, simply omit them from the recipe.

Scientific references
- "The effect of herbal medicines on the relief of irritable bowel syndrome: A systematic review" published in the World Journal of Gastroenterology, which discusses the benefits of mucilage-rich herbs like marshmallow root in managing digestive symptoms.
- "Slippery elm, its biochemistry, and use as a complementary and alternative treatment for laryngeal irritation" in the Journal of Investigational Biochemistry, highlighting the soothing properties of slippery elm, which can complement the effects of marshmallow root in digestive health.

CHAPTER 3: LIVER AND GALLBLADDER SUPPORT

For optimal liver and gallbladder support, incorporating specific herbs into your wellness routine can play a crucial role in enhancing the function of these vital organs. The liver, responsible for detoxifying harmful substances and metabolizing fats, and the gallbladder, important for storing bile produced by the liver, both benefit from herbal support to maintain their health and efficiency. The following herbs have been identified for their beneficial properties in supporting liver and gallbladder health:

Milk Thistle (Silybum marianum): Milk Thistle is renowned for its liver-protecting properties. It contains silymarin, a group of compounds said to have antioxidant and anti-inflammatory effects, which is particularly beneficial for liver health. To utilize Milk Thistle effectively, look for a standardized extract containing 70% to 80% silymarin. The recommended dosage is 100 to 200 milligrams of this extract, taken twice daily. This can help in regenerating liver cells and protecting the liver from toxic damage.

Dandelion Root (Taraxacum officinale): Dandelion root acts as a liver tonic by stimulating bile flow from the liver and gallbladder, which aids in digestion and the breakdown of fats. Prepare a dandelion root tea by simmering 1 to 2 teaspoons of the dried root in 8 ounces of water for about 10 minutes. Strain and enjoy this tea up to three times a day. Not only does it support liver function, but it also helps in the natural detoxification process.

Artichoke Leaf (Cynara scolymus): Similar to dandelion, artichoke leaf stimulates bile production, enhancing both liver and gallbladder function. It also supports the regeneration of liver tissue. Artichoke leaf can be consumed as a tea or in extract form. For the tea, steep 1 to 2 teaspoons of dried leaves in hot water for 10 minutes. If opting for an extract, the recommended dosage is 300 to 500 milligrams, taken three times daily.

Turmeric (Curcuma longa): Turmeric and its active compound, curcumin, have potent anti-inflammatory and antioxidant properties that can protect the liver. Turmeric can be incorporated into your diet by adding it to foods, or it can be taken as a supplement. When using turmeric powder, aim for 1 to 3 grams per day. If choosing a curcumin supplement, look for one with piperine (black pepper extract) to enhance absorption, with a recommended dosage of 500 to 1,000 milligrams daily.

Peppermint (Mentha piperita): Peppermint is not only soothing for the digestive tract but can also ease bile duct spasms and help with gallbladder discomfort. Peppermint tea is a gentle way to incorporate this herb into your routine. Use 1 teaspoon of dried peppermint leaves steeped in hot water for about 10 minutes. This tea can be consumed 2 to 3 times a day.

In addition to these herbs, maintaining a diet low in processed foods and high in fiber, fruits, and vegetables will support liver and gallbladder health. Regular exercise and staying hydrated are also key components of maintaining the health of these organs.

When incorporating any new supplement or herb into your routine, it's important to consult with a healthcare provider, especially if you have existing health conditions or are taking medications. Some herbs can interact with medications and may not be suitable for everyone. Monitoring your body's response to these herbal remedies and adjusting as necessary is also crucial for achieving the best results in supporting liver and gallbladder health.

Dandelion and Milk Thistle Detox

Dandelion (Taraxacum officinale) and **Milk Thistle (Silybum marianum)** are two potent herbs widely recognized for their detoxification support, particularly for the liver and gallbladder. These herbs function synergistically to enhance the body's natural detoxification processes, supporting liver function, and promoting the flow of bile from the gallbladder, which is essential for the digestion and breakdown of fats.

Dandelion, a ubiquitous weed found in many backyards, is much more than a simple nuisance. Every part of the dandelion plant is edible and packed with nutrients, but for liver support, the root is most commonly used. Dandelion root acts as a diuretic, increasing urine production and supporting the liver in eliminating toxins from the body. It also stimulates bile production, which helps the liver detoxify more efficiently.

To prepare a **Dandelion Root Detox Tea**, follow these steps:

1. **Harvesting**: Choose dandelion roots from areas that have not been treated with pesticides. Autumn is the best time for harvesting, as the roots are rich in inulin.

2. **Cleaning**: Wash the roots thoroughly to remove soil and debris.

3. **Drying**: Cut the roots into small pieces and spread them out on a clean surface to dry. This can take 3-14 days, depending on humidity levels. Alternatively, use a dehydrator set at 95°F (35°C) for about 12 hours.

4. **Roasting (Optional)**: For a richer flavor, roast the dried root pieces in an oven at 250°F (120°C) for 2 hours.

5. **Brewing**: Use 1-2 teaspoons of the dried (and optionally roasted) root per cup of water. Simmer in boiling water for 15-20 minutes, then strain.

Milk Thistle is renowned for its liver-protective effects, attributed to its active ingredient, silymarin. Silymarin acts as an antioxidant, protecting liver cells from damage by toxins and aiding in the regeneration of damaged liver tissue.

For a **Milk Thistle Seed Extract**, the process involves:

1. **Selecting Seeds**: Use whole, organic milk thistle seeds for the highest quality extract.

2. **Grinding**: Grind the seeds using a coffee grinder or mortar and pestle to increase the surface area for extraction.

3. **Soaking**: Soak the ground seeds in high-proof alcohol (vodka or brandy works well) in a ratio of 1 part seeds to 3 parts alcohol. Seal in a glass jar.

4. **Storing**: Keep the jar in a cool, dark place for 4-6 weeks, shaking it every few days to mix the contents.

5. **Straining**: After the soaking period, strain the mixture through a fine mesh strainer or cheesecloth into a clean, dark glass bottle. Store in a cool, dark place.

Combining Dandelion and Milk Thistle in a detox regimen amplifies the benefits, as both herbs work to protect and support liver function while promoting the elimination of toxins. It's important to start with small doses to assess tolerance and gradually increase to the recommended amounts. For the dandelion tea, drinking 1-2 cups daily is a good starting point, while for the milk thistle extract, following the dosage instructions on the product or consulting with a healthcare provider is advisable.

Important Considerations:
- Always source herbs from reputable suppliers to ensure purity and avoid contamination.
- While these herbs are generally considered safe, individuals with gallbladder disease, bile duct obstruction, or other medical conditions should consult with a healthcare professional before starting any new herbal regimen.
- Pregnant or nursing women should avoid these herbs unless advised otherwise by a healthcare provider.
- As with any supplement, it's crucial to monitor your body's response and consult with a healthcare provider to ensure these herbs are appropriate for your health needs.

Incorporating **Dandelion** and **Milk Thistle** into a holistic approach to wellness can provide significant benefits for liver and gallbladder health, contributing to an overall sense of well-being and vitality.

Dandelion Root Detox Tea

Beneficial effects

Dandelion Root Detox Tea is a natural and effective way to support liver and gallbladder health. Dandelion root acts as a powerful detoxifier, stimulating the liver to eliminate toxins more efficiently. It also promotes digestion and helps to balance the natural and beneficial bacteria in the intestines. This herbal tea can aid in reducing inflammation, improving bile flow, and may help in managing water retention. Its diuretic properties support the removal of excess fluids from the body, contributing to a gentle cleansing effect.

Portions

Serves 2

Preparation time

5 minutes

Cooking time

10 minutes

Ingredients

- 2 tablespoons of dried dandelion root
- 4 cups of water
- Optional: Honey or lemon to taste

Instructions

1. Measure 4 cups of water and pour it into a medium-sized pot. Place the pot on the stove and turn the heat to high, bringing the water to a boil.

2. While the water is heating, measure out 2 tablespoons of dried dandelion root. If the dandelion root is not already in a coarse powder form, use a mortar and pestle or a coffee grinder to lightly crush the roots. This increases the surface area, allowing more of the beneficial compounds to be released during brewing.

3. Once the water has reached a rolling boil, add the crushed dandelion root to the pot.

4. Reduce the heat to low, allowing the dandelion root to simmer gently for 10 minutes. This slow simmering process helps to extract the roots' beneficial compounds into the water.

5. After simmering, remove the pot from the heat. Cover the pot with a lid and let the tea steep for an additional 5 minutes. Steeping the tea covered helps to trap the volatile oils and flavors, enhancing the medicinal properties of the tea.

6. Strain the tea through a fine mesh sieve into a teapot or directly into cups, discarding the dandelion root solids.

7. If desired, add honey or a squeeze of lemon to each cup for added flavor. Stir well to ensure any added sweeteners or lemon juice are fully dissolved.

8. Serve the tea warm to enjoy its detoxifying benefits.

Variations

- For a more complex flavor, add a cinnamon stick or a few slices of fresh ginger to the pot along with the dandelion root.
- Incorporate a teaspoon of dried peppermint leaves in the last 5 minutes of simmering for a refreshing twist.
- To enhance the detoxifying effects, mix in a tablespoon of dried burdock root with the dandelion root before simmering.

Storage tips

This tea is best enjoyed fresh but can be stored in a sealed container in the refrigerator for up to 48 hours. Reheat gently on the stove or enjoy cold for a refreshing detox beverage.

Tips for allergens

For those with sensitivities, ensure the dandelion root (and any additional herbs used) are sourced from reputable suppliers to avoid cross-contamination with allergens. If honey is not suitable, consider maple syrup or agave nectar as sweetener alternatives.

Scientific references

- "The diuretic effect in human subjects of an extract of Taraxacum officinale folium over a single day" published in the Journal of Alternative and Complementary Medicine, which discusses the diuretic properties of dandelion.
- "Taraxacum—a review on its phytochemical and pharmacological profile" in the Journal of Ethnopharmacology, highlighting the detoxifying effects of dandelion root on liver function.

BOOK 15: RESPIRATORY SUPPORT WITH HERBS

CHAPTER 1: DECONGESTING AIRWAYS NATURALLY

For those seeking natural methods to clear congested airways, a variety of herbs have been traditionally used to alleviate respiratory discomfort. These herbs can be incorporated into teas, inhalations, or topical applications to help open up the airways, reduce inflammation, and soothe irritation.

Eucalyptus (Eucalyptus globulus) is renowned for its ability to clear nasal passages and bronchial congestion. The key component, eucalyptol, has a cooling effect that helps to relieve coughs and improve airflow. To harness the benefits of eucalyptus, add a few drops of eucalyptus essential oil to a bowl of hot water, cover your head with a towel, and inhale the steam for 5-10 minutes. This method helps to loosen mucus and reduce congestion.

Peppermint (Mentha piperita) contains menthol, which is effective in soothing sore throats, calming coughs, and clearing sinuses. A simple peppermint tea can be made by steeping 1 teaspoon of dried peppermint leaves in a cup of boiling water for 10 minutes. Drinking this tea 2-3 times a day can provide respiratory relief.

Thyme (Thymus vulgaris) has powerful antibacterial and antiviral properties, making it beneficial in treating respiratory infections that can lead to congestion. To make a thyme infusion, simmer 2 teaspoons of dried thyme in a cup of water for 15 minutes. Strain and drink up to three times daily. Thyme helps in loosening mucus and facilitating its expulsion.

Mullein (Verbascum thapsus) is a gentle herb known for its ability to reduce inflammation in the respiratory tract and soothe irritated mucous membranes. A mullein leaf tea can be prepared by steeping 1-2 teaspoons of dried mullein leaves in boiling water for 10-15 minutes. This tea can be consumed several times a day to help alleviate cough and clear the airways.

Licorice Root (Glycyrrhiza glabra) acts as an expectorant, helping to loosen and expel phlegm from the respiratory system. It also soothes the throat and reduces irritation. Prepare a licorice root tea by simmering 1 teaspoon of dried licorice root in a cup of water for 10 minutes. It is advisable to drink this tea once daily. Note: Licorice root should be avoided by those with high blood pressure, kidney disease, or pregnant women.

Ginger (Zingiber officinale) is another effective herb for decongesting the airways. Its anti-inflammatory properties help to reduce swelling in the nasal passages and relieve congestion. A ginger tea can be made by simmering a 1-inch piece of fresh ginger in two cups of water for 10 minutes. Adding honey and lemon not only enhances the flavor but also provides additional throat-soothing benefits.

For topical application, a chest rub made from eucalyptus and peppermint essential oils can be effective in relieving congestion. Mix 3 drops of eucalyptus oil and 2 drops of peppermint oil with 1 tablespoon of a carrier oil such as coconut or olive oil. Gently massage this blend onto the chest and back to help open up the airways. Incorporating these herbal remedies into your wellness routine can provide natural and effective relief from respiratory congestion. Always ensure the quality of the herbs and essential oils used, opting for organic and sustainably sourced products whenever possible. Additionally, it is important to consult with a healthcare provider before starting any new herbal regimen, especially for those with existing health conditions or those taking medication, to avoid potential interactions.

Thyme and Peppermint for Sinus Relief

Thyme (**Thymus vulgaris**) and Peppermint (**Mentha piperita**) are potent herbs recognized for their efficacy in providing sinus relief. These herbs function through different mechanisms to alleviate congestion, reduce inflammation, and soothe the mucous membranes of the respiratory tract.

Thyme is rich in thymol, a natural compound with strong antibacterial and antiviral properties, making it an excellent choice for treating infections that contribute to sinus congestion. To harness thyme's benefits, a tea can be prepared by steeping 2 teaspoons of dried thyme leaves in 1 cup (approximately 240 milliliters) of boiling water for 10 minutes. Strain the leaves and drink the tea warm. For enhanced sinus relief, inhale the steam from the tea as it brews, as the warm vapors can help to open nasal passages and facilitate mucus drainage.

Peppermint contains menthol, which is known for its cooling and soothing effects on the sinuses. Menthol helps to improve airflow in the nasal passages and provides a calming effect on inflamed tissues. A peppermint tea can be made by adding 1 teaspoon of dried peppermint leaves to 1 cup (approximately 240 milliliters) of boiling water and steeping for 10 minutes. Similar to thyme tea, peppermint tea can be consumed warm, and inhaling the steam can provide immediate relief from nasal congestion.

For direct sinus relief, a steam inhalation method can be employed using both thyme and peppermint. Add 2 teaspoons of dried thyme and 1 teaspoon of dried peppermint to a large bowl of boiling water. Lean over the bowl, cover your head and the bowl with a towel to trap the steam, and inhale deeply for 5-10 minutes. This method allows the therapeutic properties of both herbs to be directly absorbed by the nasal passages, providing quick relief from congestion.

Another effective approach is to prepare a nasal rinse with thyme and peppermint. Boil 2 cups (approximately 480 milliliters) of water and add 1 teaspoon of dried thyme and 1 teaspoon of dried peppermint. Allow the mixture to steep and cool to a lukewarm temperature. Strain the solution through a fine mesh to remove all plant particles, then use a neti pot to gently rinse the nasal passages. This can help to clear mucus, reduce nasal swelling, and soothe irritated mucous membranes.

When using thyme and peppermint for sinus relief, it's important to source high-quality, organic herbs to ensure the absence of pesticides and contaminants. Always ensure the water used for teas, steam inhalation, or nasal rinses is purified or distilled to avoid introducing impurities into the respiratory system.

While thyme and peppermint are generally safe for most individuals, those with allergies to plants in the Lamiaceae family should proceed with caution. Pregnant or nursing women and individuals on medication should consult with a healthcare provider before using these herbs for sinus relief.

Incorporating thyme and peppermint into your routine during times of sinus congestion can provide a natural, effective way to alleviate symptoms and support respiratory health. Whether through teas, steam inhalation, or nasal rinses, these herbs offer a holistic approach to managing sinus discomfort.

Thyme and Peppermint Steam Inhalationv

Beneficial effects

Thyme and peppermint steam inhalation harnesses the natural expectorant properties of thyme and the soothing, menthol-rich essence of peppermint to alleviate respiratory congestion. Thyme has been traditionally used to fight off respiratory infections and improve breathing by opening airways, while peppermint can cool and soothe sore throats and ease coughing. Together, they create a powerful herbal steam that can provide immediate relief for sinus congestion, colds, and respiratory discomfort.

Ingredients

- 2 tablespoons fresh thyme leaves (or 1 tablespoon dried thyme)
- 2 tablespoons fresh peppermint leaves (or 1 tablespoon dried peppermint)
- 4 cups boiling water

Instructions

1. Begin by boiling 4 cups of water in a large pot. Once boiling, remove the pot from the heat.
2. While the water is boiling, thoroughly wash the fresh thyme and peppermint leaves to remove any dirt or debris. If using dried herbs, measure out the appropriate amounts.
3. Add the fresh or dried thyme and peppermint leaves directly into the boiling water. Stir gently to ensure the herbs are fully submerged and begin to release their essential oils.
4. Cover the pot with a lid and allow the herbs to steep in the hot water for 5 minutes. This steeping process allows the medicinal properties of the herbs to infuse into the steam.
5. After 5 minutes, carefully remove the lid. Ensure the steam is not too hot to prevent burns before proceeding to the next step.
6. Drape a large towel over your head and shoulders, and lean over the pot at a safe distance, allowing the herbal steam to envelop your face. Close your eyes to avoid irritation.
7. Inhale deeply for 5 to 10 minutes, allowing the thyme and peppermint-infused steam to penetrate your respiratory system. Take breaks as needed to avoid discomfort.
8. After completing the inhalation process, gently pat your face dry with a clean towel. Drink a glass of water to stay hydrated.

Variations

- For additional antimicrobial benefits, add a teaspoon of eucalyptus leaves to the mix.
- If suffering from a headache in addition to congestion, incorporating a tablespoon of lavender flowers can provide soothing relief.
- For a stronger decongestant effect, include a slice of fresh ginger in the boiling water along with the herbs.

Storage tips

The fresh thyme and peppermint leaves should be used immediately after preparation for the best therapeutic effect. However, if you have leftover herbs, they can be stored in the refrigerator. Wrap the fresh herbs in a damp paper towel and place them inside a sealed plastic bag. They should last for several days.

Tips for allergens

Individuals with allergies to specific herbs should consult with a healthcare provider before trying this inhalation. If allergic to thyme or peppermint, consider substituting with other respiratory-supportive herbs like eucalyptus or rosemary, following the same preparation steps.

Scientific references

- "Antimicrobial properties of plant essential oils against human pathogens and their mode of action: An updated review" published in Evidence-Based Complementary and Alternative Medicine, which discusses the benefits of thyme and peppermint in fighting respiratory infections.
- "Peppermint Oil: Clinical Uses in the Treatment of Gastrointestinal Diseases" found in the Journal of Gastrointestinal and Liver Diseases, highlighting peppermint's soothing effects on the throat and its ability to ease coughing.

CHAPTER 2: STRENGTHENING THE LUNGS

Mullein (Verbascum thapsus) is renowned for its ability to strengthen and support lung health. This herb acts as an expectorant, helping to clear congestion from the lungs and improve breathing. For those looking to incorporate Mullein into their respiratory support regimen, the following detailed guide outlines the preparation of a Mullein leaf tea, a simple yet effective remedy.

Ingredients:
- 1 to 2 teaspoons of dried Mullein leaves
- 8 ounces of boiling water

Preparation Steps:
1. Begin by sourcing high-quality, organic dried Mullein leaves from a reputable supplier. This ensures the potency and safety of the herb.
2. Measure 1 to 2 teaspoons of the dried leaves. The amount can be adjusted based on personal preference and the desired strength of the tea.
3. Boil 8 ounces of water in a clean pot. Once boiling, remove the water from heat.
4. Place the dried Mullein leaves in a tea infuser or directly into the pot. If placing the leaves directly in the pot, a strainer will be needed later to remove the leaves.
5. Pour the hot water over the Mullein leaves and cover the pot with a lid. Steeping the tea covered is crucial as it preserves the volatile oils and medicinal properties of the herb.
6. Allow the tea to steep for 10 to 15 minutes. This duration extracts the therapeutic compounds from the leaves without compromising the flavor.
7. If the leaves were added directly to the pot, strain the tea using a fine mesh strainer to remove the leaves. For those using a tea infuser, simply remove the infuser from the pot.
8. The tea can be enjoyed as is or sweetened with a natural sweetener like honey, which also offers additional soothing properties for the throat.

Consumption Recommendations:
For optimal respiratory support, consume 1 to 3 cups of Mullein leaf tea daily. This regimen can be adjusted based on individual needs and responses to the herb. It is important to listen to your body and consult with a healthcare provider, especially if you are pregnant, nursing, or have existing health conditions.

Storage:
Store any unused dried Mullein leaves in a cool, dark place in an airtight container to preserve their potency. Properly stored, the leaves can last for several years.

This detailed guide to preparing and using Mullein leaf tea for lung health is designed to be accessible and straightforward, allowing individuals of varying knowledge levels and backgrounds to benefit from the healing properties of this powerful herb.

Mullein for Respiratory Health

Mullein (Verbascum thapsus) serves as a cornerstone herb in the realm of respiratory health, particularly for those dealing with chronic conditions that affect the lungs such as bronchitis, asthma, and even the common cold. This herb's efficacy lies in its ability to act as an expectorant, facilitating the expulsion of mucus from the lungs and airways, and as a demulcent, providing a soothing barrier to irritated mucous membranes. The utilization of Mullein in a therapeutic context involves a meticulous approach to preparation and dosage to ensure maximum benefit and safety.

To harness the respiratory benefits of Mullein, one can prepare a Mullein leaf infusion, which involves steeping the dried leaves in hot water. This process begins with selecting high-quality, dried Mullein leaves, preferably organic, to avoid any potential contaminants that could detract from the herb's medicinal value. For the preparation of the infusion, approximately one tablespoon of dried Mullein leaves should be added to one cup (about 8 ounces) of boiling water. It's crucial to cover the vessel during the steeping process, which should last for about 10 to 15 minutes, to prevent the escape of essential volatile oils and compounds into the air.

Straining the infusion is a critical step, as Mullein leaves are covered in fine hairs that can be irritating to the throat if ingested. A fine mesh strainer or a cloth can be employed to ensure that these hairs are removed from the final preparation. The resulting liquid can be consumed hot or cooled, depending on personal preference. For those experiencing chronic respiratory issues, drinking 2 to 3 cups of Mullein leaf infusion daily can provide significant relief. However, it's important to start with a lower dosage to gauge individual tolerance before gradually increasing to the recommended amount.

In addition to the infusion, Mullein can also be used in other forms such as tinctures or capsules, which might be preferable for some individuals seeking a more concentrated or convenient option. When using a tincture, typically, a dosage of 1/2 to 1 teaspoon (2.5 to 5 ml) taken three times a day is suggested. However, as with any herbal remedy, it's advisable to consult with a healthcare provider before incorporating Mullein into a health regimen, especially for those who are pregnant, nursing, or on medication for chronic conditions.

The storage of Mullein, whether in its dried leaf form or as a prepared infusion, tincture, or capsule, should be done with care to preserve its medicinal qualities. Dried leaves should be kept in an airtight container away from direct sunlight and moisture to prevent degradation. Prepared infusions should be consumed within a day to ensure potency, while tinctures and capsules should be stored according to the manufacturer's instructions, usually in a cool, dark place.

Incorporating Mullein into a holistic approach to respiratory health can offer a natural and effective way to manage chronic conditions, improve lung function, and enhance overall well-being. Its long history of use in herbal medicine, coupled with contemporary anecdotal and some scientific support, underscores Mullein's role as a valuable ally in the quest for respiratory health. However, as with any herbal remedy, the key to achieving the best outcomes lies in understanding the proper preparation, dosage, and application specific to one's individual health needs and circumstances.

Mullein and Nettle Tea Blend

Beneficial effects

Mullein and nettle tea blend harnesses the respiratory support properties of both herbs. Mullein is known for its ability to soothe the respiratory tract and ease coughing, making it beneficial for those with bronchitis or asthma. Nettle, on the other hand, acts as a natural antihistamine, helping to manage allergic reactions and reduce inflammation. Together, they create a powerful tea that supports lung health and eases respiratory discomfort.

Portions

Serves 2

Preparation time

5 minutes

Cooking time

10 minutes

Ingredients

- 1 tablespoon dried mullein leaves
- 1 tablespoon dried nettle leaves
- 4 cups water
- Optional: Honey or lemon to taste

Instructions

1. Begin by bringing 4 cups of water to a boil in a medium-sized pot.
2. While the water is heating, measure out 1 tablespoon of dried mullein leaves and 1 tablespoon of dried nettle leaves. Ensure the herbs are free from any debris or dust.
3. Once the water has reached a rolling boil, add both the mullein and nettle leaves to the pot.
4. Reduce the heat to low and allow the herbs to simmer gently for 10 minutes. This slow simmering process helps to extract the beneficial compounds from the herbs.
5. After 10 minutes, remove the pot from the heat. Cover the pot with a lid and allow the tea to steep for an additional 5 minutes. This steeping period enhances the strength and efficacy of the tea.
6. Strain the tea through a fine mesh sieve into a teapot or directly into cups, discarding the used herbs.
7. If desired, add honey or a squeeze of lemon to each cup for added flavor. Stir well to ensure any added sweeteners are fully dissolved.
8. Serve the tea warm to enjoy its respiratory benefits.

Variations

- For added respiratory support, include a teaspoon of dried thyme or eucalyptus leaves to the pot during the simmering process.

- Incorporate a slice of fresh ginger in the tea while simmering to add a warming, spicy flavor and additional anti-inflammatory benefits.
- To enhance the tea's soothing effects, add a teaspoon of dried chamomile flowers during the last 5 minutes of simmering.

Storage tips

This tea is best enjoyed fresh but can be stored in a sealed container in the refrigerator for up to 24 hours. Reheat gently on the stove or enjoy cold for a refreshing alternative.

Tips for allergens

For those with sensitivities, ensure the mullein and nettle leaves are sourced from reputable suppliers to avoid cross-contamination with allergens. If honey is not suitable, consider maple syrup or agave nectar as sweetener alternatives.

Scientific references

- "The role of herbal medicines in the treatment of allergic asthma: A systematic review" published in the Respiratory Medicine journal, which discusses the antihistamine properties of nettle.
- "Mullein as a medicinal plant for the treatment of the respiratory tract diseases" found in the Journal of Phytotherapy Research, highlighting mullein's effectiveness in soothing the respiratory tract and easing coughing.

BOOK 16: IMMUNE-BOOSTING HERBS

CHAPTER 1: ANTIVIRAL AND ANTIBACTERIAL HERBS

Antiviral and antibacterial herbs play a crucial role in enhancing the immune system's ability to fight off infections. These herbs contain compounds that can inhibit the growth of viruses and bacteria, offering a natural approach to preventing and managing illnesses. To effectively utilize these herbs, it's essential to understand their specific properties, how to prepare them, and the recommended dosages for optimal health benefits.

Echinacea (Echinacea spp.) is renowned for its ability to boost the immune system and fend off colds and flu. The active compounds in Echinacea, such as alkamides, have been shown to enhance immune function. For preparation, Echinacea can be taken as a tea, tincture, or capsule. A typical dosage is 1-2 grams of dried root or herb, as tea, three times a day, or 2-4 milliliters of tincture three times a day at the first sign of symptoms.

Garlic (Allium sativum) possesses potent antibacterial and antiviral properties, making it effective against various pathogens. Allicin, a compound in garlic, is responsible for its therapeutic effects. To harness the benefits of garlic, it can be consumed raw, cooked, or as aged garlic supplements. For immune support, one to two cloves of raw garlic per day or 600-1200 mg of aged garlic extract might be recommended.

Ginger (Zingiber officinale) is another powerful herb with antiviral properties, particularly effective against respiratory infections. Gingerol, the active component, helps in reducing inflammation and can combat viruses. Ginger can be consumed fresh, in teas, or as a supplement. A simple ginger tea involves simmering about 2 inches of fresh ginger root in water for 10-15 minutes, which can be consumed 2-3 times daily for immune support.

Elderberry (Sambucus nigra) is widely used for its antiviral effects against flu viruses. It works by inhibiting the virus's entry and replication in human cells. Elderberry can be taken as syrup, lozenges, or capsules. For preventive measures, 1 tablespoon (15 ml) of elderberry syrup four times a day for adults and 1 teaspoon (5 ml) four times a day for children during flu season is often suggested.

Thyme (Thymus vulgaris) contains thymol, an essential oil with strong antibacterial and antiviral properties. Thyme is beneficial in treating respiratory infections and coughs. A thyme tea can be made by steeping 1-2 teaspoons of dried thyme in boiling water for 10 minutes. This tea can be consumed 1-3 times daily to help relieve symptoms and boost immunity.

Oregano (Origanum vulgare), known for its potent antiviral and antibacterial properties, is effective against a wide range of pathogens. The active compounds, carvacrol, and thymol, are responsible for its therapeutic effects. Oregano oil can be diluted with a carrier oil and applied topically, or it can be consumed orally in capsule form. For oral consumption, it's recommended to follow the manufacturer's dosage guidelines, as oregano oil is potent.

When incorporating these antiviral and antibacterial herbs into your regimen, it's crucial to source high-quality, organic herbs to ensure their efficacy and safety. Additionally, while these herbs can offer significant health benefits, they should not replace medical treatment for serious infections. Always consult with a healthcare provider before starting any new herbal supplement, especially if you have existing health conditions or are taking medications.

Echinacea for Fighting Infections

Echinacea, a group of herbaceous plants native to North America, has been a cornerstone in herbal medicine, particularly for its immune-boosting properties. The plant's ability to fight infections is primarily attributed to its complex mix of phytochemicals, including alkamides, glycoproteins, polysaccharides, and caffeic acid derivatives. These compounds collectively enhance the body's immune response, making Echinacea a powerful ally against colds, flu, and other respiratory infections.

To harness the benefits of Echinacea for fighting infections, it's essential to understand the optimal forms and dosages. Echinacea can be consumed in several forms, including teas, capsules, tinctures, and extracts. Each form has specific preparation methods and recommended dosages to ensure efficacy and safety.

Tea Preparation:

1. Use 1-2 grams of dried Echinacea root or herb per cup of boiling water.

2. Steep the Echinacea in boiling water for 15-20 minutes. This long steeping time allows the water to extract the active compounds effectively.

3. Strain the tea and consume immediately. Drinking 2-3 cups daily at the first sign of infection can support the immune system's fight against pathogens.

Tincture Preparation:

1. A standard Echinacea tincture has a concentration of 1:5 (herb to solvent ratio), with an alcohol volume of 45-70%.

2. To consume, dilute 2-4 milliliters of tincture in water three times a day. The alcohol acts as a solvent, extracting the active compounds from the plant material.

Capsule and Extract Dosage:

1. Follow the manufacturer's recommended dosage when taking Echinacea in capsule or extract form. Typically, this might be 300-500 mg of Echinacea extract three times a day.

2. Ensure the product specifies that it contains the active constituents of Echinacea, such as alkamides, to guarantee its effectiveness.

Quality and Selection:

- Opt for organic Echinacea products to avoid pesticides and herbicides that can negate the herb's health benefits.

- Ensure the Echinacea product is sourced from reputable suppliers and contains Echinacea purpurea, Echinacea angustifolia, or a blend of both, as these species have been most researched for their immune-supportive properties.

Timing and Duration:

- Begin taking Echinacea at the first sign of an infection for the best results. The early intervention helps the immune system mount an effective response.

- Limit the use of Echinacea to no more than 8 weeks at a time to prevent overstimulation of the immune system. A break allows the body to reset.

Safety Considerations:

- While Echinacea is generally safe for most people, individuals with autoimmune diseases or those taking immunosuppressive medication should consult with a healthcare provider before use.

- Pregnant or nursing women should seek medical advice due to the lack of extensive research in these groups. Incorporating Echinacea into your wellness routine during cold and flu season or at the first sign of an infection can bolster your immune defenses, potentially reducing the severity and duration of symptoms. Remember, the key to maximizing Echinacea's benefits lies in choosing high-quality products, adhering to recommended dosages, and timing its use for optimal immune support.

Echinacea Immune Tincture

Beneficial effects

Echinacea Immune Tincture leverages the natural antiviral and antibacterial properties of Echinacea, a well-regarded herb in the realm of immune support. Echinacea is known for its ability to enhance the body's immune response, making it more efficient in fighting off infections. Regular use of this tincture can help reduce the duration and severity of colds and flu, and it may also offer preventive benefits during peak cold and flu seasons.

Portions

Makes approximately 1 cup (240 ml)

Preparation time

10 minutes (plus 4-6 weeks for steeping)

Cooking time

N/A

Ingredients

- 1/2 cup dried Echinacea purpurea root, leaves, and flowers
- 2 cups 100-proof vodka or apple cider vinegar (for a non-alcoholic version)
- A clean glass jar with a tight-fitting lid
- Cheesecloth or a fine mesh strainer
- A clean bottle for storage

Instructions

1. Begin by thoroughly washing and drying your glass jar to ensure it's free from any contaminants.
2. Place the dried Echinacea parts into the jar, breaking them into smaller pieces if necessary to fit.

3. Pour the vodka or apple cider vinegar over the Echinacea, ensuring the herbs are completely submerged. If using vinegar, ensure it is raw and contains the "mother" for added health benefits.
4. Seal the jar tightly with the lid. Shake it gently to mix the contents.
5. Label the jar with the date and contents. Store it in a cool, dark place, such as a cupboard or pantry, away from direct sunlight.
6. Allow the mixture to steep for 4-6 weeks, shaking the jar gently every few days to redistribute the contents.
7. After steeping, strain the tincture through a cheesecloth or fine mesh strainer into a clean bottle. Squeeze or press the cheesecloth to extract as much liquid as possible.
8. Label the storage bottle with the date and contents. The tincture can be stored in a cool, dark place for up to 2 years.

Variations
- For added immune support, consider adding other herbs such as astragalus or elderberry to the tincture during the steeping process.
- To improve the taste, you can add a small amount of honey to the finished tincture (note: adding honey will reduce the shelf life).

Storage tips
Store the finished tincture in a cool, dark place, ideally in a cupboard away from direct sunlight. The alcohol or vinegar acts as a preservative, ensuring the tincture remains potent and effective for up to 2 years.

Tips for allergens
For those with sensitivities to alcohol, the apple cider vinegar version provides a suitable alternative. Ensure all herbs used are sourced from reputable suppliers to avoid contamination with allergens.

Scientific references
- "Echinacea for preventing and treating the common cold" published in the Cochrane Database of Systematic Reviews, which discusses the effectiveness of Echinacea in immune system support.

CHAPTER 2: HERBS FOR LONG-TERM IMMUNITY

For bolstering long-term immunity, incorporating adaptogenic herbs into your daily regimen can be transformative. Adaptogens are a unique class of healing plants that help balance, restore, and protect the body. Unlike other herbs that target specific areas of the body, adaptogens help enhance the body's overall resilience to stress, thereby strengthening the immune system over time. Here, we delve into the specifics of using adaptogens for long-term immune support, focusing on **Astragalus** and **Reishi** mushrooms, two powerhouse herbs renowned for their immune-boosting properties.

Astragalus (Astragalus membranaceus), a staple in traditional Chinese medicine, is celebrated for its profound immune-enhancing effects. It works by increasing the body's production of white blood cells, which are crucial for fighting off infections and diseases. To incorporate Astragalus into your daily routine, consider the following:

- **Preparation of Astragalus Tea**: Start with 1 to 2 teaspoons of dried Astragalus root. Add the root to 8 ounces of water in a pot. Bring the water to a boil, then simmer for 15 to 20 minutes. This slow cooking process allows the water to extract the root's beneficial compounds. Strain the tea and enjoy it warm. You can drink this tea 2 to 3 times daily. For a more potent infusion, you can increase the amount of Astragalus or let it simmer longer.

- **Astragalus Tincture**: If you prefer a more concentrated form, Astragalus tincture is available. The recommended dosage is 1 to 2 milliliters (about 30 to 60 drops), taken three times daily. Tinctures offer a convenient way to get your daily dose of Astragalus, especially for those with a busy lifestyle.

Reishi Mushroom (Ganoderma lucidum), often referred to as the "mushroom of immortality," supports immune health by modulating the immune system and reducing inflammation. Reishi can be consumed in several forms:

- **Reishi Tea**: To make Reishi tea, slice about 5 grams of dried Reishi mushroom and add it to 8 ounces of boiling water. Simmer the mixture for 2 hours on low heat, as Reishi is tough and requires a longer extraction time to release its beneficial compounds. Strain the liquid and drink it once it's cool enough. Due to its bitter taste, you might want to add honey or mix it with other herbal teas to improve the flavor.

- **Reishi Capsules**: For those who find the taste of Reishi unpalatable, capsules are a tasteless and convenient alternative. The general recommendation is to take 1 to 2 grams of Reishi in capsule form daily. However, it's important to start with the lower end of the dosage range and gradually increase it to see how your body responds.

When integrating Astragalus and Reishi into your regimen for long-term immunity, consistency is key. These herbs work best when taken regularly over extended periods. It's also crucial to source your herbs from reputable suppliers to ensure their quality and potency.

Remember, while adaptogens like Astragalus and Reishi are powerful tools for enhancing immune function, they should be part of a holistic approach to health that includes a balanced diet, regular exercise, adequate sleep, and stress management practices. Always consult with a healthcare provider before adding new supplements to your routine, especially if you have existing health conditions or are taking medications.

Astragalus for Resilience

Astragalus (Astragalus membranaceus) is a perennial plant native to the northern and eastern regions of China as well as Mongolia and Korea. It has been a foundational herb in Traditional Chinese Medicine (TCM) for centuries, primarily used to enhance the body's natural defense mechanisms and promote overall vitality. The root of the plant is where its potent immune-boosting properties are concentrated, making it an invaluable resource for building long-term resilience against illness.

Selecting and Preparing Astragalus Root: When choosing astragalus root, look for slices of the dried root that are pale yellow to white. The roots should be firm, indicating they have been properly dried and are of good quality. To prepare a simple astragalus tea, take 3 to 5 grams of the dried root and add it to about 500 ml (roughly 2 cups) of water. Bring the mixture to a boil, then reduce the heat and simmer for 30 to 60 minutes. The longer you simmer the root, the more potent the tea will be. After simmering, strain the liquid to remove the root pieces, and the tea is ready to drink.

Incorporating Astragalus into Your Diet: Beyond tea, astragalus can be incorporated into soups and broths. Adding 10 to 15 grams of astragalus root to your favorite soup recipe not only imbues it with a sweet, slightly earthy flavor but also turns your meal into an immune-boosting powerhouse. Simmer the root with the rest of your ingredients, removing it before serving. This method allows the astragalus to slowly release its beneficial compounds into the broth, making it an easy and effective way to consume the herb regularly.

Astragalus Tincture: For those who prefer a more concentrated form or are looking for convenience, astragalus tincture is an excellent option. You can either purchase a pre-made tincture or make your own by soaking the dried root in alcohol. To use a tincture, the typical dosage is 1 to 2 milliliters (about 20 to 40 drops), taken three times daily. Tinctures are particularly useful for consistent, long-term use as they have a long shelf life and can be easily carried and consumed throughout the day.

Dosage and Safety: While astragalus is considered safe for most people, it's important to start with a lower dose to see how your body reacts, especially if you are new to using herbal supplements. Pregnant or nursing women and individuals on immunosuppressive drugs should consult a healthcare professional before adding astragalus to their regimen due to its potent effects on the immune system.

Quality Matters: As with all herbal remedies, the efficacy of astragalus is directly related to the quality of the herb. Ensure you are purchasing astragalus from reputable sources that provide organic, sustainably harvested roots. High-quality astragalus should have a sweet, slightly grassy smell and a beige to yellow color, indicating proper drying and preservation of the root's beneficial compounds.

By integrating astragalus into your daily wellness routine, you can support your body's immune system, enhance your energy levels, and build resilience against stress and disease. Whether through teas, soups, or tinctures, this powerful herb offers a natural and effective way to maintain health and vitality throughout the year.

Astragalus and Reishi Immune Tonic

Beneficial effects

Astragalus and Reishi Immune Tonic is a powerful blend designed to strengthen the immune system over time. Astragalus is known for its ability to increase the body's production of white blood cells, which are crucial for fighting off infections. Reishi mushroom, often referred to as the "mushroom of immortality," supports immune health and helps reduce stress, which can weaken the immune response. Together, these herbs work synergistically to build long-term immune resilience, making this tonic an excellent addition to a holistic health regimen.

Portions

Makes approximately 2 cups (480 ml)

Preparation time

24 hours for soaking, 2 hours for simmering

Cooking time

2 hours

Ingredients

- 1/4 cup dried astragalus root slices
- 1/4 cup dried reishi mushroom slices
- 4 cups of water
- 1/2 cup raw honey (optional, for taste)

Instructions

1. Begin by placing the dried astragalus root slices and dried reishi mushroom slices in a large glass bowl. Cover the herbs with 4 cups of cold water. Allow them to soak for 24 hours. This soaking process helps to soften the hard, woody textures of the roots and mushrooms, making it easier to extract their beneficial compounds during the simmering process.

2. After soaking, transfer the astragalus, reishi, and the water they were soaked in into a large pot. Slowly bring the mixture to a gentle boil over medium heat. Once boiling, reduce the heat to the lowest setting, allowing the mixture to simmer gently.

3. Cover the pot with a lid, leaving a small gap to prevent overflow. Simmer the mixture for approximately 2 hours. This slow cooking process helps to extract the maximum amount of beneficial compounds from the astragalus and reishi.

4. After 2 hours, remove the pot from the heat. Allow the tonic to cool slightly before handling.

5. Strain the tonic through a fine mesh sieve or cheesecloth into a large, clean glass jar or bottle, discarding the solid pieces of astragalus and reishi. If desired, stir in 1/2 cup of raw honey to the warm tonic until fully dissolved. The honey adds a natural sweetness and additional antibacterial properties to the tonic.

6. Once the tonic has cooled to room temperature, seal the jar or bottle with a tight-fitting lid.

Variations
- For added flavor and immune support, consider adding a cinnamon stick or a few slices of fresh ginger to the pot during the simmering process.
- Incorporate a splash of apple cider vinegar to the finished tonic for added digestive benefits.

Storage tips
Store the Astragalus and Reishi Immune Tonic in the refrigerator for up to 2 weeks. Always use a clean spoon or cup when serving to maintain freshness and prevent contamination.

Tips for allergens
Individuals with mushroom allergies should avoid this tonic due to the presence of reishi mushrooms. For those allergic to honey, the sweetener can be omitted or substituted with maple syrup for a vegan-friendly version.

Scientific references
- "Effects of Astragalus on Cardiac Function and Immune System" published in the American Journal of Chinese Medicine, which discusses the immune-boosting properties of astragalus.
- "Ganoderma lucidum (Reishi mushroom) for cancer treatment" in the Cochrane Database of Systematic Reviews, highlighting the immune-modulating effects of reishi mushrooms.

BOOK 17: HERBAL SKINCARE AND BEAUTY

CHAPTER 1: HERBS FOR SKIN HEALTH

Calendula, known scientifically as Calendula officinalis, stands out for its potent anti-inflammatory and antimicrobial properties, making it an excellent choice for treating various skin conditions. To harness these benefits, one can prepare a Calendula-infused oil. Begin by selecting high-quality, dried Calendula flowers, ensuring they are free from moisture to prevent mold growth in the oil. Place the dried flowers in a clean, dry jar, filling it halfway. Pour a carrier oil, such as jojoba or sweet almond oil, over the flowers until the jar is nearly full, ensuring the flowers are completely submerged to prevent air pockets, which could lead to spoilage. Seal the jar tightly and place it in a warm, sunny spot for 4 to 6 weeks, shaking it gently every few days to distribute the plant's properties evenly throughout the oil. After the infusion period, strain the oil through a fine mesh sieve or cheesecloth into a clean, dry bottle, pressing the flowers to extract as much oil as possible. Label the bottle with the date and contents. This Calendula-infused oil can be applied directly to the skin to soothe irritations, rashes, and other conditions, or used as a base for salves and creams.

Chamomile, with its species Matricaria chamomilla (German chamomile) and Chamaemelum nobile (Roman chamomile), is renowned for its calming and soothing effects on the skin, making it ideal for sensitive or irritated skin. To create a Chamomile facial steam, bring a pot of water to a gentle boil and add a handful of dried Chamomile flowers. Remove the pot from heat and allow it to cool slightly. Drape a towel over your head and lean over the pot at a comfortable distance, allowing the steam to envelop your face for 5-10 minutes. This method opens the pores and facilitates the delivery of Chamomile's soothing properties directly to the skin, making it a simple yet effective treatment for calming inflammation and reducing redness.

Aloe Vera, or Aloe barbadensis miller, is widely recognized for its healing and moisturizing properties, particularly after sun exposure. For a simple Aloe Vera gel, carefully slice open a fresh Aloe Vera leaf to expose the inner gel. Using a spoon, scrape the gel into a blender, being careful to avoid the yellow latex which can cause irritation for some people. Blend the gel until smooth, then transfer it to a clean container. For an extra soothing effect, you can mix the Aloe gel with a few drops of Lavender essential oil before applying it to the skin. This mixture can be stored in the refrigerator for a cooling effect upon application, providing immediate relief for sunburned or irritated skin.

Witch Hazel, Hamamelis virginiana, is valued for its astringent and anti-inflammatory properties, making it an excellent ingredient for facial toners or acne treatments. To create a Witch Hazel toner, combine equal parts of Witch Hazel extract and distilled water in a clean bottle. If desired, add a few drops of Tea Tree essential oil for its antimicrobial benefits, which can be particularly helpful for acne-prone skin. Shake the bottle to mix the ingredients thoroughly. Apply the toner to the face with a cotton ball after cleansing, avoiding the eye area. This toner can be used daily to help reduce inflammation, tighten pores, and balance the skin's natural oils.

These detailed preparations and applications of herbs for skin health offer natural, effective ways to address various skin concerns, from inflammation and irritation to hydration and toning. By incorporating these herbal remedies into your skincare routine, you can leverage the healing power of nature to maintain healthy, radiant skin.

Calendula and Chamomile for Skin

Calendula officinalis, commonly known as Calendula, and Matricaria chamomilla, known as Chamomile, are two herbs celebrated for their soothing and healing properties, particularly when it comes to skin irritations. These plants have been used for centuries in traditional medicine to treat a variety of skin issues, from minor cuts and scrapes to burns, rashes, and eczema. Their effectiveness lies in their anti-inflammatory, antimicrobial, and skin-regenerative properties, making them invaluable ingredients in natural skincare.

To harness the benefits of Calendula for skin irritations, one can prepare a Calendula-infused oil. This process begins by sourcing high-quality, dried Calendula flowers. It's crucial to ensure the flowers are completely dry to prevent the growth of mold once they are submerged in oil. Fill a clean, dry jar halfway with the dried flowers, then pour a carrier oil—such as jojoba, sweet almond, or even olive oil—over the flowers until the jar is nearly full. The choice of carrier oil depends on personal preference or specific skin needs, as each oil brings its own benefits to the infusion. Jojoba oil is very similar to the skin's natural sebum, making it an excellent choice for most skin types, while sweet almond oil is particularly nourishing for dry skin. Seal the jar tightly and place it in a warm, sunny spot, such as a windowsill, for 4 to 6 weeks. This spot should receive direct sunlight for the majority of the day to facilitate the infusion process. Every few days, gently shake the jar to ensure the oil extracts the healing properties of the Calendula evenly. After the infusion period, strain the oil through a fine mesh sieve or cheesecloth into a clean, dry bottle, making sure to press the flowers to extract as much oil as possible. This Calendula-infused oil can be applied directly to the skin to soothe irritations, or it can be used as a base for creating salves, creams, or lotions.

Chamomile, on the other hand, is best utilized for its calming effects on the skin in the form of a gentle steam or a soothing tea that can be applied topically. For a Chamomile steam, bring a pot of water to a boil and add a generous amount of dried Chamomile flowers. Remove the pot from the heat and allow it to cool for a moment before leaning over it with a towel draped over your head to capture the steam. Ensure the steam is not too hot as to avoid scalding the skin; it should be a comfortable warmth that feels soothing. Stay under the towel for about 5 to 10 minutes, allowing the Chamomile steam to penetrate and soothe the skin. This method is particularly beneficial for calming inflammation, reducing redness, and hydrating the skin. For a topical application, brew a strong Chamomile tea, let it cool, then apply it to the skin using a clean cloth or cotton pad. This can be especially soothing for irritated skin or sunburns, providing a cooling and calming effect.

Both Calendula and Chamomile can be grown in a home garden, requiring moderate sunlight and well-drained soil, making them accessible for those interested in creating their own herbal remedies. When growing these herbs, choose an area that receives at least six hours of direct sunlight daily and has soil that retains moisture without becoming waterlogged. Regular harvesting of the flowers encourages continued blooming throughout the growing season, ensuring a steady supply of fresh materials for your herbal preparations.

Incorporating Calendula and Chamomile into your skincare routine offers a natural, effective way to soothe and heal skin irritations. Whether used separately or combined, these herbs provide a gentle yet powerful solution for maintaining healthy, resilient skin.

Calendula and Chamomile Healing Cream

Beneficial effects

Calendula and Chamomile Healing Cream combines the soothing properties of chamomile with the healing capabilities of calendula, making it an excellent remedy for skin irritations, minor cuts, and burns. Chamomile is known for its calming effect on the skin, reducing redness and inflammation, while calendula promotes wound healing and improves skin hydration. This cream harnesses the natural power of these herbs to support skin regeneration and provide a protective barrier against environmental stressors.

Portions

Makes approximately 1 cup (240 ml)

Preparation time

15 minutes

Cooking time

30 minutes

Ingredients

- 1/4 cup dried calendula petals
- 1/4 cup dried chamomile flowers
- 1/2 cup coconut oil
- 1/4 cup shea butter
- 2 tablespoons beeswax pellets
- 1 teaspoon vitamin E oil
- 10 drops lavender essential oil (optional for added soothing properties)

Instructions

1. Begin by combining the dried calendula petals and chamomile flowers in a double boiler over low heat. If you don't have a double boiler, place a heat-safe bowl over a pot of simmering water.

2. Add the coconut oil and shea butter to the herbs, stirring gently until the mixture is fully melted and combined. The gentle heat will help infuse the oil with the healing properties of the herbs.

3. Once the oils are melted and well mixed with the herbs, sprinkle the beeswax pellets into the mixture. Continue to stir until the beeswax is completely melted, creating a smooth consistency.

4. Remove the mixture from the heat and allow it to cool slightly for about 5 minutes. Avoid letting it solidify.

5. As the mixture begins to cool but remains liquid, stir in the vitamin E oil and lavender essential oil. Vitamin E acts as a natural antioxidant, preserving the cream and supporting skin healing, while lavender adds a calming scent and additional anti-inflammatory benefits.

6. Carefully pour the mixture through a fine mesh strainer or cheesecloth into a clean, dry container to remove the solid herb particles. Press or squeeze the herbs to extract as much oil as possible.

7. Allow the cream to cool completely. As it cools, it will thicken and set into a creamy consistency.

8. Once cooled and set, seal the container with a lid. Label the container with the date and contents.

Variations
- For extra moisturizing properties, add a tablespoon of almond oil or jojoba oil to the mixture before adding the beeswax.
- If you prefer a vegan version, substitute the beeswax with an equal amount of candelilla wax or soy wax.
- For sensitive skin, omit the lavender essential oil or substitute it with chamomile essential oil for its hypoallergenic properties.

Storage tips
Store the healing cream in a cool, dark place. The cream should remain effective for up to 6 months if stored properly. If the cream changes color, smell, or texture, it should be discarded.

Tips for allergens
For those with allergies to beeswax, using a plant-based wax as suggested in the variations can provide a suitable alternative. Always patch test a small amount of the cream on your skin before full application to ensure there is no allergic reaction, especially if you have sensitive skin or are prone to allergies.

Scientific references
- "Anti-inflammatory and skin barrier repair effects of topical application of some plant oils" published in the International Journal of Molecular Sciences, which discusses the benefits of plant oils, including coconut oil, for skin health.
- "Wound healing and anti-inflammatory effect in animal models of Calendula officinalis L. growing in Brazil" found in the Evidence-Based Complementary and Alternative Medicine journal, highlighting the wound-healing properties of calendula.
- "Chamomile: A herbal medicine of the past with a bright future" published in Molecular Medicine Reports, which reviews the soothing and anti-inflammatory effects of chamomile on the skin.

CHAPTER 2: HERBAL ANTI-AGING SOLUTIONS

Rosehip, scientifically known as Rosa canina, is celebrated for its high vitamin C content, making it a powerful ally in promoting collagen production for skin elasticity and strength. To create a Rosehip facial serum, begin by sourcing high-quality, dried Rosehip berries. These should be finely ground using a coffee grinder or mortar and pestle to increase the surface area for oil infusion, enhancing the extraction of nutrients. Choose a carrier oil that is beneficial for aging skin, such as argan oil, known for its hydrating properties and ability to improve skin elasticity, or jojoba oil, which closely mimics the skin's natural sebum and is excellent for all skin types. Combine one part ground Rosehip berries with ten parts carrier oil in a clean, dry jar. Seal the jar tightly and place it in a dark, cool place for 4 to 6 weeks, shaking it gently every few days to mix the contents. After the infusion period, strain the oil through a fine mesh sieve or cheesecloth into a clean, dry bottle, pressing the berries to extract as much oil as possible. For enhanced anti-aging benefits, add a few drops of vitamin E oil and frankincense essential oil to the strained Rosehip oil. Vitamin E acts as a natural preservative and antioxidant, while frankincense is known for its ability to reduce the appearance of wrinkles and fine lines. Label the bottle with the date and contents. Apply a few drops of this serum to the face and neck each night after cleansing, gently massaging it into the skin in upward motions.

Ginseng, particularly Panax ginseng, is revered for its potent antioxidant properties that can combat free radical damage, a key factor in skin aging. To incorporate Ginseng into an anti-aging skincare routine, prepare a Ginseng-infused water to use as a facial toner or mist. Start by simmering one tablespoon of dried Ginseng root in two cups of water for 15 minutes, allowing the water to draw out the Ginseng's beneficial compounds. Strain the mixture and let it cool. Transfer the Ginseng water into a clean spray bottle, adding a few drops of lavender essential oil for its soothing aroma and skin-calming benefits. Store the toner in the refrigerator to maintain freshness and provide a cooling sensation upon application. Use this Ginseng toner in the morning and evening after cleansing by spraying it directly onto the face or applying it with a cotton pad, avoiding the eye area. This toner can help tighten and revitalize the skin, leaving it feeling refreshed and rejuvenated.

For targeting fine lines and promoting skin hydration, Hyaluronic Acid (HA) is a non-herbal but essential ingredient that can be combined with herbal preparations to enhance skin moisture retention. While HA is not directly derived from herbs, its inclusion in a DIY herbal skincare regimen can significantly amplify the anti-aging effects of herbal treatments. To create a hydrating herbal face mask, mix one teaspoon of green tea powder, known for its antioxidant properties, with enough aloe vera gel to form a paste. Aloe vera, or Aloe barbadensis miller, provides a soothing and moisturizing base for the mask. Add a quarter teaspoon of Hyaluronic Acid serum to the mixture for its moisture-binding properties, ensuring deep hydration. Apply the mask to clean, dry skin and leave it on for 15-20 minutes before rinsing off with warm water. This mask can be used once or twice a week to help maintain a plump, youthful complexion.

Incorporating these detailed herbal preparations into your skincare routine can offer a natural, effective approach to combating the signs of aging. By harnessing the power of Rosehip, Ginseng, and complementary ingredients like Hyaluronic Acid, you can create potent anti-aging treatments that nourish and rejuvenate the skin.

Rosehip and Ginseng for Skin Vitality

Rosehip, known scientifically as **Rosa canina**, is a powerhouse of nutrients beneficial for skin vitality, including **vitamin C**, **vitamin A** (in the form of beta-carotene), and essential fatty acids. These components collectively work to promote **collagen production**, **skin regeneration**, and **moisture retention**, making Rosehip an excellent ingredient for anti-aging skincare products. To harness these benefits, one can prepare a Rosehip oil serum. Start by sourcing high-quality, **organic dried Rosehip berries**. Using a coffee grinder, grind the berries into a fine powder to increase the surface area for better infusion into the carrier oil. For the carrier oil, select **argan oil** for its hydrating properties or **jojoba oil** for its compatibility with most skin types. Combine one tablespoon of the ground Rosehip powder with approximately eight ounces of the carrier oil in a clean, dry glass jar. Seal the jar tightly and store it in a cool, dark place, shaking it daily for 4 to 6 weeks. After the infusion period, strain the oil using a fine mesh sieve or cheesecloth into another clean, dry bottle. For enhanced skin benefits, consider adding a few drops of **vitamin E oil** to the strained Rosehip oil to act as a natural preservative and antioxidant.

Ginseng, particularly **Panax ginseng**, is revered for its potent antioxidant properties, which help combat free radical damage, a significant factor in the skin aging process. Ginseng's bioactive compounds, including **ginsenosides**, have been shown to boost skin hydration, diminish rough texture, and help reduce the appearance of fine lines and wrinkles. To incorporate Ginseng into your skincare routine, prepare a Ginseng root decoction. Begin by thinly slicing approximately one inch of fresh Ginseng root. Add the slices to two cups of water in a small saucepan and bring to a simmer. Allow the mixture to gently simmer for about 20 minutes, reducing the liquid by half to concentrate the extract. Strain the decoction and let it cool. The resulting Ginseng water can be used as a facial toner or added to homemade face masks. For a simple Ginseng toner, transfer the cooled decoction into a clean spray bottle. You can enhance its skin-soothing properties by adding a few drops of **lavender essential oil**. Store the toner in the refrigerator and use it within one week for maximum freshness. Spritz the Ginseng toner on your face after cleansing, morning and evening, to rejuvenate and revitalize the skin.

Combining Rosehip and Ginseng in your skincare regimen offers a synergistic approach to enhancing skin vitality and combating the signs of aging. Both ingredients are rich in antioxidants and nutrients that support skin health, repair, and rejuvenation. For those looking to create a comprehensive anti-aging skincare routine, incorporating these potent botanicals can provide a natural, effective way to maintain youthful, radiant skin. Remember, consistency is key when using natural remedies. Regular use of Rosehip and Ginseng, along with a balanced diet and adequate hydration, can significantly improve skin texture, tone, and overall appearance.

Rosehip Facial Serum for Radiant Skin

Creating a Rosehip facial serum for radiant skin involves a meticulous process that harnesses the natural potency of Rosehip berries, renowned for their high levels of vitamin C, essential fatty acids, and antioxidants. These components are crucial for promoting collagen production, enhancing skin elasticity, and combating signs of aging such as fine lines and wrinkles. To begin, source high-quality, organic dried Rosehip berries. The integrity of your ingredients directly influences the efficacy of your serum, so choosing organic ensures that the berries are free from pesticides and other harmful chemicals.

First, grind the dried Rosehip berries into a fine powder using a coffee grinder or mortar and pestle. This increases the surface area of the berries, allowing for a more efficient infusion into your carrier oil and ensuring maximum extraction of the berries' beneficial properties. For the carrier oil, argan oil is an excellent choice due to its hydrating properties and ability to improve skin elasticity. Alternatively, jojoba oil can be used for its similarity to the skin's natural sebum, making it suitable for all skin types.

Measure one tablespoon of the finely ground Rosehip powder and mix it with approximately eight ounces of your chosen carrier oil in a clean, dry glass jar. The ratio of Rosehip powder to carrier oil is crucial for achieving the right concentration of nutrients in your serum. Seal the jar tightly to prevent any moisture from entering, which could spoil the mixture.

Store the jar in a cool, dark place, such as a cupboard or a drawer, where it is protected from direct sunlight and temperature fluctuations. This environment helps to preserve the active compounds in the Rosehip powder during the infusion process. Shake the jar gently once a day to ensure the Rosehip powder is evenly distributed throughout the carrier oil, facilitating a consistent infusion.

After four to six weeks, the infusion process will be complete. Strain the oil through a fine mesh sieve or cheesecloth into another clean, dry bottle to remove the Rosehip powder particles. Pressing the remnants in the sieve or cheesecloth will help extract as much oil as possible, ensuring you don't waste any of the nutrient-rich serum.

To further enhance the anti-aging benefits of your Rosehip facial serum, add a few drops of vitamin E oil and frankincense essential oil to the strained mixture. Vitamin E oil serves as a natural preservative and antioxidant, extending the shelf life of your serum and providing additional protection against free radical damage. Frankincense essential oil is celebrated for its ability to reduce the appearance of wrinkles and fine lines, promoting a more youthful and radiant complexion.

Label your bottle with the date of production and the ingredients used. This not only helps you keep track of the serum's freshness but also ensures you remember the specific formulation you created. Apply a few drops of the serum to your face and neck each night after cleansing, gently massaging it into the skin in upward motions. The serum's rich composition nourishes the skin deeply, supporting cell regeneration overnight and leaving you with a glowing, revitalized complexion by morning.

Remember, the effectiveness of your Rosehip facial serum relies on the quality of the ingredients and the precision of the process. By following these detailed steps, you can create a potent, natural anti-aging serum that harnesses the transformative power of Rosehip for radiant, youthful skin.

BOOK 18: ADVANCED HERBAL FERMENTATION

CHAPTER 1: HERBAL KOMBUCHA AND PROBIOTICS

Kombucha, a fermented tea beverage, has gained popularity for its probiotic content and potential health benefits. The process of making kombucha involves fermenting sweetened tea with a symbiotic culture of bacteria and yeast (SCOBY). This fermentation process produces a drink rich in various acids, enzymes, and, most importantly, probiotics, which are beneficial for gut health. To infuse kombucha with the added benefits of medicinal herbs, one can incorporate herbal teas or tinctures during the brewing process. This section will guide you through the steps to create your own herbal kombucha, focusing on selecting appropriate herbs, preparing the infusion, and ensuring safety during fermentation.

Selecting Herbs for Kombucha:
Choose herbs known for their health benefits and compatibility with kombucha's fermentation process. Popular choices include ginger for its digestive benefits, chamomile for its calming properties, and hibiscus for its high vitamin C content and refreshing flavor. When selecting herbs, consider their flavor profile and how they will complement the natural tartness of kombucha. It's essential to use organic herbs to avoid introducing pesticides into your brew.

Preparing the Herbal Infusion:
1. Start by brewing a strong herbal tea. Use about 2 tablespoons of dried herbs per quart of water. If using fresh herbs, increase the amount to 4 tablespoons, as fresh herbs are less concentrated than dried ones.
2. Boil water and pour it over the herbs in a heat-proof container. Allow the herbs to steep for 15 to 20 minutes. The goal is to create a potent infusion that will not be diluted too much once added to the kombucha.
3. Strain the herbs from the infusion, ensuring no plant material remains, as it could interfere with the fermentation process.

Integrating the Herbal Infusion into the Kombucha Brew:
After preparing your sweetened tea base and allowing it to cool to room temperature, mix in the herbal infusion. Add the SCOBY and cover the container with a breathable cloth, securing it with a rubber band. This setup allows air to flow while keeping contaminants out.

Fermentation Time and Conditions:
Place your kombucha in a warm, dark place, away from direct sunlight, at a temperature between 68-78°F. The fermentation time can vary depending on the desired level of sweetness and acidity, usually ranging from 7 to 14 days. Taste your kombucha periodically to determine when it has reached the perfect balance for your palate.

Bottling and Second Fermentation:
Once the initial fermentation is complete, you can bottle your kombucha for a second fermentation. This step is optional but can enhance the kombucha's effervescence and flavor. Add a few pieces of fresh herbs or a splash of the herbal infusion to each bottle before sealing. Allow the bottles to ferment at room temperature for 2 to 3 days, then refrigerate to stop the fermentation process.

Safety Tips:
- Always use clean, sterilized equipment to prevent contamination.
- Inspect your SCOBY regularly for signs of mold or unusual odors. A healthy SCOBY is essential for a successful fermentation.
- If you're new to brewing kombucha, start with small batches to experiment with flavors and fermentation times.
By incorporating medicinal herbs into your kombucha, you can enjoy the combined benefits of probiotics and herbal remedies. This process allows for creativity and personalization in crafting a beverage that supports your health and wellness goals. Whether you're seeking digestive support, stress relief, or a refreshing, healthful drink, herbal kombucha offers a versatile and enjoyable solution.

Infusing Kombucha with Herbs

Infusing kombucha with medicinal herbs transforms this already healthful beverage into a potent tonic, tailored to address specific wellness goals. The process begins with selecting high-quality, organic herbs known for their therapeutic properties. For instance, incorporating ginger can enhance the digestive benefits of kombucha, while lavender can add a calming effect. It's crucial to source these herbs from reputable suppliers to ensure they are free from contaminants and have been handled properly for medicinal use.

Once you have selected your herbs, the next step is to prepare them for infusion. This typically involves drying and grinding the herbs to increase the surface area that will be in contact with the kombucha, thereby maximizing the transfer of beneficial compounds. For herbs that are already dried, a coarse grind using a mortar and pestle or a coffee grinder set to a coarse setting is sufficient. Fresh herbs, on the other hand, should be washed, patted dry, and chopped finely before drying in a dehydrator or a low oven to preserve their medicinal qualities.

The timing of adding these herbs to your kombucha is critical for achieving the desired flavor and therapeutic effect. Adding the herbs during the first fermentation process, where the kombucha culture (SCOBY) is active, can alter the fermentation dynamics. The SCOBY may consume some of the herbal compounds, which can change the taste and potency of the final product. Therefore, it's generally recommended to infuse herbs during the second fermentation process, after the SCOBY has been removed. This stage allows the kombucha to absorb the herbal essences without the interference of the SCOBY, enhancing both the flavor and the medicinal properties of the brew.

To infuse the herbs, place the prepared herbal material into a clean, airtight fermentation bottle. Pour the finished kombucha over the herbs, ensuring there is enough space left at the top of the bottle to avoid overflow during carbonation. Seal the bottle tightly and store it in a dark, room-temperature spot for a period ranging from a few days to a week, depending on the desired strength of the infusion. It's important to burp the bottles daily to release excess pressure and prevent the risk of explosion.

After the infusion period, strain the kombucha to remove all herbal residues. This can be done using a fine mesh strainer or cheesecloth. The strained kombucha should then be transferred to clean bottles for storage or immediate consumption. The final product will be a uniquely flavored, herbal-infused kombucha that not only tastes great but also carries the enhanced health benefits of the chosen herbs.

For those looking to experiment with flavors and health benefits, consider starting with simple, well-known herbs like mint for its refreshing qualities or chamomile for its soothing effects on the digestive system and nerves. As you become more familiar with the process and the effects of different herbs, you can begin to create more complex blends tailored to specific health needs or flavor profiles.

Remember, the key to successful herbal infusion in kombucha is patience and attention to detail. From selecting and preparing the herbs to timing the infusion and carefully monitoring the fermentation process, each step contributes to creating a healthful and enjoyable beverage. As with any herbal remedy, it's advisable to consult with a healthcare professional before consuming, especially for those with underlying health conditions or those who are pregnant or breastfeeding, to ensure safety and efficacy.

Ginger and Hibiscus Kombucha

Beneficial effects

Ginger and Hibiscus Kombucha combines the digestive benefits of ginger with the antioxidant properties of hibiscus, creating a refreshing and health-boosting fermented drink. Ginger is known for its ability to soothe the stomach and reduce nausea, while hibiscus has been shown to lower blood pressure and support liver health. Together, they create a kombucha that not only tastes great but also supports overall wellness.

Portions

Makes approximately 1 gallon

Preparation time

30 minutes (plus 7-14 days for fermentation)

Cooking time

N/A

Ingredients

- 1 gallon filtered water
- 1 cup organic sugar
- 8 bags black tea (or 2 tablespoons loose leaf)
- 1 cup starter tea from a previous batch of kombucha
- 1 SCOBY (Symbiotic Culture Of Bacteria and Yeast)
- 1 cup fresh ginger, peeled and thinly sliced
- 1 cup dried hibiscus flowers

Instructions

1. Begin by bringing the gallon of filtered water to a boil in a large pot. Once boiling, remove the pot from the heat.

2. Add the organic sugar to the hot water, stirring until completely dissolved. This creates the sweet tea base that the kombucha will ferment.

3. Add the black tea bags or loose leaf tea to the sugar water. Allow the tea to steep until the water has completely cooled to room temperature. This can take several hours. It's crucial that the water is at room temperature to avoid harming the SCOBY.

4. Once the tea is cooled, remove the tea bags or strain out the loose leaf tea. Pour the sweet tea into a clean, gallon-sized glass jar.

5. Add the cup of starter tea to the jar. The starter tea helps to acidify the batch, creating an environment where the SCOBY can thrive.

6. Gently place the SCOBY into the jar. The SCOBY may float, sink, or sit sideways, which is perfectly normal.

7. Cover the mouth of the jar with a few layers of tightly woven cloth, coffee filter, or paper towel. Secure it with a rubber band. This covering allows air to flow into the jar while keeping out contaminants.

8. Store the jar in a warm, dark place (around 70-75°F) where it won't be disturbed. Allow the tea to ferment for 7 to 14 days, checking the taste periodically after the first week. The longer it ferments, the less sweet and more vinegary it will taste.

9. Once the kombucha has reached your desired level of tartness, remove the SCOBY and 1 cup of kombucha to use as starter tea for your next batch.

10. Add the fresh ginger slices and dried hibiscus flowers to the kombucha and cover again with the cloth. Allow it to ferment for an additional 2-3 days for the flavors to infuse.

11. After the flavor infusion period, strain out the ginger slices and hibiscus flowers. Bottle the kombucha in clean, airtight bottles, leaving about an inch of headspace to avoid excessive carbonation buildup.

12. Store the bottled kombucha in the refrigerator to slow down the fermentation process. Chill before serving.

Variations
- For a spicier kick, increase the amount of ginger or allow it to infuse for a longer period.
- Add a few sprigs of fresh mint or a teaspoon of vanilla extract during the second fermentation for a different flavor profile.

Storage tips
Keep the bottled kombucha refrigerated and consume within a month for the best taste and carbonation. Always burp the bottles every few days to release excess pressure and avoid over-carbonation.

Tips for allergens
For those sensitive to caffeine, decaffeinated black tea can be used as an alternative, though it may affect the SCOBY's health over time. Always ensure the SCOBY and starter tea come from a reputable source to avoid contamination.

Scientific references
- "Ginger in gastrointestinal disorders: A systematic review of clinical trials" published in Food Science & Nutrition, highlighting ginger's digestive benefits.
- "Hibiscus sabdariffa L. in the treatment of hypertension and hyperlipidemia: A comprehensive review of animal and human studies" found in Fitoterapia, discussing the health benefits of hibiscus.

CHAPTER 2: HERBAL VINEGARS AND OXYMELS

Herbal vinegars and oxymels offer a delightful and effective way to incorporate the healing properties of herbs into your daily routine. These preparations harness the acidic environment of vinegar to extract vital minerals and phytonutrients from herbs, making them more bioavailable to the body. Oxymels, a traditional blend of vinegar and honey, combine the potent extraction capabilities of vinegar with the soothing, antimicrobial properties of honey, creating a balanced remedy that is both potent and palatable.

Choosing Your Vinegar: For herbal vinegars, apple cider vinegar is often preferred due to its own health benefits, including supporting digestion and balancing pH levels. Ensure the vinegar is raw and contains the "mother" to maximize health benefits. White wine or red wine vinegars are also suitable and can be chosen based on personal taste preferences or the characteristics of the herbs being used.

Selecting Herbs: Almost any herb can be used to make an herbal vinegar or oxymel, but some popular choices include rosemary for its circulatory benefits, dandelion leaves for detoxification, and thyme for respiratory health. Fresh herbs are ideal for their vitality and potency, but dried herbs can also be used effectively. When using dried herbs, ensure they are of high quality and have been stored properly to preserve their medicinal properties.

Preparation of Herbal Vinegars: Begin by filling a clean, dry jar about halfway with your chosen herbs. If using fresh herbs, slightly bruise or chop them to expose more surface area. Cover the herbs with vinegar, ensuring they are completely submerged to prevent mold growth. Seal the jar with a plastic lid or place parchment paper under a metal lid to prevent corrosion from the vinegar. Label the jar with the date and contents. Store the jar in a cool, dark place for 3 to 6 weeks, shaking it every few days to encourage extraction. After the infusion period, strain the vinegar through a fine mesh sieve or cheesecloth into a clean bottle. Compost the herbs and label the vinegar with its intended use and date.

Creating an Oxymel: To make an oxymel, follow the same process as for an herbal vinegar, but add honey to the mixture. A common ratio is 3 parts vinegar to 1 part honey, but this can be adjusted based on personal taste preferences and the desired sweetness. After combining the vinegar, honey, and herbs in a jar, shake well to dissolve the honey. Allow the mixture to infuse for 2 to 4 weeks, shaking regularly. Strain the oxymel into a clean bottle, label, and store.

Usage: Herbal vinegars can be used in salad dressings, marinades, or taken by the spoonful as a dietary supplement. Oxymels can be enjoyed as is, diluted in water, or added to tea. They are particularly soothing during cold and flu season for their expectorant properties and ability to soothe sore throats.

Considerations: Always use clean, sterilized equipment to prevent contamination. Be mindful of the shelf life of your preparations; while vinegar acts as a preservative, the addition of fresh plant material can introduce water, potentially shortening the shelf life. Store your finished vinegars and oxymels in a cool, dark place, and monitor them for any signs of spoilage.

By incorporating herbal vinegars and oxymels into your wellness practices, you can enjoy the myriad health benefits of herbs in a delicious and convenient form. Whether you're looking to boost your immune system, support your digestive health, or simply add more flavor to your meals, these ancient remedies offer something for everyone.

Preserving Herbs with Apple Cider Vinegar

Preserving herbs with apple cider vinegar is a method that not only extends the shelf life of your herbs but also enhances their medicinal properties, making them more bioavailable to the body. Apple cider vinegar, known for its health benefits such as aiding digestion and balancing pH levels, serves as an excellent medium for herb preservation. The process involves a few straightforward steps, ensuring that the herbs' essence is captured in the vinegar, ready to be used for culinary or medicinal purposes.

Firstly, select high-quality, organic apple cider vinegar that contains the "mother," a cloudy sediment at the bottom of the bottle indicating the presence of beneficial enzymes and probiotics. This type of vinegar ensures that you're starting with a product that is as beneficial and nutrient-rich as possible.

When choosing herbs for preservation, consider both fresh and dried varieties. Fresh herbs should be harvested just before use, ensuring they are free from moisture to prevent mold growth in the vinegar. Popular choices for preservation include rosemary, known for its circulatory benefits; dandelion leaves, which support detoxification; and thyme, beneficial for respiratory health. If using dried herbs, verify their quality and freshness, as this significantly impacts the potency of your herbal vinegar.

To begin the preservation process, thoroughly wash and pat dry your fresh herbs to remove any dirt or contaminants. If you're using fresh herbs, slightly bruise or chop them to expose more surface area, which will facilitate the extraction of their medicinal properties into the vinegar. For dried herbs, ensure they are loosely broken up to allow the vinegar to penetrate the plant material.

Fill a clean, dry jar about halfway with your chosen herbs. Pour the apple cider vinegar over the herbs until they are completely submerged. This step is crucial as any herbs exposed to air could potentially mold, compromising the quality of your herbal vinegar. If using a metal lid, place a piece of parchment paper between the jar and the lid to prevent corrosion caused by the vinegar. Alternatively, use a plastic lid for a tighter seal and to avoid any reaction with the vinegar.

Label the jar with the date and contents, then store it in a cool, dark place. A pantry or cupboard away from direct sunlight is ideal. Shake the jar every few days to mix the herbs and vinegar, ensuring a thorough extraction. Allow the mixture to infuse for 3 to 6 weeks, depending on the desired strength. The longer it sits, the more potent the vinegar will become.

After the infusion period, strain the vinegar through a fine mesh sieve or cheesecloth into a clean bottle. Press or squeeze the herbs to extract as much liquid as possible. Compost the leftover herb material. Label the finished vinegar with its intended use and date, then store it in a cool, dark place. Herbal vinegars can be used in salad dressings, marinades, or taken by the spoonful as a dietary supplement, offering a convenient way to incorporate the healing properties of herbs into your daily routine.

This method of preserving herbs with apple cider vinegar not only extends the shelf life of your herbs but also creates a versatile, health-promoting product that can be easily incorporated into your wellness practices. Whether used for culinary purposes or as a medicinal tonic, herbal vinegars offer a delightful way to enjoy the benefits of herbs year-round.

Elderberry and Thyme Oxymel

Beneficial effects
Elderberry and Thyme Oxymel combines the immune-boosting properties of elderberries with the antiseptic and cough-suppressant qualities of thyme. Elderberries are rich in vitamins and antioxidants, known to enhance immune function and alleviate cold and flu symptoms. Thyme, with its compounds like thymol, acts as a natural cough remedy. This oxymel, a traditional blend of vinegar and honey, offers a palatable way to harness these benefits, supporting respiratory health and immune defense.

Portions
Makes approximately 2 cups

Preparation time
15 minutes (plus 4-6 weeks for infusion)

Cooking time
N/A

Ingredients
- 1 cup fresh elderberries (or 1/2 cup dried)
- 1/4 cup fresh thyme leaves
- 1 cup raw apple cider vinegar
- 1 cup raw honey

Instructions
1. If using fresh elderberries, carefully remove the berries from the stems. For dried elderberries, ensure they are free from any debris or dust.
2. Place the elderberries and thyme leaves into a clean, dry quart-sized glass jar.
3. Pour the apple cider vinegar over the elderberries and thyme, ensuring the ingredients are completely submerged. If necessary, use a spoon to press down the elderberries and thyme to release their flavors and make room for the vinegar.
4. Seal the jar with a plastic lid or place a piece of parchment paper under a metal lid to prevent corrosion from the vinegar. Shake the jar gently to mix the contents.
5. Label the jar with the date and contents. Store it in a cool, dark place, shaking it daily for the first week to help the infusion process.

6. After 4-6 weeks, strain the mixture through a fine mesh sieve or cheesecloth into a clean bowl, pressing or squeezing the solids to extract as much liquid as possible.

7. Measure the infused vinegar and pour it into a clean jar or bottle. For every cup of infused vinegar, add an equal amount of raw honey.

8. Stir or shake the mixture until the honey is completely dissolved into the vinegar.

9. Transfer the finished oxymel into a clean bottle or jar, sealing it with a lid.

Variations

- For a spicier kick, add a small piece of fresh ginger or a few peppercorns to the jar during the infusion process.

- Incorporate a cinnamon stick or a few cloves for additional warming and antimicrobial properties.

Storage tips

Store the elderberry and thyme oxymel in a cool, dark place for up to 6 months. Refrigeration is not necessary but can extend the shelf life.

Tips for allergens

For those with honey allergies, substitute the honey with an equal amount of vegetable glycerin or a simple syrup made from sugar and water for a vegan version. However, this may alter the traditional benefits associated with raw honey.

Scientific references

- "Antiviral effect of flavonoids on human viruses" published in the Journal of Medical Virology, which discusses the antiviral properties of compounds found in elderberries.

- "Thymol, thyme, and other plant sources: Health and potential uses" in the Phytotherapy Research journal, highlighting the health benefits of thymol found in thyme.

BOOK 19: HERBAL ADAPTOGENS FOR STRESS

CHAPTER 1: UNDERSTANDING ADAPTOGENS

Adaptogens are a unique class of herbal remedies known for their ability to help the body resist stressors of all kinds, whether physical, chemical, or biological. These herbs and roots have been used for centuries in Chinese and Ayurvedic healing traditions, but they are only now becoming a part of mainstream wellness practices in the West. Adaptogens work by normalizing and balancing the body, enhancing its ability to maintain homeostasis and fight off stress and fatigue. They are particularly beneficial because they adapt their function according to the specific needs of your body, which is why they are called adaptogens.

Ashwagandha (Withania somnifera), for instance, is renowned for its ability to reduce anxiety and stress, improve sleep, and enhance endurance. When incorporating Ashwagandha into your daily routine, it's advisable to start with a small dose, such as 300-500 mg of a root extract, to assess your body's response. It can be taken in capsule form or as a powder mixed into beverages or food. Consistency is key, as the benefits of Ashwagandha build over time, with optimal effects usually observed after 6 to 8 weeks of regular use.

Rhodiola Rosea is another powerful adaptogen known for its fatigue-fighting properties. It works by increasing the body's resistance to stress, thereby improving energy levels, mood, and cognitive function. For Rhodiola, a typical dose ranges from 100-600 mg per day of an extract standardized to contain 3% rosavins and 1% salidroside, the active compounds. It's most effective when taken on an empty stomach, ideally 30 minutes before breakfast and lunch.

Holy Basil (Ocimum sanctum), also known as Tulsi, is revered in Ayurveda for its ability to foster clear thoughts, relaxation, and a sense of well-being. To incorporate Holy Basil into your regimen, consider drinking 1-2 cups of Tulsi tea daily, especially during times of high stress. Alternatively, Holy Basil supplements can be taken, with a common dosage being 300-600 mg of an extract, once or twice daily.

Cordyceps, a type of medicinal mushroom, offers benefits like improved energy levels, enhanced endurance, and better stress response. For those interested in trying Cordyceps, it's available in powder form that can be added to coffee, tea, or smoothies. A typical dose ranges from 1-3 grams per day. Since Cordyceps can stimulate the immune system, it's best to consult with a healthcare provider before starting, especially for those with autoimmune conditions.

Ginseng (Panax ginseng), perhaps one of the most well-known adaptogens, has been shown to help fight fatigue, enhance mental performance, and support immune function. When using Ginseng, look for a product that contains at least 5% ginsenosides, and consider a dosage of 200-400 mg per day. It's often recommended to take Ginseng in cycles, such as 2-3 weeks on, followed by a break of 1-2 weeks.

Adaptogen blends are also available, combining multiple adaptogenic herbs into one formula. These blends are designed to provide a synergistic effect, enhancing the individual benefits of each herb. When choosing an adaptogen blend, ensure it comes from a reputable source and follows the recommended dosages for each included herb.

Incorporating adaptogens into your daily wellness routine requires patience and attentiveness to your body's signals. Start with lower doses to see how you respond, and adjust as needed. Always consult with a healthcare professional before adding new supplements to your regimen, especially if you have existing health conditions or are taking other medications. Remember, the key to benefiting from adaptogens lies in their consistent use over time, allowing your body to gradually adapt and harness their stress-resilient properties.

What Makes an Herb an Adaptogen?

Adaptogens are a specialized group of herbs that support the body's natural ability to deal with stress. They help stabilize and balance various physiological processes, enhancing the body's resilience to physical, emotional, and environmental stressors. The criteria that define an herb as an adaptogen are specific and scientifically grounded. These herbs must be non-toxic to the recipient in normal therapeutic doses, offer widespread support to the body, and help return the body to a state of equilibrium, known as homeostasis.

Non-toxicity: An essential characteristic of adaptogens is their safety. They must be safe for long-term use and cause minimal side effects. This criterion ensures that adaptogens can be taken regularly to support health without causing harm or significant adverse reactions. For example, **Ashwagandha (Withania somnifera)** is widely recognized for its safety profile when used within the recommended dosage range, making it a staple in stress management protocols.

Generalized Support: Adaptogens work on a wide range of physiological systems rather than targeting a specific organ or system. They exert a normalizing effect, improving the function of multiple body systems simultaneously. This broad action is crucial because stress affects the body in a generalized way, impacting everything from the immune system to energy metabolism. **Rhodiola Rosea**, for instance, influences the nervous, hormonal, and immune systems, enhancing overall resilience to stress.

Homeostasis: The ability to help the body maintain or return to homeostasis is perhaps the most defining feature of adaptogens. Homeostasis is the body's internal balance, a state where physiological processes operate optimally despite external changes or challenges. Adaptogens aid in modulating the body's stress response systems, such as the hypothalamic-pituitary-adrenal (HPA) axis and the sympathoadrenal system, helping to reduce overactivity or stimulate underactivity as needed. For example, **Holy Basil (Ocimum sanctum)** has been shown to modulate cortisol levels, a key hormone involved in the stress response, helping to maintain a more balanced state.

To incorporate adaptogens into a wellness routine, it's important to select high-quality, organically sourced herbs. Starting with lower doses and gradually increasing as needed allows individuals to gauge their response and adjust accordingly. Adaptogens can be consumed in various forms, including teas, tinctures, capsules, and powders. For instance, to use **Ashwagandha**, one might start with a capsule containing 300-500 mg of root extract, taken with meals to enhance absorption. Consistency is key, as the benefits of adaptogens accumulate over time, with noticeable effects often observed after several weeks of regular use.

When selecting an adaptogen, consider the specific stress-related challenges being faced. For energy and mental clarity, **Siberian Ginseng (Eleutherococcus senticosus)** might be beneficial, offering support for those experiencing fatigue and cognitive fog due to stress. Alternatively, for improved sleep and relaxation, **Ashwagandha** or **Holy Basil** could be more appropriate, targeting the underlying stress that disrupts restful sleep.

In summary, adaptogens are a unique class of herbs that support the body's ability to manage stress, characterized by their non-toxicity, generalized support across multiple body systems, and ability to help the body maintain equilibrium. By carefully selecting and incorporating these herbs into one's wellness routine, it's possible to enhance resilience to stress, improve overall well-being, and support optimal health.

Adaptogen Energy Powder Recipe

Creating an Adaptogen Energy Powder requires a thoughtful selection of adaptogenic herbs known for their stress-resilient properties and energy-boosting capabilities. This recipe is designed to be easily incorporated into your daily routine, offering a natural way to enhance vitality and manage stress. The following steps and ingredients ensure a potent blend, leveraging the synergistic effects of multiple adaptogens.

Ingredients:
- 1/4 cup Ashwagandha powder (Withania somnifera): Renowned for its stress-reducing and energy-enhancing properties.
- 1/4 cup Rhodiola Rosea powder: Known for fighting fatigue and enhancing mental performance.
- 1/4 cup Holy Basil (Tulsi) powder (Ocimum sanctum): Valued for its ability to uplift mood and support cognitive function.
- 1/4 cup Cordyceps powder: A medicinal mushroom that boosts energy levels and supports endurance.
- 1/4 cup Maca root powder: Aids in increasing stamina and energy.
- 2 tablespoons Ginseng powder (Panax ginseng): Promotes energy production and combats fatigue.
- Optional: 1 tablespoon Cacao powder for flavor and a boost of antioxidants.

Tools:
- Mixing bowl
- Whisk or spoon for stirring
- Airtight container for storage
- Measuring cups and spoons

Instructions:
1. Begin by ensuring all your adaptogenic herbs are in powdered form. This increases the surface area for absorption, making the blend more effective. If you have whole dried herbs, use a coffee grinder or mortar and pestle to grind them into a fine powder.
2. In a clean, dry mixing bowl, combine the Ashwagandha, Rhodiola Rosea, Holy Basil, Cordyceps, Maca root, and Ginseng powders. If you choose to include Cacao powder for its flavor and antioxidant properties, add it now.

3. Use a whisk or spoon to thoroughly mix the powders. Ensure the blend is uniform in color and texture, indicating that the ingredients are well distributed throughout the mixture. This step is crucial for achieving a consistent dosage of each adaptogen in every serving.

4. Once mixed, carefully transfer the adaptogen energy powder into an airtight container. Label the container with the contents and date of creation. Storing the powder in a cool, dry place away from direct sunlight will help preserve its potency and extend its shelf life.

5. To use, incorporate a teaspoon of the adaptogen energy powder into your daily routine. It can be added to smoothies, mixed into a glass of water, or blended into your morning oatmeal. Starting with a smaller dose allows you to gauge your body's response and adjust accordingly.

6. Consistency is key when using adaptogenic herbs. Incorporate the adaptogen energy powder into your daily regimen for at least 6 to 8 weeks to observe the full benefits. Adjust the dosage as needed, but do not exceed the recommended amount of each adaptogen to avoid potential adverse effects.

7. For individuals new to adaptogens, it's advisable to consult with a healthcare professional before starting, especially if you have underlying health conditions or are taking medications. This ensures the adaptogen blend complements your health regimen without interfering with other treatments.

This Adaptogen Energy Powder recipe harnesses the collective power of adaptogenic herbs to support your body's stress response system, enhance energy levels, and promote overall well-being. By incorporating this blend into your daily wellness routine, you can take a proactive step towards managing stress and boosting vitality naturally.

CHAPTER 2: DAILY ADAPTOGEN USE

Incorporating adaptogens into your daily routine can significantly enhance your body's resilience to stress and improve overall well-being. Adaptogens, a unique class of herbs, help balance, restore, and protect the body by increasing its resistance to stressors. To effectively use adaptogens daily, it's essential to understand their properties and how to integrate them into your lifestyle seamlessly.

Ashwagandha (Withania somnifera), known for its stress-reducing effects, can be taken in capsule form or as a powder. A recommended starting dose is 300-500 mg of a standardized extract or 1-2 teaspoons of the powdered root daily. It's best consumed with meals or a glass of water. Ashwagandha works well when taken consistently over time, with many users reporting a noticeable decrease in stress levels after several weeks of regular use.

Rhodiola (Rhodiola rosea) is another potent adaptogen, particularly effective for combating fatigue and enhancing mental performance. For Rhodiola, a typical dose ranges from 100-400 mg of a standardized extract, taken 30 minutes before breakfast and lunch to avoid potential insomnia. Due to its energizing effects, it's advisable not to take Rhodiola late in the day.

Incorporating these adaptogens into your daily regimen requires attention to timing, dosage, and consistency. For instance, starting with a lower dose and gradually increasing it allows your body to adapt without adverse effects. Additionally, since adaptogens work synergistically with the body, their benefits are more pronounced with long-term use. Therefore, patience and consistency are key.

To ensure optimal absorption and effectiveness, consider the form in which you take adaptogens. Capsules and powders are the most common, but tinctures are also an option for those who prefer a liquid form. When using powders, they can be easily incorporated into smoothies, teas, or even certain foods, making them a versatile choice for daily use.

Moreover, combining adaptogens with a healthy lifestyle amplifies their benefits. A balanced diet, regular exercise, and adequate sleep all support the body's ability to manage stress, creating a solid foundation for adaptogens to work more effectively.

Lastly, while adaptogens are generally safe for most people, it's crucial to consult with a healthcare provider before starting any new supplement regimen, especially for those with existing health conditions or those taking medications. This ensures that adaptogens will not interact negatively with your health status or any medications you may be taking.

By integrating adaptogens like Ashwagandha and Rhodiola into your daily routine, you can enhance your body's natural resilience to stress, improve mental clarity and energy levels, and support overall health and well-being. Remember, the key to success with adaptogens lies in consistent use, proper dosing, and patience as your body adjusts and responds to these powerful natural allies.

Ashwagandha and Rhodiola for Energy

Ashwagandha (Withania somnifera) and Rhodiola (Rhodiola rosea) stand out as two powerful adaptogens that play a pivotal role in energy balance and stress management. When used thoughtfully, these herbs can significantly enhance your body's resilience to stress and contribute to sustained energy levels throughout the day. To harness their full potential, it's crucial to understand their distinct properties and how to incorporate them into your daily regimen effectively.

Ashwagandha, often referred to as Indian ginseng, has a rich history in Ayurvedic medicine for its remarkable stress-reducing and rejuvenating properties. It functions by moderating the body's response to stress, regulating the production of cortisol, which is the body's primary stress hormone. For optimal results, consider taking 300-500 mg of a standardized extract of Ashwagandha root, preferably in capsule form, twice daily with meals. This dosage ensures adequate absorption and minimizes the risk of gastrointestinal discomfort, which can occur when taken on an empty stomach. If you prefer a more traditional approach, 1-2 teaspoons of Ashwagandha powder can be mixed into warm milk or water, incorporating a pinch of cinnamon or honey for flavor enhancement. This method not only facilitates ease of consumption but also promotes a calming nighttime routine, aiding in relaxation and sleep.

Rhodiola, native to the cold, mountainous regions of Europe and Asia, is celebrated for its ability to enhance mental performance, endurance, and resistance to high-altitude sickness. Unlike Ashwagandha, Rhodiola provides a stimulating effect, making it particularly beneficial for combating fatigue and enhancing concentration and stamina. To leverage Rhodiola's energizing properties, start with 100-400 mg of a standardized extract, taken approximately 30 minutes before breakfast and lunch. This timing is strategic, capitalizing on the body's natural cortisol rhythm, thereby supporting optimal alertness and energy levels during the day while avoiding interference with sleep patterns at night.

It's important to note that while both Ashwagandha and Rhodiola are generally well-tolerated, individual responses can vary. Starting with the lower end of the recommended dosage and gradually increasing it allows you to gauge your body's reaction and adjust accordingly. Consistency is key; adaptogens yield the most significant benefits when used regularly over time. However, patience is essential, as the full effects may take several weeks to manifest.

Furthermore, integrating Ashwagandha and Rhodiola into your daily routine should be accompanied by a holistic approach to wellness. This includes maintaining a balanced diet rich in nutrients, engaging in regular physical activity, and ensuring adequate sleep, all of which are foundational elements that support the body's stress response system and overall vitality.

Lastly, while Ashwagandha and Rhodiola offer a natural pathway to enhancing energy and managing stress, it's imperative to consult with a healthcare provider before introducing any new supplements into your regimen, especially if you have underlying health conditions or are taking medications. This precautionary step ensures that the adaptogens complement your health without adverse interactions, paving the way for a balanced and energized state of well-being.

Adaptogen Morning Elixir

Beneficial effects

The Adaptogen Morning Elixir is designed to kick-start your day with a boost of energy and resilience. Adaptogens, such as ashwagandha and rhodiola, are known for their ability to help the body resist stressors of all kinds, whether physical, chemical, or biological. These herbs have been studied for their effects on enhancing mental performance, reducing fatigue, and supporting adrenal health, making this elixir an ideal start to a busy day. Ashwagandha is particularly noted for its ability to combat stress and improve concentrations of vitality, while rhodiola is celebrated for its fatigue-fighting and energy-enhancing properties.

Portions

Makes approximately 2 servings

Preparation time

10 minutes

Cooking time

N/A

Ingredients

- 1 teaspoon ashwagandha powder
- 1 teaspoon rhodiola powder
- 1 cup hot water (not boiling, to preserve the adaptogens' properties)
- 1 tablespoon honey (preferably raw and organic)
- 1 tablespoon lemon juice (freshly squeezed)
- A pinch of cinnamon (for flavor and additional health benefits)

Instructions

1. Start by heating the water to a temperature just below boiling. Aim for around 160°F to 180°F, as too high of a temperature can degrade the beneficial properties of the adaptogens.
2. In a heat-resistant mug or glass, combine the ashwagandha and rhodiola powders.
3. Pour the hot water over the adaptogen powders in the mug, stirring well to ensure they are fully dissolved.
4. Allow the mixture to steep for about 5 minutes. This time allows the water to become infused with the adaptogens, creating a potent brew.
5. Stir in the tablespoon of honey, ensuring it's completely dissolved for a touch of natural sweetness and to add its own health benefits, including antioxidants and soothing properties.
6. Add the tablespoon of freshly squeezed lemon juice, mixing well. The lemon juice not only adds a refreshing zest but also vitamin C, aiding in immune support and providing a gentle detoxifying effect.
7. Sprinkle a pinch of cinnamon into the elixir and stir. Cinnamon is not only flavorful but also adds its own benefits, including blood sugar regulation and anti-inflammatory properties.

8. Taste the elixir and adjust any ingredients as needed to suit your preference. Some may prefer more honey for sweetness or additional lemon for tartness.

Variations

- For a cold version, allow the elixir to cool to room temperature, then add ice cubes for a refreshing adaptogen-infused drink.
- Incorporate other adaptogens like ginseng or maca powder for additional energy-boosting effects. Start with a small amount (about 1/4 teaspoon) as these can have strong flavors.
- Mix in a shot of espresso or a tablespoon of matcha powder for a caffeinated version of the elixir, enhancing its energizing properties.

Storage tips

It's best to consume the Adaptogen Morning Elixir fresh to benefit from its full potency. However, if you need to store it, keep it in the refrigerator for up to 24 hours. Be sure to stir or shake well before consuming as the powders may settle.

Tips for allergens

For those with sensitivities to honey, substitute it with maple syrup or agave nectar as a vegan-friendly sweetener. Ensure all adaptogen powders are certified organic and sourced from reputable suppliers to avoid contamination with allergens or pollutants.

Scientific references

- "A Prospective, Randomized Double-Blind, Placebo-Controlled Study of Safety and Efficacy of a High-Concentration Full-Spectrum Extract of Ashwagandha Root in Reducing Stress and Anxiety in Adults" published in the Indian Journal of Psychological Medicine shows the stress-relief benefits of ashwagandha.
- "The effects of Rhodiola rosea L. extract on anxiety, stress, cognition and other mood symptoms" published in Phytotherapy Research highlights rhodiola's positive impact on reducing fatigue and improving mood.

BOOK 20: SEASONAL HERBAL REMEDIES

CHAPTER 1: SPRING CLEANSING

Spring cleansing is a tradition rooted in the idea of renewing and rejuvenating the body after the long winter months. This process often involves the use of specific herbs known for their detoxifying and revitalizing properties. To effectively engage in a spring cleansing regimen, it's crucial to understand which herbs are most beneficial for this purpose and how to use them correctly.

Dandelion (Taraxacum officinale) is widely recognized for its liver-supporting and detoxifying benefits. The entire plant can be used; the leaves are often added to salads or brewed into a tea, while the roots can be dried, roasted, and ground into a coffee substitute. For a cleansing dandelion tea, steep 1-2 teaspoons of dried dandelion leaves in boiling water for 10 minutes. This tea can be consumed 2-3 times daily. Dandelion supports the liver in filtering toxins from the blood, promoting overall health and vitality.

Nettle (Urtica dioica), another powerful cleansing herb, is known for its ability to support kidney function and flush toxins from the body. Nettle leaves can be steeped to make a nutrient-rich tea. Use 1 tablespoon of dried nettle leaves per cup of boiling water, allowing it to steep for about 10-15 minutes. Drinking 2 cups daily can significantly enhance the body's detoxification processes during spring cleansing.

Burdock Root (Arctium lappa) is esteemed for its blood-purifying properties. It can be incorporated into your diet by adding it to soups or stews, or by drinking it as a tea. To prepare burdock root tea, simmer one tablespoon of dried root in two cups of water for about 15 minutes. Strain and drink the tea twice a day. Burdock root works by promoting increased circulation to the skin, helping to detoxify the epidermal tissues.

Milk Thistle (Silybum marianum) is perhaps best known for its protective effects on the liver, an essential organ for detoxification. Milk thistle can be taken in capsule form, with a recommended dosage of 140 milligrams of silymarin (the active ingredient in milk thistle) 2-3 times daily. This herb not only supports liver function but also aids in the regeneration of liver cells.

Lemon Balm (Melissa officinalis), while often used for its calming effects, can also play a role in a spring cleansing regimen by supporting digestive health and detoxification. Lemon balm tea can be made by steeping 1-2 teaspoons of dried lemon balm leaves in boiling water for about 10 minutes. Drinking this tea 2-3 times a day can help soothe the digestive tract and promote the elimination of toxins.

Incorporating these herbs into your spring cleansing routine can significantly aid in the body's natural detoxification processes, leading to increased energy, improved digestion, and a greater sense of well-being. It's important to source high-quality, organic herbs whenever possible to ensure the maximum benefit and to reduce the intake of additional toxins. Always consult with a healthcare provider before starting any new herbal regimen, especially if you have existing health conditions or are taking medications, to avoid any potential interactions.

Dandelion and Burdock Detox

Dandelion (**Taraxacum officinale**) and Burdock (**Arctium lappa**) stand out as two potent herbs widely utilized in spring detoxification processes. Their combined use leverages dandelion's liver-supporting properties and burdock's blood-purifying abilities to create an effective detox regimen. Here's a detailed guide on how to harness these herbs for a comprehensive spring cleanse.

Dandelion, a ubiquitous plant, is revered for its diuretic effect, which aids the kidneys in eliminating toxins through increased urine production. Its roots and leaves are rich in vitamins A, C, and K, along with minerals such as iron, potassium, and zinc, contributing to overall health and supporting liver function. To prepare a dandelion detox tea, use the following steps:

1. **Harvesting**: Choose young, tender dandelion leaves or roots. Ensure they are from a pesticide-free area.
2. **Preparation**: For the leaves, rinse thoroughly and chop finely. For the roots, clean, chop, and then dry roast them until they turn a dark brown color.
3. **Brewing**: Steep 1 tablespoon of fresh dandelion leaves or 1 teaspoon of roasted dandelion root in 8 ounces of boiling water for about 10 minutes. Strain the mixture to remove the plant matter.
4. **Dosage**: Drink 2-3 cups of dandelion tea daily during the detox period.

Burdock Root is celebrated for its blood-cleansing and anti-inflammatory properties. It contains inulin, a prebiotic that promotes healthy gut flora, and is rich in antioxidants that support detoxification pathways in the liver. To make a burdock root detox tea, follow these instructions:

1. **Sourcing**: Obtain dried burdock root from a reputable health food store or herbalist to ensure quality.

2. **Preparation**: Use about 1 tablespoon of dried burdock root per 2 cups of water. Rinse the root under cold water before use.

3. **Decoction**: Place the burdock root in a pot with water. Bring to a boil, then simmer for about 15 minutes to extract its beneficial compounds.

4. **Dosage**: Consume 1 cup of burdock tea twice daily.

For an enhanced detox effect, consider combining dandelion and burdock in a single tea. This combination not only amplifies the detoxifying benefits but also provides a comprehensive approach to cleansing the liver and blood. To create this blend:

1. **Mix equal parts of dried dandelion root and burdock root.**
2. **Use 2 tablespoons of the blend per 4 cups of water.**
3. **Follow the decoction method by boiling and simmering for 15 minutes.**
4. **Strain and enjoy 1-2 cups daily.**

When integrating dandelion and burdock into your spring detox regimen, it's crucial to stay hydrated by drinking plenty of water throughout the day. This aids in flushing out toxins and supports the kidneys in the detoxification process. Additionally, consider incorporating other detox-supportive practices such as dry brushing, which stimulates the lymphatic system, and engaging in regular physical activity to promote sweat and toxin elimination.

Remember, while dandelion and burdock are generally safe for most individuals, those with certain medical conditions or those taking medications should consult with a healthcare provider before starting any new herbal detox program. This ensures safety and avoids potential interactions with medications or conditions.

Spring Detox Tea with Dandelion and Nettle

Beneficial effects

Spring Detox Tea with Dandelion and Nettle is crafted to support the body's natural detoxification processes, particularly as we transition from winter to spring. Dandelion root is celebrated for its liver-supportive and diuretic properties, helping to flush toxins from the body and improve digestion. Nettle leaves are rich in nutrients and antioxidants, known for their anti-inflammatory benefits and ability to support kidney function and circulatory health. Together, these herbs create a potent tea that aids in cleansing the body, boosting energy levels, and supporting overall wellness.

Portions

Makes approximately 4 cups

Preparation time

10 minutes

Cooking time

15 minutes

Ingredients

- 1 tablespoon dried dandelion root
- 1 tablespoon dried nettle leaves
- 4 cups of water
- Optional: 1 teaspoon of honey or lemon juice for flavor

Instructions

1. Begin by bringing the 4 cups of water to a boil in a medium-sized pot.

2. Once the water is boiling, add 1 tablespoon of dried dandelion root to the pot.

3. Reduce the heat to a simmer and cover the pot. Allow the dandelion root to simmer for 10 minutes. This slow simmering process helps to extract the root's beneficial compounds.

4. After 10 minutes, add 1 tablespoon of dried nettle leaves to the pot. Cover again and simmer for an additional 5 minutes. Adding the nettle leaves after the dandelion root ensures that their delicate nutrients are preserved during the brewing process.

5. Remove the pot from the heat. Let the tea steep, covered, for 5 more minutes to enhance the infusion.

6. Strain the tea through a fine mesh sieve or cheesecloth into a teapot or directly into cups, removing the dandelion root and nettle leaves.

7. If desired, add a teaspoon of honey or a squeeze of lemon juice to each cup for added flavor.

Variations

- For a cooling summer drink, allow the tea to cool to room temperature, then refrigerate to serve cold.
- Add a slice of fresh ginger during the simmering process for an extra digestive boost and a warming flavor.

- Incorporate other detoxifying herbs such as burdock root or milk thistle seed for a more comprehensive detox blend.

Storage tips

Store any leftover tea in a glass container in the refrigerator for up to 2 days. Reheat gently on the stove or enjoy cold for a refreshing detox beverage.

Tips for allergens

For those with allergies or sensitivities to dandelion or nettle, consider substituting with chamomile or peppermint, which are gentle on the stomach and still offer digestive benefits. Always consult with a healthcare provider before adding new herbs to your regimen, especially if you have existing health conditions or are taking medications.

Scientific references

- "The diuretic effect in human subjects of an extract of Taraxacum officinale folium over a single day" published in the Journal of Alternative and Complementary Medicine, which discusses the diuretic properties of dandelion.
- "Stinging nettle: A modern view on an ancient healing plant" in the HerbalGram, the journal of the American Botanical Council, highlights the anti-inflammatory and nutrient-rich profile of nettle leaves.

CHAPTER 2: SUMMER COOLING HERBS

In the sweltering heat of summer, the body seeks relief and cooling, not just from external sources but also through the foods and beverages we consume. Herbs play a pivotal role in providing this much-needed cooling effect from the inside out. Among the most effective summer cooling herbs are **Peppermint (Mentha piperita)** and **Hibiscus (Hibiscus sabdariffa)**, both renowned for their refreshing and cooling properties.

Peppermint is a versatile herb that can be grown in your garden or sourced from a local health food store. Its menthol content is responsible for its cooling sensation, making it an excellent choice for reducing body heat. To prepare a Peppermint Iced Tea, follow these steps:

1. Boil 4 cups of water and remove from heat.
2. Add 1/4 cup of fresh peppermint leaves or 2 tablespoons of dried peppermint to the hot water.
3. Cover and steep for 10-15 minutes. The longer it steeps, the stronger the mint flavor.
4. Strain the leaves from the infusion and let it cool to room temperature.
5. Once cooled, add ice cubes and sweeten with honey or a natural sweetener of your choice. For an extra refreshing twist, add slices of cucumber or lemon.

Hibiscus, with its vibrant color and tart flavor, not only makes for a visually appealing drink but is also effective in cooling the body during hot weather. Hibiscus is rich in vitamin C and antioxidants, making it beneficial for overall health beyond just its cooling effects. For a Hibiscus Iced Tea:

1. Bring 4 cups of water to a boil and add 1/4 cup of dried hibiscus flowers.
2. Turn off the heat and let it steep for 15-20 minutes. Hibiscus has a tart flavor, so the steeping time can be adjusted according to taste preference.
3. Strain the flowers and let the tea cool to room temperature.
4. Sweeten with honey or agave syrup to balance the tartness. Serve over ice and garnish with a slice of lime or lemon for an added citrusy note.

Both Peppermint and Hibiscus teas can be prepared in large batches and stored in the refrigerator, ensuring a refreshing and cooling beverage is always on hand during the summer months. Additionally, these herbs can be combined in a single brew, offering a unique flavor profile along with enhanced cooling benefits.

When preparing these teas, it's essential to use filtered or spring water for the best taste. The quality of water can significantly affect the final flavor of herbal teas. Furthermore, while these herbs are generally safe for most people, it's advisable to consume them in moderation. Peppermint, for instance, may not be suitable for individuals with GERD (Gastroesophageal Reflux Disease) as it can relax the sphincter between the stomach and esophagus, potentially worsening symptoms.

Incorporating Peppermint and Hibiscus into your summer diet is a natural and effective way to stay cool and hydrated. Beyond their cooling effects, these herbs offer a range of health benefits, including digestive support and a boost in antioxidants. As with any herbal remedy, listening to your body and adjusting consumption based on individual health conditions and needs is crucial.

Peppermint and Hibiscus for Heat Relief

Peppermint (Mentha piperita) and Hibiscus (Hibiscus sabdariffa) are two potent herbs that offer significant cooling effects on the body, especially beneficial during the hot summer months. The mechanism through which these herbs impart their cooling sensation and the method of preparing beverages from them for heat relief are rooted in both their chemical makeup and traditional uses.

Peppermint contains menthol, a compound that activates the cold-sensitive TRPM8 receptors in the skin and mucosal tissues. This activation sends signals to the brain that the body is experiencing a cooling sensation. When consumed, the menthol in peppermint can help to slightly lower the body's internal temperature, providing a refreshing feeling. For optimal use, peppermint leaves should be harvested in the morning when the essential oil content, including menthol, is highest. To prepare a cooling peppermint tea, use about one tablespoon of fresh peppermint leaves or one teaspoon of dried leaves per cup of boiling water. Allow the leaves to steep in the water for 10-15 minutes before straining. This tea can be served over ice for an enhanced cooling effect. Adding a slice of lemon or lime not only adds a pleasant citrus flavor but also contributes vitamin C, enhancing the drink's health benefits.

Hibiscus, on the other hand, is known for its deep red color and tart flavor, which comes from organic acids such as hibiscus acid, a hydroxycitric acid derivative. These acids induce a refreshing sensation upon consumption, similar to the effect of consuming citrus fruits. Hibiscus also has a mild diuretic effect, promoting the elimination of heat from the body through urination. To prepare hibiscus tea, steep about one-quarter cup of dried hibiscus flowers in four cups of boiling water for 15-20 minutes. This will result in a tart, cranberry-flavored tea that can be sweetened with honey or sugar if desired. Like peppermint tea, hibiscus tea can be served over ice to maximize its cooling effect. For an added twist, mix hibiscus and peppermint teas together in equal parts to create a beverage that is not only refreshing but also aesthetically pleasing, with the deep red of the hibiscus contrasting beautifully with the bright green of the peppermint leaves.

When serving these teas, consider the presentation, which can enhance the overall enjoyment of the drink. Use clear glasses to showcase the vibrant color of the hibiscus tea and the garnishes used. Adding fresh mint leaves, slices of cucumber, or citrus fruits as garnishes can make the drinks more inviting and add to their cooling properties.

It's important to note that while peppermint and hibiscus teas are generally safe for most people, they should be consumed in moderation. Peppermint may interact with certain medications and is not recommended for individuals with GERD, as it can relax the lower esophageal sphincter, potentially worsening symptoms. Hibiscus tea may lower blood pressure and should be used with caution by those with hypotension or those taking antihypertensive medications.

Incorporating peppermint and hibiscus into your summer diet offers a natural and effective way to combat the heat. These herbs not only provide a cooling sensation but also bring a host of other health benefits, including digestive support and a boost in antioxidants. As with any herbal remedy, listening to your body and adjusting consumption based on individual health conditions and needs is crucial.

Peppermint and Hibiscus Iced Tea

Peppermint and Hibiscus Iced Tea combines the cooling effects of peppermint with the tart, refreshing taste of hibiscus, making it an ideal beverage for hot summer days. To prepare this invigorating drink, you will need:
- 1/4 cup of dried hibiscus flowers, known for their deep red color and rich in antioxidants.
- 1/4 cup of fresh peppermint leaves, recognized for their cooling properties and ability to soothe digestive ailments.
- 4 cups of boiling water, which will be used to steep the herbs and extract their flavors and beneficial compounds.
- Honey or agave syrup, according to taste, to add a natural sweetness that complements the tartness of the hibiscus and the freshness of the peppermint.
- Ice cubes, to chill the tea and make it more refreshing.
- Optional: slices of lemon or lime, for an added citrusy zest that enhances the overall flavor profile of the tea.

Begin by placing the dried hibiscus flowers and fresh peppermint leaves in a large heatproof pitcher. Pour the boiling water over the herbs, ensuring they are fully submerged. Cover the pitcher with a lid or a clean cloth and let the mixture steep for about 15-20 minutes. This duration allows the hot water to fully extract the flavors and beneficial properties of the hibiscus and peppermint.

After steeping, strain the tea to remove the hibiscus flowers and peppermint leaves, ensuring a smooth beverage. While the tea is still warm, stir in honey or agave syrup to your desired level of sweetness. This step is crucial as it allows the sweetener to dissolve completely, creating a harmonious blend of flavors.

Allow the tea to cool to room temperature before refrigerating it for at least an hour. This chilling process not only cools the tea but also intensifies its flavors, making it more refreshing.

To serve, fill glasses with ice cubes and pour the chilled peppermint and hibiscus tea over them. If desired, garnish with slices of lemon or lime for an extra burst of flavor. This drink not only quenches thirst but also offers a delightful sensory experience, making it a perfect addition to any summer day.

BOOK 21: HERBAL REMEDIES FOR ATHLETES

CHAPTER 1: PRE-WORKOUT ENERGY BOOSTERS

For athletes looking to enhance their performance and energy levels before a workout, incorporating herbal remedies can be a game-changer. Ginseng and beetroot stand out as two potent herbs that naturally boost stamina and endurance. Here's a detailed breakdown of how to harness these herbs in a pre-workout drink. **Ginseng**, known for its ability to fight fatigue and enhance physical activity, can be prepared as follows: Start by selecting a high-quality ginseng root, preferably American ginseng (Panax quinquefolius) for its mild stimulant effect. Use about 1 gram of dried ginseng root per cup of water. Slice the root thinly to increase the surface area, which helps in extracting its active components. Simmer the sliced ginseng in water for about 15-20 minutes over low heat. Strain the decoction and let it cool to room temperature.

Beetroot is renowned for its high nitrate content, which the body converts into nitric oxide. This process enhances blood flow and oxygen delivery to muscles, improving endurance. For the beetroot component, use fresh beetroot juice for the best results. Wash and peel one medium-sized beetroot, then cut it into small chunks. Using a juicer, extract the juice from the beetroot chunks. If a juicer is not available, blend the beetroot with a little water and strain the mixture to obtain the juice.

To make the **Beetroot and Ginseng Pre-Workout Drink**, you will need:
- 1 cup of freshly prepared beetroot juice
- 1 cup of ginseng decoction
- Honey or another natural sweetener to taste
- A pinch of sea salt to replenish electrolytes lost during exercise
- Optional: a squeeze of lemon for added flavor and vitamin C

Mix the beetroot juice and ginseng decoction in a large glass. Add honey to sweeten the drink according to your preference. The addition of a pinch of sea salt not only enhances the taste but also provides essential electrolytes necessary for an intense workout. For a refreshing twist, squeeze a bit of lemon into the drink.

It's best to consume this **Beetroot and Ginseng Pre-Workout Drink** about 30 minutes before starting your exercise routine. This timing allows your body to absorb the nutrients and for the nitric oxide levels to increase, ensuring you get the maximum benefit during your workout.

Remember, while ginseng and beetroot offer significant pre-workout benefits, it's crucial to listen to your body and adjust the quantities based on personal tolerance and response. Some individuals may find they need less ginseng to avoid overstimulation. Similarly, starting with a smaller amount of beetroot juice and gradually increasing it can help your body adjust to the increased nitrate intake.

Incorporating this herbal pre-workout drink into your routine can provide a natural and effective way to boost your energy and performance, leveraging the power of ginseng and beetroot to support your athletic endeavors.

Ginseng and Beetroot for Stamina

For athletes and fitness enthusiasts aiming to naturally enhance their stamina and endurance, incorporating **ginseng** and **beetroot** into their pre-workout regimen offers a powerful solution. Both these ingredients have been scientifically recognized for their ability to improve physical performance, but they must be prepared and consumed correctly to reap the maximum benefits.

Ginseng, particularly the American ginseng (**Panax quinquefolius**), is prized for its energy-boosting and fatigue-fighting properties. To prepare a ginseng infusion, begin by thinly slicing approximately 1 gram of dried ginseng root to maximize the surface area for extraction. Place the slices in a pot and add about 8 ounces (approximately 1 cup) of water. Heat the mixture on a low simmer for 15-20 minutes, which allows the water to become infused with ginseng's active components. After simmering, strain the liquid to remove the ginseng slices, and allow the infusion to cool to room temperature. This ginseng decoction serves as the base for the energy-boosting drink.

Beetroot is another key ingredient, celebrated for its high levels of dietary nitrates that convert into nitric oxide in the body, enhancing blood flow and oxygen delivery to muscles. For the freshest and most potent beetroot juice, select one medium-sized beetroot. Wash and peel the beetroot, then chop it into small pieces to facilitate juicing. Using a juicer, process the beetroot chunks to extract the juice. If a juicer is not available, the beetroot can be blended with a small amount of water, then strained through a fine mesh to collect the juice. One cup of this juice is needed for the pre-workout drink.

To assemble the **Beetroot and Ginseng Pre-Workout Drink**, combine the cooled ginseng decoction with an equal amount of fresh beetroot juice in a large glass or shaker bottle. If desired, sweeten the mixture with honey, which provides a natural source of carbohydrates for energy. Additionally, a pinch of sea salt can be added to replenish electrolytes lost during exercise. For those who enjoy a tangy flavor, a squeeze of lemon juice not only enhances the taste but also contributes vitamin C, aiding in the absorption of the nutrients.

This drink should be consumed approximately 30 minutes before beginning a workout to allow the body sufficient time to process the nitrates and for the energy-boosting properties of ginseng to take effect. It's important to start with small quantities of both ginseng and beetroot juice to assess tolerance, as some individuals may experience gastrointestinal discomfort or overstimulation from these potent ingredients. Adjust the proportions based on personal response and preferences.

By integrating this **Beetroot and Ginseng Pre-Workout Drink** into a fitness routine, athletes can leverage the natural properties of these ingredients to support increased stamina and endurance, without the need for synthetic supplements. This not only aligns with a holistic approach to health and wellness but also offers a sustainable and accessible method for enhancing physical performance.

Beetroot and Ginseng Pre-Workout Drink

Beneficial effects
The Beetroot and Ginseng Pre-Workout Drink is designed to enhance physical performance and endurance. Beetroot is rich in nitrates, which the body converts into nitric oxide. This process helps widen blood vessels, improving blood flow and oxygen delivery to muscles during exercise. Ginseng is known for its energy-boosting properties and ability to reduce fatigue, making it an excellent addition to a pre-workout regimen. Together, these ingredients provide a natural way to support increased stamina and energy levels, making your workout more effective.

Portions
Makes approximately 2 servings

Preparation time
10 minutes

Cooking time
N/A

Ingredients
- 1 large beetroot, peeled and chopped
- 1 teaspoon of ginseng powder
- 1 cup of water
- 1 tablespoon of lemon juice
- 1 tablespoon of honey (optional, for sweetness)
- A pinch of sea salt (to replenish electrolytes)

Instructions
1. Start by thoroughly washing the beetroot to remove any dirt. Peel the beetroot using a vegetable peeler and chop it into small pieces to ensure it blends smoothly.
2. Place the chopped beetroot into a high-speed blender. Add 1 teaspoon of ginseng powder to the blender.
3. Pour 1 cup of water into the blender. This will help to liquefy the ingredients, making the drink easier to consume.
4. Blend the mixture on high speed for about 1-2 minutes or until the mixture is smooth and there are no large chunks of beetroot remaining.
5. Strain the mixture using a fine mesh sieve or cheesecloth over a bowl or large measuring cup. Press or squeeze the pulp to extract as much liquid as possible. Discard the pulp or save it for use in compost or other recipes.
6. Return the liquid to the blender. Add 1 tablespoon of lemon juice to the liquid. The lemon juice adds a refreshing taste and vitamin C, which can help with the absorption of the nutrients.
7. If desired, add 1 tablespoon of honey to the mixture for sweetness. This is optional and can be adjusted based on personal preference.
8. Add a pinch of sea salt to the mixture. This will not only enhance the flavor but also help to replenish electrolytes lost during exercise.
9. Blend the mixture again for about 30 seconds to ensure all the ingredients are well combined.

10. Pour the drink into serving glasses and consume immediately for the best results, ideally 30 minutes before beginning your workout.

Variations
- For an extra kick of energy, add a small piece of ginger (about 1 inch) to the blender with the beetroot. Ginger can help improve circulation and add a spicy flavor to the drink.
- Substitute water with coconut water for additional electrolytes and a tropical flavor.
- Add a scoop of your favorite protein powder for a protein boost.

Storage tips
It's best to consume the Beetroot and Ginseng Pre-Workout Drink fresh. However, if you need to store it, keep it in an airtight container in the refrigerator for up to 24 hours. Shake well before consuming as the ingredients may settle.

Tips for allergens
For those with allergies or sensitivities to honey, substitute it with maple syrup or agave nectar as a vegan-friendly sweetener. Ensure the ginseng powder is pure and does not contain fillers that could trigger allergies.

Scientific references
- "Dietary nitrate supplementation reduces the O2 cost of low-intensity exercise and enhances tolerance to high-intensity exercise in humans," published in the Journal of Applied Physiology, discusses the benefits of beetroot juice in enhancing physical performance.
- "Effects of Panax ginseng extract on exercise-induced oxidative stress," found in the Journal of Sports Science and Medicine, highlights ginseng's role in reducing fatigue and improving endurance.

CHAPTER 2: POST-WORKOUT RECOVERY

After an intense workout, the body requires specific nutrients and care to recover properly and to maximize the benefits of your exercise routine. Herbal remedies can play a crucial role in this recovery process, offering natural ways to reduce inflammation, replenish lost nutrients, and soothe muscle soreness. Here, we focus on two key aspects of post-workout recovery: **Herbal Anti-Inflammatory Solutions** and **Herbal Hydration and Nutrient Replenishment**.

Herbal Anti-Inflammatory Solutions

Inflammation is a natural response of the body to exercise, especially after a strenuous workout. However, excessive inflammation can lead to prolonged muscle soreness and delayed recovery times. Incorporating anti-inflammatory herbs into your post-workout routine can help mitigate these effects.

1. **Turmeric**: Known for its active compound, curcumin, turmeric is a powerful anti-inflammatory herb. For a post-workout recovery drink, blend 1 teaspoon of turmeric powder with a glass of almond milk, a pinch of black pepper (to enhance absorption), and a teaspoon of honey. The black pepper increases the bioavailability of curcumin, making this drink an effective way to reduce inflammation.

2. **Ginger**: Another potent anti-inflammatory herb, ginger can be used fresh or dried. A simple way to incorporate ginger into your recovery is by making a ginger tea. Slice about an inch of fresh ginger root and steep it in boiling water for 10-15 minutes. You can add honey or lemon for taste. Ginger not only helps with inflammation but also aids in digestion and can help soothe gastrointestinal distress that sometimes accompanies intense physical activity.

Herbal Hydration and Nutrient Replenishment

Rehydrating and replenishing lost nutrients is crucial after a workout. While water is the best way to hydrate, adding herbs can enhance the rehydration process by providing additional nutrients and electrolytes.

1. **Peppermint**: Peppermint tea can be a refreshing way to rehydrate while also providing a natural muscle relaxant effect. To prepare, steep fresh or dried peppermint leaves in hot water for 5-7 minutes. This tea can be enjoyed hot or cooled down with ice for a refreshing post-workout drink.

2. **Nettle**: Rich in iron, magnesium, and potassium, nettle is an excellent herb for replenishing lost nutrients. Nettle tea can be made by steeping dried nettle leaves in boiling water for 10-15 minutes. It's recommended to drink nettle tea after it has cooled down to room temperature to maximize nutrient absorption.

For athletes and fitness enthusiasts, integrating these herbal remedies into your post-workout routine can significantly enhance recovery, reduce muscle soreness, and prepare your body for the next session. Remember, while these herbs are generally safe, it's important to listen to your body and adjust quantities based on personal tolerance. Additionally, individuals with specific health conditions or those on medication should consult with a healthcare provider before incorporating new herbal remedies into their regimen.

Turmeric and Arnica for Inflammation

In the realm of post-workout recovery, managing inflammation is paramount for athletes to ensure quick and effective healing. Two herbs stand out for their anti-inflammatory properties: **turmeric** and **arnica**. These herbs can be utilized separately or in tandem to create potent remedies that address inflammation and muscle soreness.

Turmeric, known scientifically as Curcuma longa, contains an active compound called **curcumin**. Curcumin is highly regarded for its anti-inflammatory and antioxidant effects. To harness the benefits of turmeric for post-workout recovery, one effective method is to prepare a turmeric paste. Begin by mixing 2 tablespoons of turmeric powder with 1 tablespoon of coconut oil and a small amount of black pepper. The black pepper contains piperine, which significantly enhances the absorption of curcumin by the body. Apply this paste to sore muscles or areas experiencing inflammation, but ensure the skin is not broken or irritated. For internal use, blend 1 teaspoon of turmeric powder into a smoothie or a warm glass of milk (dairy or plant-based) with a pinch of black pepper. This drink can be consumed once daily to aid recovery and reduce inflammation from within.

Arnica, specifically Arnica montana, is another powerful herb for combating inflammation, particularly suited for external application. Arnica is available in several forms, including creams, gels, and oils. For athletes, applying an arnica-based product directly to the affected area can help alleviate pain, reduce swelling, and speed up the recovery process. It is crucial to follow the product's instructions for application and to avoid using arnica on broken skin, as it is intended for topical use only.

When combining **turmeric** and **arnica** for a comprehensive approach to inflammation, consider the following regimen: Internally, incorporate turmeric into your diet as described, focusing on its systemic anti-inflammatory benefits. Externally, apply an arnica product to specifically targeted areas to address localized pain and swelling. This dual approach allows athletes to benefit from both the systemic and localized properties of these herbs.

For those preparing their own remedies, ensure that all ingredients are of high quality and sourced from reputable suppliers. When making a turmeric paste, opt for organic turmeric powder to avoid contaminants and achieve the best results. Similarly, when selecting an arnica product, look for items with a high concentration of Arnica montana extract to ensure potency.

Remember, while turmeric is generally safe for internal and external use, arnica should be used with caution and never ingested unless in a homeopathic dilution recommended by a healthcare professional. As with any herbal remedy, individual responses can vary, and it's essential to monitor your body's reaction to these treatments. If you are taking any medications or have underlying health conditions, consult with a healthcare provider before incorporating these herbs into your recovery regimen.

Turmeric and Arnica Recovery Salve

Beneficial effects

Turmeric and Arnica Recovery Salve combines the powerful anti-inflammatory properties of turmeric with the healing effects of arnica. Turmeric contains curcumin, a compound known for its ability to reduce inflammation and pain, making it ideal for post-workout recovery. Arnica has been traditionally used to soothe muscle aches, reduce swelling, and speed up the healing of bruises. Together, these herbs create a potent salve that can help alleviate soreness and promote muscle recovery after intense physical activity.

Portions

Makes approximately 1 cup

Preparation time

15 minutes

Cooking time

1 hour

Ingredients

- 1/2 cup coconut oil
- 1/4 cup beeswax pellets
- 2 tablespoons turmeric powder
- 2 tablespoons arnica flowers
- 1/4 cup olive oil
- 10 drops lavender essential oil (for its soothing and anti-inflammatory properties)
- 5 drops peppermint essential oil (optional, for a cooling effect)

Instructions

1. Begin by setting up a double boiler. Fill a pot with a few inches of water and place it on the stove over medium heat. Place a heat-resistant bowl on top of the pot, ensuring the bottom of the bowl does not touch the water.

2. Add the coconut oil and beeswax pellets to the bowl. Stir occasionally as they melt together, forming a uniform mixture.

3. Once the beeswax and coconut oil have melted, add the turmeric powder and arnica flowers. Stir the mixture continuously for 5 minutes to ensure the turmeric and arnica are well incorporated.

4. Reduce the heat to low and let the mixture simmer gently for 30 minutes. This slow infusion process helps to extract the beneficial compounds from the turmeric and arnica.

5. After 30 minutes, carefully remove the bowl from the heat. Strain the mixture through a cheesecloth or fine mesh sieve into a clean bowl to remove the arnica flowers and any large particles of turmeric.

6. While the mixture is still warm, but not too hot, add the olive oil and essential oils. Stir well to ensure all ingredients are thoroughly combined.

7. Pour the warm salve into small glass jars or tins. Allow the salve to cool and solidify at room temperature.

8. Once cooled, seal the jars or tins with lids. Label each container with the name and date.

Variations

- For extra pain relief, add 5 drops of eucalyptus essential oil to the mixture.
- If beeswax pellets are unavailable, use the same amount of grated beeswax.

Storage tips
Store the salve in a cool, dark place. The salve should last for up to 1 year if stored properly. If the salve becomes too soft in warm temperatures, refrigerate it for a short time to harden.

Tips for allergens
For those with allergies to beeswax, substitute it with an equal amount of candelilla wax or soy wax for a vegan-friendly version. Always perform a patch test on a small area of skin before applying the salve extensively, especially if you have sensitive skin or are prone to allergies.

Scientific references
- "Curcumin: A Review of Its' Effects on Human Health," published in Foods, highlights the anti-inflammatory and pain-relief properties of curcumin found in turmeric.
- "Arnica montana L. - a plant of healing: review," published in the Journal of Pharmacy and Pharmacology, discusses the therapeutic effects of arnica on bruises, swelling, and muscle soreness.

CHAPTER 3: LONG-TERM ATHLETIC SUPPORT

For athletes aiming to maintain peak performance over the long term, integrating a regimen of adaptogenic herbs can be transformative. Adaptogens, by their nature, support the body's ability to handle stress, whether physical, chemical, or biological, enhancing overall stamina and endurance. This section delves into specific adaptogenic herbs that are pivotal for long-term athletic support, detailing their benefits, preparation methods, and optimal consumption practices.

Cordyceps (Cordyceps sinensis) is renowned for its ability to increase oxygen uptake and boost mitochondrial energy production, which is crucial for endurance athletes. To incorporate cordyceps into your regimen, start with a high-quality, powdered form of the mushroom. A daily dose of 3-5 grams mixed into a pre-workout smoothie or tea can help enhance aerobic capacity and delay fatigue. For those preferring a more direct approach, cordyceps capsules are available, with dosages following the manufacturer's recommendations.

Nettle (Urtica dioica) is not traditionally categorized as an adaptogen but offers significant benefits in the form of iron and mineral replenishment, vital for athletes who engage in rigorous training schedules. A simple way to utilize nettle is by preparing a nettle leaf tea. Steep 1-2 teaspoons of dried nettle leaves in boiling water for 10-15 minutes. Drinking 1-2 cups daily can aid in recovery by replenishing essential minerals lost through sweat.

Ashwagandha (Withania somnifera) supports endurance by modulating stress responses, thereby enhancing recovery times and reducing the risk of overtraining. For ashwagandha, a daily intake of 300-500 mg of a root extract, preferably in capsule form, is recommended. Taking this supplement in the morning or evening can help improve sleep quality, another critical factor in athletic recovery and performance.

Rhodiola Rosea is another potent adaptogen with a strong affinity for enhancing physical performance and mental focus, reducing fatigue, and improving recovery times. A standardized extract of Rhodiola Rosea, containing 3% rosavins and 1% salidroside, taken in doses of 200-400 mg about 30 minutes before physical activity, can provide an energy boost and enhance endurance.

Eleuthero (Siberian Ginseng, Eleutherococcus senticosus) is beneficial for increasing stamina and reducing recovery times. A daily dose of 300-1200 mg of Eleuthero root extract can support sustained energy levels and athletic performance. It's best consumed in the morning or early afternoon to avoid potential interference with sleep patterns.

Incorporating these adaptogens requires attention to timing, dosage, and consistency to achieve the best results. Begin with lower doses to assess tolerance and gradually increase to the recommended levels as your body adapts. It's also crucial to cycle the use of adaptogens, taking breaks every 6-8 weeks to prevent your body from becoming accustomed to their effects, which can diminish their benefits over time.

For athletes, the integration of adaptogens into their daily routine should be viewed as one component of a holistic approach to health and performance. This includes a balanced diet, adequate hydration, regular exercise, and sufficient rest. Consulting with a healthcare provider before adding any new supplements to your regimen is also advisable, especially for those with underlying health conditions or those taking other medications.

By following these guidelines, athletes can leverage the power of adaptogens to support their long-term performance goals, ensuring they remain at the top of their game, both physically and mentally, for years to come.

Cordyceps and Nettle for Strength

Cordyceps and nettle stand out as two potent herbs that can significantly enhance strength and endurance, especially beneficial for athletes seeking long-term athletic support. Integrating these herbs into a daily regimen can offer a natural boost to physical performance and recovery.

Cordyceps, a type of fungus that grows on the larvae of insects, has been used in traditional Chinese medicine for centuries to increase energy and vitality. Its ability to improve oxygen uptake and boost cellular energy (ATP) production makes it an excellent supplement for athletes. To incorporate cordyceps into your diet, consider using a high-quality cordyceps extract. Start with a dosage of 500mg to 1000mg per day, taken with meals to enhance absorption. It's available in both powder and capsule forms, allowing for flexibility in how you consume it. For those who prefer a more direct approach, adding cordyceps powder to a morning smoothie or post-workout shake can provide a convenient and effective energy boost.

Nettle, or Urtica dioica, is rich in vitamins and minerals, particularly iron, which is crucial for maintaining energy levels and supporting muscle recovery. Nettle can be consumed in several forms, including tea, capsules, or tinctures. For athletes, drinking 1-2 cups of nettle tea daily can help replenish minerals lost through sweat and support overall vitality. To prepare nettle tea, steep 1-2 teaspoons of dried nettle leaves in boiling water for 10-15 minutes. This method extracts the plant's beneficial compounds, offering a nourishing drink that can be enjoyed throughout the day. Alternatively, nettle capsules can provide a more concentrated dose of the herb's nutrients, typically taken 1-2 times daily with water.

Combining **cordyceps and nettle** offers a synergistic effect that can enhance athletic performance. The increased oxygen utilization from cordyceps, paired with the mineral-rich profile of nettle, creates a foundation for improved endurance and strength. For those looking to integrate both herbs into their regimen, consider starting your day with a cordyceps supplement taken with breakfast, followed by nettle tea in the afternoon to support recovery and hydration.

When sourcing these herbs, opt for organic and sustainably harvested products to ensure purity and potency. Reputable brands that provide third-party testing results can offer additional assurance of the product's quality.

Incorporating cordyceps and nettle into your daily routine requires consistency for optimal benefits. As with any supplement, it's advisable to consult with a healthcare provider before beginning any new herbal regimen, especially for those with existing health conditions or those taking medication. With the right approach, cordyceps and nettle can be powerful allies in achieving long-term athletic goals, enhancing both performance and recovery.

Cordyceps and Nettle Tonic
Beneficial effects
The Cordyceps and Nettle Tonic is designed to support long-term athletic performance and endurance. Cordyceps, a type of medicinal mushroom, has been shown to increase oxygen uptake and boost cellular energy (ATP), which can significantly enhance stamina and reduce fatigue. Nettle, rich in iron and vitamins, supports blood health and provides anti-inflammatory benefits, aiding in recovery and overall vitality. This tonic is an excellent addition to any athlete's regimen, aiming to improve performance, support recovery, and maintain energy levels.

Portions
Makes approximately 4 servings

Preparation time
10 minutes

Cooking time
N/A

Ingredients
- 1 teaspoon cordyceps mushroom powder
- 2 tablespoons dried nettle leaves
- 4 cups of filtered water
- 1 tablespoon raw honey (optional, for sweetness)
- Juice of 1 lemon (for added vitamin C and flavor)
- A pinch of sea salt (to replenish electrolytes lost during exercise)

Instructions
1. Begin by bringing the 4 cups of filtered water to a gentle boil in a medium-sized pot.
2. Once the water is boiling, reduce the heat to a simmer and add the 2 tablespoons of dried nettle leaves. Cover the pot and allow the nettle leaves to steep for about 5 minutes.
3. After 5 minutes, remove the pot from the heat. Add 1 teaspoon of cordyceps mushroom powder to the pot, stirring well to ensure it's fully dissolved in the hot water.
4. Allow the mixture to cool for a few minutes. Once it's cool enough to handle but still warm, strain the tonic through a fine mesh sieve or cheesecloth into a large pitcher or jar, discarding the nettle leaves.
5. Stir in 1 tablespoon of raw honey to the warm tonic (if using), ensuring it dissolves completely. This step is optional and can be adjusted based on personal preference for sweetness.

6. Squeeze the juice of 1 lemon into the tonic, adding a refreshing flavor and a boost of vitamin C, which can help with the absorption of the iron from the nettle leaves.

7. Finish by adding a pinch of sea salt to the tonic, mixing well to ensure it's evenly distributed. This will help replenish electrolytes, especially beneficial after intense workouts or training sessions.

8. Serve the tonic warm, or allow it to cool completely and refrigerate for a refreshing cold beverage. Consume one serving of the tonic daily, preferably in the morning or before a workout, to maximize its benefits.

Variations

- For an extra energy boost, add a teaspoon of matcha powder to the tonic during step 3 for its antioxidant properties and natural caffeine content.
- Incorporate a slice of fresh ginger or turmeric during the steeping process for additional anti-inflammatory benefits and a warming flavor.
- Replace honey with maple syrup for a vegan-friendly sweetener option.

Storage tips

Store any leftover tonic in an airtight container in the refrigerator for up to 3 days. Shake well before consuming, as natural separation may occur.

Tips for allergens

For those with sensitivities or allergies to mushrooms, consider consulting a healthcare provider before adding cordyceps to your diet. Nettle leaves are generally well-tolerated, but it's always best to start with a small amount to ensure no adverse reactions for those new to using nettle.

Scientific references

- "Cordyceps as a Herbal Drug" in the book *Herbal Medicine: Biomolecular and Clinical Aspects*, which discusses the energy-boosting and performance-enhancing effects of cordyceps mushrooms.
- "The iron and vitamin content of nettle" published in the *Journal of the Science of Food and Agriculture*, highlighting the nutritional benefits of nettle leaves, particularly in supporting blood health and reducing inflammation.

BOOK 22: HERBAL FIRST AID

CHAPTER 1: EMERGENCY WOUND CARE

When dealing with **emergency wound care**, the primary goal is to prevent infection and promote healing. Utilizing herbs in this context can be incredibly beneficial due to their natural antiseptic, anti-inflammatory, and healing properties. Here are detailed steps and recommendations for treating cuts and scrapes with **Yarrow (Achillea millefolium)** and **Plantain (Plantago major)**, two potent herbs known for their wound-healing capabilities.

Yarrow, known for its ability to stop bleeding and disinfect wounds, should be your first go-to herb in case of a fresh cut. To use Yarrow effectively:

1. **Clean the Wound**: Gently rinse the wound with clean water to remove any debris. Avoid using hydrogen peroxide or alcohol as these can damage tissue and delay healing.
2. **Prepare Yarrow**: If you have fresh Yarrow leaves, crush them between your hands or use a mortar and pestle to release the juices. For dried Yarrow, a quick poultice can be made by mixing the powdered herb with a small amount of water to form a paste.
3. **Apply Yarrow**: Place the crushed or poulticed Yarrow directly onto the wound. If the wound is bleeding, the fresh Yarrow leaves can help promote clotting more quickly.
4. **Secure with a Bandage**: Cover the Yarrow with a clean gauze or cloth and secure it with medical tape. If possible, elevate the wound above the heart to reduce bleeding.

Plantain, abundant in many lawns and gardens, is excellent for its soothing, anti-inflammatory, and infection-preventing qualities. After initial bleeding has stopped and the wound has been cleaned, Plantain can be applied:

1. **Prepare Plantain**: Similar to Yarrow, fresh Plantain leaves can be crushed or chewed to release their healing juices. Dried Plantain can be rehydrated with a bit of water to make a paste.
2. **Apply Plantain**: Apply the prepared Plantain directly to the wound or on top of the Yarrow if used in conjunction. Plantain works well to soothe the area and reduce inflammation.
3. **Reapply as Needed**: Change the Plantain application two to three times a day. Always clean the wound gently before reapplying to prevent infection.

For both herbs, it's crucial to **monitor the wound** for signs of infection, such as increased redness, warmth, swelling, or pus. While these herbs are beneficial for minor wounds, seek professional medical attention for deep cuts, punctures, or if signs of infection arise.

Materials Needed:
- Fresh or dried Yarrow leaves
- Fresh or dried Plantain leaves
- Clean water for rinsing the wound
- Gauze or clean cloth
- Medical tape
- Mortar and pestle (optional, for making poultices)

Recommendations:
- Always use **clean materials** to avoid introducing bacteria into the wound.
- **Test** the herbs on a small area of skin before applying to wounds to ensure there are no allergic reactions.
- **Harvest** Yarrow and Plantain from areas free of pesticides and pollution for the safest application.
- **Educate** yourself on the identification of these herbs to ensure the correct plants are used.

Incorporating Yarrow and Plantain into your first aid kit as dried herbs or tinctures ensures you're prepared to handle minor wounds effectively with natural remedies. Remember, the key to successful herbal first aid is prompt and proper care, and while these herbs offer excellent support for minor injuries, they do not replace professional medical treatment for serious or infected wounds.

Yarrow and Plantain for Cuts

Yarrow (Achillea millefolium) and Plantain (Plantago major) are two potent herbs known for their exceptional wound-healing properties, making them indispensable in the realm of herbal first aid for treating cuts and scrapes. The efficacy of these plants lies in their natural antiseptic, anti-inflammatory, and hemostatic (bleeding-stopping) qualities, which can significantly accelerate the healing process while minimizing the risk of infection.

To effectively utilize Yarrow in the case of a fresh cut, the first step involves ensuring the wound is clean. This is crucial for preventing infection and should be done by gently rinsing the area with clean, preferably sterile, water. It's important to avoid using substances like hydrogen peroxide or alcohol for cleaning as they can damage the tissue and impede healing. Once the wound is clean, if you have access to fresh Yarrow leaves, you should crush them to release the juices that contain the plant's medicinal properties. This can be done by hand or with a mortar and pestle. For those using dried Yarrow, you can create a quick poultice by mixing the powdered herb with a small amount of sterile water to form a thick paste. This paste or the crushed fresh leaves should then be applied directly to the wound. Yarrow's natural ability to stop bleeding will be beneficial if the wound is still bleeding. After applying Yarrow, cover the area with a clean gauze or cloth and secure it with medical tape, ensuring to elevate the wound above the heart level if possible to reduce bleeding.

Following the application of Yarrow, Plantain can be used as a secondary treatment to soothe the wound and reduce inflammation. Plantain leaves, whether fresh or dried, should be prepared in a similar manner to Yarrow. Fresh leaves can be crushed or chewed to release their beneficial juices, while dried leaves can be rehydrated with a bit of sterile water to make a paste. This preparation should then be applied directly to the wound or over the Yarrow application. It's beneficial to change the Plantain application two to three times a day, cleaning the wound gently each time before reapplication to prevent infection.

For both Yarrow and Plantain, monitoring the wound for signs of infection is critical. Signs to watch for include increased redness, warmth, swelling, or the presence of pus. While these herbs are highly effective for minor wounds, professional medical attention should be sought for deep cuts, punctures, or if any signs of infection arise.

Materials needed for this process include fresh or dried Yarrow leaves, fresh or dried Plantain leaves, clean water for rinsing the wound, gauze or a clean cloth for covering the wound, and medical tape for securing the dressing. Optionally, a mortar and pestle can be used for making poultices.

When harvesting Yarrow and Plantain, it's essential to choose plants from areas free of pesticides and pollution to ensure the safest application. Additionally, familiarizing yourself with the correct identification of these herbs is crucial to avoid using the wrong plants. Testing the herbs on a small skin area before application can also help ensure there are no allergic reactions.

Incorporating Yarrow and Plantain into your first aid kit, whether as dried herbs or tinctures, equips you with natural remedies that are effective for handling minor wounds. This approach underscores the importance of prompt and proper care in herbal first aid, highlighting that while these herbs provide excellent support for minor injuries, they do not replace the need for professional medical treatment in the case of serious or infected wounds.

Yarrow and Plantain Healing Poultice
Beneficial effects
The Yarrow and Plantain Healing Poultice is a time-honored remedy known for its potent anti-inflammatory, antiseptic, and healing properties. Yarrow, with its ability to staunch bleeding and reduce inflammation, pairs effectively with plantain, which is renowned for its wound healing and antibacterial benefits. This poultice can be particularly beneficial for minor cuts, scrapes, insect bites, and skin irritations, promoting faster healing and reducing the risk of infection.

Portions
This recipe yields enough poultice for 1-2 small wounds or bites.

Preparation time
5 minutes

Cooking time
N/A

Ingredients
- 1 tablespoon fresh yarrow leaves (or 1 teaspoon dried)
- 1 tablespoon fresh plantain leaves (or 1 teaspoon dried)
- A small amount of water (to form a paste)
- Optional: A clean cloth or gauze for application

Instructions
1. If using fresh leaves, thoroughly wash the yarrow and plantain leaves to remove any dirt or debris. Pat them dry with a clean towel.

2. Using a mortar and pestle, crush the yarrow and plantain leaves together until they form a coarse paste. If you don't have a mortar and pestle, you can chop the leaves finely with a knife and then mash them with the back of a spoon or a fork.

3. Gradually add a few drops of water to the crushed leaves, just enough to form a paste that will stick to the skin without dripping.

4. If the wound is open, ensure it has been cleaned properly before applying the poultice. For closed skin irritations or bites, you can proceed directly to application.

5. Apply the paste directly to the affected area. If preferred, spread the paste onto a clean piece of cloth or gauze first, then place the cloth or gauze over the skin.

6. Secure the poultice in place with a bandage or medical tape if it's on a spot that moves a lot or if clothing might rub against it.

7. Leave the poultice on the skin for up to an hour, checking periodically to ensure it doesn't dry out completely. If using on an open wound, shorter durations of 15-30 minutes are advisable to prevent any plant matter from sticking to the wound.

8. Gently wash the area with warm water to remove the poultice. Pat dry with a clean towel.

Variations
- For added antimicrobial properties, a teaspoon of honey can be mixed into the paste before application.
- To enhance the soothing effects, especially for burns or stings, aloe vera gel can be blended with the yarrow and plantain paste.

Storage tips
It's best to prepare the yarrow and plantain poultice fresh for each use. However, if you have leftover paste, it can be stored in a small, airtight container in the refrigerator for up to 24 hours. Note that the paste may discolor or lose potency over time.

Tips for allergens
Individuals with sensitivities to Asteraceae/Compositae family plants (such as yarrow) should perform a patch test before applying the poultice broadly. Substitute with chamomile or calendula if yarrow is not suitable.

Scientific references
- "Anti-inflammatory and wound healing activity of a growth substance in Aloe vera," published in the Journal of the American Podiatric Medical Association, highlights the healing properties of aloe vera, which can be beneficial when combined with yarrow and plantain.
- "Antibacterial activity of Plantago major leaves," found in the Journal of Ethnopharmacology, supports the use of plantain for its antibacterial benefits in wound care.

CHAPTER 2: BURNS AND SKIN DAMAGE

For treating **burns and skin damage** with herbal remedies, it's crucial to understand the severity of the burn before applying any treatment. Burns are categorized into three types: first-degree (superficial burns that affect only the outer layer of skin), second-degree (burns that affect both the outer layer and the underlying layer of skin, causing blisters), and third-degree (burns that penetrate the full thickness of the skin, potentially damaging tissues underneath). Herbal treatments can be particularly beneficial for first and some second-degree burns to promote healing, reduce pain, and prevent infection.

Aloe Vera is widely recognized for its soothing and healing properties on burns. To use Aloe Vera effectively on a first or mild second-degree burn, follow these steps:

1. **Cool the Burn**: Immediately run cool (not cold) water over the burn for several minutes. Avoid using ice as it can restrict blood flow, which can impede the healing process.

2. **Apply Aloe Vera Gel**: Use pure Aloe Vera gel directly from the plant if possible. Break off a leaf and squeeze the gel onto the burn. If using store-bought Aloe Vera, ensure it's 100% pure Aloe without added ingredients.

3. **Reapply as Needed**: Aloe Vera can be applied 2-3 times a day. For extra soothing effects, the gel can be refrigerated before application.

Lavender Essential Oil is another excellent remedy for burns due to its antiseptic and pain-relieving properties. To use:

1. **Dilute Lavender Oil**: Mix 1-2 drops of Lavender essential oil with a tablespoon of a carrier oil, such as coconut or almond oil. Never apply essential oils directly to the skin without dilution.

2. **Apply to the Burn**: Gently dab the diluted Lavender oil on the affected area using a clean cotton pad or ball. Avoid rubbing or putting pressure on the burn.

3. **Cover Lightly**: If needed, cover the burn with a loose, sterile gauze bandage to protect the area. Do not wrap tightly.

Honey has been used for centuries to treat burns and wounds due to its natural antibacterial and anti-inflammatory properties. To use honey on a burn:

1. **Clean the Area**: After cooling the burn, gently pat the area dry with a clean cloth.

2. **Apply Honey**: Spread a thin layer of raw, unpasteurized honey over the burn.

3. **Cover with Gauze**: Place a piece of sterile gauze over the honey-applied area. Change the dressing once a day.

Calendula, known for its ability to reduce inflammation and promote skin healing, can be used in the form of a cream or ointment for burns.

1. **Prepare Calendula**: If using Calendula flowers, create an infusion by pouring boiling water over the flowers and letting it steep for about 10 minutes. Strain and cool the infusion.

2. **Apply Calendula**: Soak a clean cloth in the Calendula infusion and apply it as a compress to the burn. Alternatively, apply Calendula cream directly to the area 2-3 times a day.

Materials Needed:
- Aloe Vera plant or 100% pure Aloe Vera gel
- Lavender essential oil and carrier oil (coconut, almond)
- Raw, unpasteurized honey
- Calendula flowers (for homemade infusion) or Calendula cream
- Clean water for rinsing and making infusions
- Sterile gauze and clean cloths for application and coverings

Recommendations:
- Always perform a patch test when using a new product or plant on the skin to ensure there are no allergic reactions.
- For severe burns, or if there is no improvement within a few days, seek medical attention.
- Keep the burn clean and monitor for signs of infection, such as increased pain, redness, fever, swelling, or oozing.
- Ensure all materials and herbs used are clean and free from contaminants.

Using these herbal remedies can aid in the healing process of minor burns and skin damage, offering natural alternatives to promote recovery and comfort.

Aloe Vera and Lavender for Burns

Aloe Vera, known scientifically as Aloe barbadensis miller, stands out for its exceptional soothing and healing properties, particularly when it comes to treating burns. The gel found inside the leaves of the Aloe Vera plant contains compounds that provide pain relief, reduce inflammation, and stimulate skin regeneration, making it an indispensable remedy for first and mild second-degree burns. To harness the full potential of Aloe Vera, it's crucial to use it correctly. Begin by sourcing a fresh Aloe Vera leaf, preferably from an organically grown plant to ensure it's free from harmful pesticides. Using a clean knife, slice off a section of the leaf and carefully peel away the green outer layer to reveal the translucent gel inside. For a burn treatment, gently apply a generous layer of this fresh gel directly onto the affected area. The coolness of the gel provides immediate soothing relief. If fresh Aloe Vera is not available, opt for a store-bought gel that is 100% pure Aloe Vera, ensuring it doesn't contain alcohol, fragrances, or coloring agents, which could irritate the burn.

Lavender essential oil, Lavandula angustifolia, is renowned for its antiseptic and analgesic properties, making it another excellent choice for burn care. Its ability to alleviate pain while preventing infection is why Lavender oil is a staple in natural burn treatment. However, it's imperative to dilute the essential oil before application to avoid any potential skin irritation. Create a blend by adding 1-2 drops of Lavender essential oil to a tablespoon of carrier oil, such as coconut oil or sweet almond oil, both of which have their own skin-soothing benefits. Apply a small amount of this mixture to the burn, dabbing it gently with a clean cotton pad or a soft cloth. This not only helps in reducing the pain but also in accelerating the healing process without leaving the skin greasy or clogged.

In the immediate aftermath of a burn, the first step should always be to cool the area under running tap water for several minutes to reduce the heat and prevent further damage to the skin. After patting the skin dry with a clean towel, Aloe Vera can be applied followed by the diluted Lavender oil. This combination not only soothes the burn but also creates an environment conducive to healing. For ongoing care, Aloe Vera gel can be reapplied 2-3 times a day, with the Lavender oil blend used once daily to keep the area sanitized and support skin repair.

When preparing and applying these remedies, ensure all utensils, containers, and your hands are clean to prevent introducing any bacteria to the burn. It's also advisable to perform a patch test on a small, unaffected area of skin before applying these substances to a burn, especially if you have sensitive skin or are prone to allergies. This helps ascertain your skin's tolerance to Aloe Vera and Lavender oil, minimizing the risk of an adverse reaction.

Materials needed for this treatment include a fresh Aloe Vera leaf or 100% pure Aloe Vera gel, Lavender essential oil, a carrier oil of your choice, a clean knife for cutting the Aloe leaf, and sterile gauze if covering the burn is necessary. Remember, while these herbal remedies can be incredibly effective for minor burns, they are not a substitute for professional medical advice. Severe burns, characterized by extensive damage, blisters, or signs of infection, require immediate attention from a healthcare provider.

Aloe and Lavender Burn Gel

Beneficial effects

Aloe and Lavender Burn Gel harnesses the soothing and healing properties of aloe vera combined with the calming and anti-inflammatory benefits of lavender essential oil. Aloe vera is widely recognized for its ability to support skin regeneration and provide a cooling effect on burns, reducing pain and inflammation. Lavender essential oil not only enhances the gel's soothing effect but also offers antimicrobial properties, helping to prevent infection in minor burns. This natural remedy is ideal for first aid treatment of minor kitchen burns, sunburns, or other skin irritations that do not require medical attention.

Portions

Makes approximately 1 cup

Preparation time

10 minutes

Cooking time

N/A

Ingredients

- 1 cup pure aloe vera gel
- 10-15 drops lavender essential oil
- 1 tablespoon vitamin E oil (optional, for added skin healing and preservation)
- 1 clean, sterilized jar with lid for storage

Instructions

1. Start by ensuring your work area and utensils are clean to prevent any contamination of the gel.

2. In a medium-sized bowl, carefully measure out 1 cup of pure aloe vera gel. Aloe vera gel should be clear to slightly golden in color, indicating it is pure and free from added colors or fillers.

3. Add 10-15 drops of lavender essential oil to the aloe vera gel. The amount can be adjusted based on personal preference for fragrance strength, but it's important not to exceed 15 drops to avoid skin irritation.

4. If using, add 1 tablespoon of vitamin E oil to the mixture. Vitamin E oil acts as an antioxidant that can help extend the shelf life of the gel and support skin healing.

5. Using a clean spoon or spatula, gently mix the ingredients together until well combined. The mixture should be homogenous, with no oil droplets visible.

6. Carefully transfer the gel into a clean, sterilized jar. Using a funnel can help prevent spills and ensure all the gel makes it into the jar.

7. Seal the jar with its lid tightly to prevent any air or contaminants from getting in.

8. Label the jar with the contents and date of preparation.

Variations

- For extra cooling effects, refrigerate the gel for at least 1 hour before applying to the skin.
- Add 5 drops of tea tree oil for its antiseptic properties, especially if the gel will be used on cuts or abrasions.

Storage tips

Store the aloe and lavender burn gel in the refrigerator to maintain its freshness and enhance the cooling effect upon application. The gel can be kept for up to 1 month when stored properly. Always check the gel before use for any signs of spoilage, such as an off smell or discoloration.

Tips for allergens

Individuals with sensitive skin or allergies to aloe vera or lavender should perform a patch test on a small area of skin before applying the gel extensively. If irritation occurs, discontinue use immediately. For those allergic to aloe vera, a chamomile-infused gel can be a soothing alternative, though it will not have the same skin-healing properties as aloe.

Scientific references

- "Aloe vera: A short review," published in the Indian Journal of Dermatology, discusses the skin healing and anti-inflammatory properties of aloe vera.
- "Lavender oil in the treatment of acute burn injuries," featured in the journal Burns, highlights the efficacy of lavender oil in soothing burns and promoting healing.

BOOK 23: ALOE AND LAVENDER BURN GEL

CHAPTER 1: HERBS FOR JOINT AND BONE HEALTH

Turmeric and Boswellia are renowned for their anti-inflammatory properties, making them ideal for addressing joint pain and promoting bone health. To harness these benefits, creating a **Turmeric and Boswellia Anti-Inflammatory Tonic** is an effective remedy. This tonic combines the potent anti-inflammatory compounds found in both herbs, curcumin from turmeric and boswellic acids from Boswellia, to help reduce inflammation and pain associated with conditions like arthritis and osteoporosis.

Ingredients:
- 1 teaspoon of ground turmeric
- 1/2 teaspoon of Boswellia powder
- 1 tablespoon of honey (preferably raw and organic)
- A pinch of black pepper (to enhance turmeric absorption)
- 2 cups of water

Instructions:

1. **Prepare the Water Base:** Begin by boiling the 2 cups of water in a small saucepan. The use of water as a base for this tonic helps in the easy assimilation of the herbs into the body.

2. **Add Turmeric and Boswellia:** Once the water reaches a rolling boil, reduce the heat to a simmer and add the ground turmeric and Boswellia powder. The simmering process aids in the extraction of the active compounds from the herbs, making them more bioavailable.

3. **Simmer:** Allow the mixture to simmer gently for 10 minutes. This duration is crucial as it ensures that the compounds are adequately extracted without destroying the delicate oils and components of the herbs.

4. **Enhance Absorption:** After simmering, turn off the heat and stir in a pinch of black pepper. Black pepper contains piperine, a compound that significantly enhances the absorption of curcumin by the body, making the tonic more effective.

5. **Sweeten:** Add a tablespoon of honey to the mixture. Honey not only improves the taste but also brings its own anti-inflammatory and antimicrobial properties to the tonic, complementing the effects of turmeric and Boswellia.

6. **Strain and Serve:** Strain the tonic through a fine mesh sieve into a cup. This step is important to remove any undissolved particles of turmeric and Boswellia, ensuring a smooth drinking experience.

7. **Consume Warm:** Drink the tonic while it is still warm. Consuming the tonic warm increases its soothing effect on the throat and enhances digestion, facilitating the absorption of the active ingredients.

Recommendations:
- For best results, consume this tonic once daily, preferably in the morning on an empty stomach. This timing allows the body to absorb the tonic's compounds more efficiently, maximizing its anti-inflammatory effects throughout the day.
- It is advisable to consult with a healthcare provider before adding this tonic to your routine, especially for those on medication or with existing health conditions, to avoid any potential interactions.

By following these detailed steps, individuals can create a powerful Turmeric and Boswellia Anti-Inflammatory Tonic at home, leveraging the natural healing properties of these herbs to support joint and bone health.

Turmeric and Boswellia for Inflammation

Turmeric and Boswellia, both revered for their potent anti-inflammatory properties, offer a natural approach to managing inflammation and pain, particularly in the context of joint and bone health. The active compound in turmeric, curcumin, and the boswellic acids found in Boswellia work synergistically to modulate the body's inflammatory response, providing relief from conditions such as arthritis and osteoporosis. To effectively utilize these herbs, it's crucial to understand their mechanisms and how to incorporate them into a daily regimen for maximum benefit.

When preparing a Turmeric and Boswellia Anti-Inflammatory Tonic, the selection of high-quality, organic ingredients ensures the purity and potency of the remedy. Ground turmeric should be bright yellow and aromatic, indicating its freshness and curcumin content. Similarly, Boswellia powder should be finely ground, allowing for better dissolution and absorption. The addition of a pinch of black pepper is not merely a flavor enhancer; it contains piperine, a compound that significantly increases the bioavailability of curcumin, making the tonic far more effective.

The process of simmering the mixture for 10 minutes is critical. This gentle heat allows for the extraction of the active compounds without compromising their integrity. It's a delicate balance to maintain the therapeutic properties of the herbs while making them readily available for absorption by the body. Straining the tonic ensures a smooth texture, removing any gritty particles that could detract from the drinking experience. The warmth of the tonic not only makes it more palatable but also aids in the digestive process, facilitating the absorption of the anti-inflammatory compounds.

Consumption guidelines are equally important for achieving the desired therapeutic effect. Drinking the tonic on an empty stomach maximizes absorption, as there are no other foods to interfere with the digestive process. This timing leverages the body's natural circadian rhythms, optimizing the anti-inflammatory response. Regular, daily consumption reinforces the cumulative effect of the herbs, gradually reducing inflammation and improving joint and bone health over time.

Consultation with a healthcare provider is advisable to ensure compatibility with existing health conditions and medications. This precautionary step is crucial to prevent any potential interactions and to tailor the remedy to individual health needs, ensuring safety and efficacy.

Incorporating Turmeric and Boswellia into one's daily routine as an Anti-Inflammatory Tonic represents a proactive approach to managing inflammation naturally. By understanding the specific properties of these herbs, their preparation, and optimal consumption practices, individuals can harness the healing power of nature to support their joint and bone health, embodying a holistic approach to wellness that aligns with the body's natural processes.

Turmeric and Boswellia Anti-Inflammatory Tonic
Beneficial effects
Turmeric and Boswellia Anti-Inflammatory Tonic leverages the potent anti-inflammatory properties of both turmeric, with its active compound curcumin, and Boswellia, also known as Indian frankincense. Turmeric has been widely studied for its ability to reduce inflammation and support joint health, while Boswellia has been shown to decrease inflammation related to chronic conditions like osteoarthritis and rheumatoid arthritis. This tonic is designed to provide a natural way to manage inflammation and support overall wellness.

Portions
Makes approximately 4 servings
Preparation time
5 minutes
Cooking time
N/A
Ingredients
- 4 cups of filtered water
- 2 tablespoons of turmeric powder
- 1 tablespoon of Boswellia powder
- 1 teaspoon of ground black pepper (to enhance curcumin absorption)
- 1 tablespoon of honey (optional, for sweetness)
- Juice of 1 lemon

Instructions
1. Pour 4 cups of filtered water into a large pitcher or jar.
2. Add 2 tablespoons of turmeric powder and 1 tablespoon of Boswellia powder to the water. Stir thoroughly to combine. The powders may not fully dissolve, creating a suspension.
3. Incorporate 1 teaspoon of ground black pepper into the mixture. Black pepper contains piperine, which significantly enhances the absorption of curcumin by the body, making the tonic more effective.
4. If desired, add 1 tablespoon of honey to the mixture for sweetness. Stir well until the honey is completely dissolved. Adjust the sweetness according to taste.
5. Squeeze the juice of 1 lemon into the pitcher or jar, adding a refreshing flavor and vitamin C, which can also aid in the absorption of the tonic's beneficial compounds.
6. Stir the tonic thoroughly one last time to ensure all ingredients are well mixed.

7. Serve the tonic immediately, or for a chilled version, refrigerate for at least 1 hour before serving. Shake or stir well before pouring into glasses due to the natural settling of the powders.

Variations

- For a warming drink, gently heat the tonic in a saucepan over low heat until warm but not boiling, and consume as a warm tea.
- Add a slice of fresh ginger for additional anti-inflammatory benefits and a spicy flavor profile.
- Substitute honey with maple syrup for a vegan-friendly sweetener option.

Storage tips

Store any leftover tonic in the refrigerator for up to 3 days. Ensure the pitcher or jar is sealed tightly to maintain freshness. The tonic should be shaken or stirred well before each use as the turmeric and Boswellia powders will settle to the bottom.

Tips for allergens

Individuals with allergies to turmeric, Boswellia, or black pepper should avoid this tonic. For those with sensitivities to honey, using maple syrup or simply omitting the sweetener can be a suitable alternative.

Scientific references

- "Curcumin: A Review of Its' Effects on Human Health," published in Foods, discusses the anti-inflammatory and health benefits of curcumin found in turmeric.
- "Boswellia serrata, A Potential Antiinflammatory Agent: An Overview," published in the Indian Journal of Pharmaceutical Sciences, highlights the anti-inflammatory properties of Boswellia.

CHAPTER 2: COGNITIVE SUPPORT WITH HERBS

Ginkgo Biloba and Rosemary are two potent herbs known for their cognitive-enhancing properties. These herbs have been used traditionally to improve memory, focus, and overall brain health. The following recipes provide a method to incorporate these herbs into a daily routine for cognitive support.

Ginkgo Biloba is renowned for its ability to improve blood circulation to the brain, which in turn enhances memory and cognitive speed. To prepare a **Ginkgo Biloba Tea**, you will need:
- 1-2 teaspoons of dried Ginkgo Biloba leaves
- 8 ounces of boiling water

Place the Ginkgo Biloba leaves in a tea infuser or teapot. Pour boiling water over the leaves and allow them to steep for 10 minutes. Straining the tea into a cup, it's ready to be enjoyed. Drinking this tea in the morning can help kickstart your day with improved mental clarity.

Rosemary, on the other hand, has been linked to improved concentration and memory retention, possibly due to its antioxidant properties and its ability to increase blood flow. For a **Rosemary Infused Water**, you will need:
- A sprig of fresh rosemary
- 16 ounces of water

Place the fresh rosemary sprig in a jar or bottle of water and let it infuse for at least an hour. For a stronger flavor and more potent cognitive effects, you can let it infuse overnight in the refrigerator. Drinking rosemary-infused water throughout the day can help maintain focus and alertness.

For those looking to combine the benefits of both herbs, a **Ginkgo and Rosemary Cognitive Support Tincture** can be made. You will need:
- 1/4 cup dried Ginkgo Biloba leaves
- 1/4 cup dried rosemary leaves
- 1 pint of vodka or apple cider vinegar (for those avoiding alcohol)

Combine the herbs in a glass jar and cover them with the vodka or vinegar, ensuring that the herbs are completely submerged. Seal the jar tightly and place it in a cool, dark place for 4 to 6 weeks, shaking it daily. After the infusion period, strain the tincture through a cheesecloth into another clean, dark glass bottle. A standard dose is 1-2 droppers full, taken 1-2 times daily. This tincture combines the circulatory benefits of Ginkgo Biloba with the antioxidative properties of rosemary for a powerful cognitive boost.

When preparing and using these herbal remedies, it's important to source high-quality, organic herbs to ensure the absence of pesticides and contaminants that could detract from their health benefits. Additionally, while these herbs are generally considered safe for most people, it's advisable to consult with a healthcare provider before starting any new herbal regimen, especially for those with pre-existing conditions or those taking medications, as herbs can interact with some medications.

Incorporating Ginkgo Biloba and Rosemary into your daily routine can be a simple yet effective way to support cognitive health and enhance mental performance. Whether through tea, infused water, or a tincture, these herbs offer a natural means to boost brain function.

Ginkgo Biloba and Rosemary for Memory

Ginkgo Biloba and Rosemary, when utilized together, create a potent combination for enhancing memory and cognitive function. The efficacy of Ginkgo Biloba in improving blood circulation, particularly to the brain, is well-documented. This increased blood flow is crucial for delivering oxygen and nutrients to brain cells, thereby enhancing memory, focus, and overall cognitive speed. To harness the benefits of Ginkgo Biloba, it's recommended to use 1-2 teaspoons of dried Ginkgo Biloba leaves per 8 ounces of boiling water. The leaves should be steeped in boiling water for approximately 10 minutes to ensure the active compounds are adequately extracted. This tea can be consumed once daily, preferably in the morning, to support cognitive function throughout the day.

Rosemary, on the other hand, is not only celebrated for its aromatic qualities but also for its cognitive-enhancing properties. The compound 1,8-cineole, found in Rosemary, has been linked to improved memory retention and concentration. This is believed to be due to its antioxidant properties and its ability to increase blood flow, similar to Ginkgo Biloba, but through different mechanisms. For daily cognitive support, incorporating a sprig of fresh Rosemary into 16 ounces of water, allowing it to infuse for at least an hour or overnight in the refrigerator, creates a refreshing drink that can help maintain focus and alertness throughout the day.

For individuals seeking to combine the cognitive benefits of both Ginkgo Biloba and Rosemary, creating a tincture may provide a more concentrated and convenient option. This involves combining 1/4 cup of dried Ginkgo Biloba leaves and 1/4 cup of dried Rosemary leaves in a pint of vodka or apple cider vinegar, for those avoiding alcohol. The mixture should be stored in a cool, dark place for 4 to 6 weeks, with daily shaking to promote extraction. After the infusion period, the liquid is strained and stored in a dark glass bottle. The recommended dosage is 1-2 droppers full, taken 1-2 times daily. This tincture leverages the circulatory benefits of Ginkgo Biloba along with the antioxidative properties of Rosemary for a synergistic effect on cognitive function.

When preparing these remedies, sourcing high-quality, organic herbs is paramount to ensure the absence of pesticides and contaminants, which could detract from their health benefits. Furthermore, while Ginkgo Biloba and Rosemary are generally safe for most people, consulting with a healthcare provider before starting any new herbal regimen is advisable, especially for those with pre-existing conditions or those taking medications, to avoid potential interactions.

Incorporating Ginkgo Biloba and Rosemary into one's daily routine represents a natural and effective strategy for supporting cognitive health. Whether through tea, infused water, or a tincture, these herbs offer a holistic approach to enhancing memory and focus.

Rosemary and Ginkgo Brain Tea

Beneficial effects

Rosemary and Ginkgo Brain Tea is crafted to enhance cognitive function, memory, and overall brain health. Rosemary is renowned for its ability to improve concentration and memory recall by increasing blood flow to the brain. Ginkgo Biloba, on the other hand, is celebrated for its neuroprotective effects and ability to enhance cognitive performance, particularly in tasks related to memory and attention. Together, these herbs create a potent blend that supports mental clarity and cognitive longevity.

Portions

Makes approximately 4 cups

Preparation time

10 minutes

Cooking time

15 minutes

Ingredients

- 4 cups of water
- 2 tablespoons of dried rosemary leaves
- 2 tablespoons of dried ginkgo biloba leaves
- Honey or stevia (optional, for sweetness)
- Lemon slice (optional, for flavor)

Instructions

1. Begin by bringing 4 cups of water to a boil in a medium-sized saucepan.
2. Once the water reaches a rolling boil, reduce the heat to low and add 2 tablespoons of dried rosemary leaves.
3. Add 2 tablespoons of dried ginkgo biloba leaves to the saucepan, stirring the mixture gently to ensure the herbs are fully submerged in the water.
4. Cover the saucepan with a lid and allow the mixture to simmer gently for 15 minutes. This slow simmering process helps to extract the active compounds from the herbs, maximizing the tea's cognitive benefits.
5. After 15 minutes, remove the saucepan from the heat. Let the tea steep, covered, for an additional 5 minutes to further enhance its flavor and potency.
6. Strain the tea through a fine mesh sieve or cheesecloth into a teapot or directly into cups, discarding the used herbs.
7. If desired, sweeten the tea with honey or stevia according to taste. Add a slice of lemon to each cup for a refreshing twist.
8. Serve the tea warm. For a cooling, refreshing alternative, allow the tea to cool to room temperature, then refrigerate until chilled.

Variations

- For a stronger cognitive boost, add a teaspoon of dried peppermint leaves to the blend. Peppermint can enhance mental alertness and energy.
- Incorporate a slice of fresh ginger during the simmering process for additional anti-inflammatory benefits and a spicy kick.

Storage tips

Store any leftover tea in a glass pitcher or jar in the refrigerator for up to 2 days. Reheat gently on the stove or enjoy cold for a revitalizing drink.

Tips for allergens

Individuals with allergies to plants in the daisy family should consult with a healthcare provider before consuming ginkgo biloba, as it may cause allergic reactions in sensitive individuals. Similarly, those with a sensitivity to rosemary should proceed with caution and consider consulting a healthcare professional.

Scientific references

- "Pharmacological Effects of Rosa Damascena" published in the Iranian Journal of Basic Medical Sciences, which discusses the therapeutic benefits of rosemary, including improved memory and cognitive function.
- "Ginkgo Biloba for Cognitive Improvement and Memory" featured in the Journal of the American Medical Association, highlights the cognitive benefits of Ginkgo Biloba, including enhanced memory and brain function.

CHAPTER 3: SKIN AND HAIR VITALITY

Rosehip and Horsetail are two potent herbs known for their remarkable benefits for skin and hair health, especially as we age. These natural ingredients are packed with vitamins, minerals, and antioxidants that can help to rejuvenate and restore vitality to aging skin and hair. Here's how to create a **Rosehip and Horsetail Beauty Elixir** that harnesses these benefits.

Ingredients:
- 1/4 cup dried rosehip berries, known for their high vitamin C content and ability to boost collagen production, leading to firmer, more youthful skin.
- 1/4 cup dried horsetail, chosen for its silica content which strengthens hair and nails and improves skin elasticity.
- 2 cups of boiling water, used to extract the active compounds from the herbs.
- 1 tablespoon of honey, optional, for its moisturizing and antibacterial properties.

Instructions:
1. **Prepare the Herbs:** Begin by measuring out the dried rosehip berries and horsetail. Ensure that the herbs are finely chopped or crushed to increase the surface area for better extraction of their beneficial compounds.
2. **Boil Water:** Heat 2 cups of water in a kettle or saucepan until it reaches a rolling boil. The use of boiling water is crucial as it helps to extract the vitamins, minerals, and other phytonutrients from the herbs effectively.
3. **Steep the Herbs:** Place the rosehip berries and horsetail in a heat-resistant container or teapot. Pour the boiling water over the herbs, making sure they are fully submerged. Cover the container with a lid or a small plate to prevent the escape of steam, which contains essential volatile compounds.
4. **Allow to Infuse:** Let the mixture steep for at least 20 minutes. This duration is necessary to ensure that the water becomes saturated with the active ingredients from the rosehip and horsetail, creating a potent infusion.
5. **Strain the Elixir:** After steeping, strain the liquid through a fine mesh sieve or cheesecloth into another container. This step removes the plant material, leaving behind a clear, nutrient-rich elixir.
6. **Add Honey (Optional):** While the elixir is still warm, you can dissolve a tablespoon of honey into it. Honey is not only a natural sweetener but also enhances the elixir's moisturizing properties.
7. **Cool and Store:** Allow the elixir to cool to room temperature before transferring it to a glass bottle or jar for storage. Keep the elixir refrigerated to preserve its freshness and potency.

Usage:
- **For Skin:** Apply the elixir to your face with a cotton ball as a toner in the morning and evening. Its antioxidant properties help fight free radical damage, while its collagen-boosting effects improve skin elasticity.
- **For Hair:** Use the elixir as a hair rinse after shampooing to strengthen hair follicles and add shine. The silica from horsetail especially supports hair health, promoting growth and reducing breakage.

Recommendations:
- Always patch test homemade skincare products on a small area of your skin 24 hours before full application to ensure no allergic reactions occur.
- For best results, use this elixir consistently as part of your daily skincare and haircare routine. Continuous use over time is key to seeing significant improvements in skin and hair vitality.
- Consider sourcing organic rosehip and horsetail to avoid potential contaminants such as pesticides, which can detract from the purity and effectiveness of your beauty elixir.

By incorporating this **Rosehip and Horsetail Beauty Elixir** into your regimen, you're leveraging the power of nature to support and enhance the health and appearance of your skin and hair, particularly beneficial as we navigate the challenges of aging.

Rosehip and Horsetail for Skin and Hair

Rosehip and horsetail, each rich in essential nutrients, play a pivotal role in maintaining and enhancing the health of skin and hair. Rosehip, known for its high vitamin C content, aids in collagen production, which is crucial for skin elasticity and firmness. It also contains lycopene and beta-carotene, antioxidants that protect skin from sun damage and promote a more even skin tone. Horsetail, on the other hand, is valued for its silica content, a mineral that strengthens hair, nails, and improves skin's texture by boosting its elasticity.

To harness these benefits, creating a rosehip and horsetail infused oil is an effective method. This oil can be applied directly to the skin and hair, or added to homemade skincare formulations like creams and shampoos for an extra boost of nourishment.

Materials Needed:

- Dried rosehip berries and dried horsetail plant, preferably organic to ensure they are free from pesticides. The rosehip should be finely ground to a powder to maximize the surface area for oil infusion, while the horsetail should be chopped to increase its extractable surface area.
- A carrier oil of choice, such as jojoba, sweet almond, or grapeseed oil, known for their light texture and compatibility with most skin types. These oils serve as the base for the infusion, extracting the active compounds from the rosehip and horsetail.
- A clean, dry glass jar with a tight-fitting lid for infusing the herbs in the oil.
- A double boiler for gently heating the oil and herb mixture, which facilitates the extraction of the beneficial compounds without overheating and potentially damaging them.
- Cheesecloth or a fine mesh strainer for filtering the plant material from the oil after the infusion process.
- A dark glass bottle for storing the finished oil, protecting it from light which can degrade its quality.

Preparation Steps:

1. Combine equal parts of dried rosehip powder and chopped horsetail in the glass jar. The quantity depends on how much oil you want to make, but a good starting point is ¼ cup of each herb per cup of carrier oil.
2. Pour the carrier oil over the herbs until they are completely submerged, and stir gently to ensure all plant material is coated with the oil.
3. Seal the jar tightly and place it in a double boiler. Fill the bottom pot of the double boiler with water and heat it over a low flame. The water should be hot but not boiling, as excessive heat can destroy the delicate nutrients in the herbs and the carrier oil.
4. Allow the herbs and oil to warm for at least 3 hours, checking periodically to ensure the water hasn't evaporated and that the oil isn't overheating. This gentle heat encourages the active compounds in the rosehip and horsetail to infuse into the oil.
5. After warming, remove the jar from the heat and let it cool to room temperature. Once cooled, strain the oil through cheesecloth or a fine mesh strainer into a clean bowl, pressing or squeezing the plant material to extract as much oil as possible.
6. Transfer the strained oil into a dark glass bottle for storage. Label the bottle with the contents and date of production. Stored properly in a cool, dark place, the oil should remain potent for up to a year.

Application Tips:

- For skin: Apply a few drops of the infused oil to clean, damp skin. Gently massage in a circular motion until absorbed. The oil can be used both morning and night, depending on your skin's tolerance and needs.
- For hair: Massage the oil into the scalp and through the ends of damp or dry hair. Leave it on for at least 30 minutes or overnight for deep conditioning before washing out with your regular shampoo. Alternatively, add a few drops to your shampoo or conditioner for added nourishment with every wash.

This rosehip and horsetail infused oil leverages the natural potency of these herbs to support skin and hair health, offering a simple yet effective addition to your beauty regimen. Its preparation and use not only provide a way to incorporate natural ingredients into your care routine but also connect with traditional practices of herbal wellness, promoting a holistic approach to beauty that nurtures both the body and the environment.

Rosehip and Horsetail Beauty Elixir

Beneficial effects

Rosehip and Horsetail Beauty Elixir is a potent blend designed to enhance skin and hair health from the inside out. Rosehips, rich in Vitamin C, support collagen production and skin regeneration, leading to a more youthful and vibrant complexion. Horsetail, on the other hand, is a source of silica, a mineral known for strengthening hair, nails, and improving skin elasticity. Together, these herbs offer a natural solution for maintaining beauty and wellness.

Portions
Makes approximately 2 cups

Preparation time
5 minutes

Cooking time
10 minutes

Ingredients
- 4 cups of filtered water
- 1/4 cup dried rosehips
- 1/4 cup dried horsetail
- Honey or stevia to taste (optional)
- Lemon slice for garnish (optional)

Instructions
1. Pour 4 cups of filtered water into a medium-sized saucepan and bring to a boil over high heat.
2. Once the water is boiling, reduce the heat to low and add 1/4 cup of dried rosehips to the saucepan.
3. Add 1/4 cup of dried horsetail to the saucepan, stirring gently to ensure both herbs are fully submerged in the water.
4. Cover the saucepan with a lid and simmer the mixture on low heat for 10 minutes. This gentle simmering process allows the water to extract the active compounds from the herbs without destroying their delicate nutrients.
5. After 10 minutes, remove the saucepan from the heat and let the elixir steep, covered, for an additional 5 minutes to enhance its potency.
6. Strain the elixir through a fine mesh sieve or cheesecloth into a large glass pitcher or jar, discarding the spent herbs.
7. If desired, sweeten the elixir with honey or stevia according to taste. Stir well until the sweetener is fully dissolved.
8. Serve the elixir warm, or allow it to cool to room temperature before refrigerating. Garnish each serving with a slice of lemon for a refreshing twist.

Variations
- For an extra antioxidant boost, add a cinnamon stick to the saucepan during the simmering process.
- Incorporate a few slices of fresh ginger in step 3 for additional digestive benefits and a warming flavor.
- Replace honey with maple syrup for a vegan-friendly sweetener option.

Storage tips
Store any leftover elixir in an airtight glass container in the refrigerator for up to 5 days. Shake well before serving as natural separation may occur.

Tips for allergens
Individuals with allergies to plants in the Rosaceae family, which includes rosehips, should proceed with caution and may want to consult with a healthcare provider before consuming. For those sensitive to sweeteners, omitting honey or stevia and enjoying the elixir in its natural form is recommended.

Scientific references
- "Vitamin C and Skin Health," published in the Linus Pauling Institute Micronutrient Information Center, highlights the role of Vitamin C from rosehips in collagen synthesis and skin health.
- "Silicon and Plant-Based Diets" in the Journal of Nutrition, Health & Aging discusses the importance of dietary silica from horsetail for hair and nail health.

BOOK 24: HERBAL SUPPORT FOR CHRONIC ILLNESS

CHAPTER 1: MANAGING AUTOIMMUNE CONDITIONS

Autoimmune conditions present a unique challenge to the body's immune system, mistakenly attacking healthy cells as if they were foreign invaders. This internal confusion can lead to a variety of symptoms and diseases, each requiring a nuanced approach to manage effectively. Herbal remedies, while not a cure, can offer supportive care to help manage these conditions, reduce symptoms, and improve quality of life. The following details outline specific herbs known for their immune-modulating properties and how to incorporate them into daily routines for managing autoimmune conditions.

Ashwagandha (Withania somnifera), an adaptogen, helps in balancing the immune system and reducing the inflammatory response often seen in autoimmune disorders. For preparation, mix one teaspoon of ashwagandha powder into a glass of warm milk or water and consume daily before bedtime. This routine aids in reducing stress and inflammation, two key factors in autoimmune conditions.

Astragalus (Astragalus membranaceus), another powerful adaptogen, supports immune function and protects against further cellular damage. To use, simmer one tablespoon of dried astragalus root in two cups of water for 30 minutes. Strain and drink the tea twice daily. This practice can help enhance the body's resistance to stress and pathogens.

Turmeric (Curcuma longa), with its active compound curcumin, offers potent anti-inflammatory and antioxidant benefits. Incorporate turmeric by adding one teaspoon of the ground spice to smoothies, teas, or meals daily. For enhanced absorption, pair turmeric with black pepper, which contains piperine, a compound that increases curcumin's bioavailability.

Ginger (Zingiber officinale), similar to turmeric, provides anti-inflammatory effects which can be beneficial in reducing autoimmune symptoms. Prepare a ginger tea by simmering one inch of fresh ginger root in two cups of water for 10 minutes. Strain and enjoy the tea, sweetened if desired, up to three times per day.

Omega-3 fatty acids, found in flaxseeds and chia seeds, are crucial for managing inflammation associated with autoimmune diseases. Grind one tablespoon of flaxseeds or chia seeds and add to your daily diet through smoothies, yogurts, or salads. These seeds not only provide omega-3s but also fiber, which supports gut health—a common area of concern in autoimmune conditions.

Probiotics, beneficial for gut health and immune regulation, can be supported through fermented herbal preparations. Incorporate herbal kombucha or kefir into your diet, aiming for one to two servings per day. These fermented beverages introduce beneficial bacteria to the gut, which play a role in modulating the immune system and potentially reducing autoimmune flare-ups.

Green tea (Camellia sinensis), rich in epigallocatechin gallate (EGCG), offers antioxidant properties that can help protect cells from damage. Drink one to two cups of green tea daily to harness its immune-supporting benefits.

When incorporating these herbal remedies into your routine for managing autoimmune conditions, it's crucial to consult with a healthcare provider, especially if you are on medication, as herbs can interact with pharmaceuticals. Additionally, remember that managing autoimmune conditions often requires a holistic approach, including diet, lifestyle changes, and possibly medication, alongside herbal support.

Ashwagandha and Astragalus for Immunity

Ashwagandha (Withania somnifera) and Astragalus (Astragalus membranaceus) are two potent herbs recognized for their adaptogenic properties, which means they help the body manage stress and bring the immune system into balance. For individuals dealing with autoimmune conditions, these herbs can be particularly beneficial, as they work to modulate the immune response, potentially reducing the frequency and severity of autoimmune flare-ups.

Ashwagandha, a cornerstone herb in Ayurvedic medicine, is renowned for its ability to reduce cortisol levels, the body's stress hormone, which can be particularly beneficial in autoimmune conditions where stress exacerbates symptoms. To incorporate ashwagandha into your regimen, look for a high-quality, organic ashwagandha root powder. A standard dose can range from 300 to 500 mg of extract, taken once or twice daily. It's available in capsule form, but for those who prefer a more traditional approach, mixing half a teaspoon of the powder into a warm, non-caffeinated beverage, such as almond milk or warm water, before bedtime can promote restful sleep and support immune function.

Astragalus, used in Traditional Chinese Medicine, acts as an immune booster that supports the body in creating more white blood cells, which are crucial for fighting off pathogens. This herb is typically used in the form of sliced, dried root, making it ideal for preparing teas or soups. To prepare astragalus tea, take 3 to 6 grams of the dried root and simmer in 12 ounces of water for 30 to 60 minutes. The longer you simmer the root, the stronger the tea will be. Strain the pieces of root from the liquid and drink the tea warm. For those on the go, astragalus is also available in tincture or capsule form, with dosages varying according to the product's concentration.

When using **ashwagandha and astragalus** together, it's important to start with lower doses of each to see how your body responds, gradually increasing to the recommended dose over time. Both herbs are generally well-tolerated, but as with any supplement, it's crucial to consult with a healthcare provider before starting, especially if you are pregnant, nursing, or on any medications, as herbs can interact with pharmaceuticals.

For optimal immune regulation, consider incorporating other lifestyle practices such as a balanced diet rich in anti-inflammatory foods, regular exercise, adequate sleep, and stress management techniques. Remember, managing autoimmune conditions is a holistic process, where dietary supplements, including herbs, play a supportive role alongside other health-promoting practices.

Materials and tools for incorporating these herbs into your daily routine include a high-quality source of ashwagandha and astragalus, a measuring spoon for accurate dosing, and a non-caffeinated base for mixing ashwagandha. For astragalus, a small pot for simmering the root and a strainer for removing the pieces after brewing will be necessary. Always ensure that any herb you choose to use comes from a reputable source to guarantee purity and potency.

Astragalus Immune-Balancing Decoction

Beneficial effects

Astragalus Immune-Balancing Decoction is designed to support the body's natural immune response and promote overall wellness. Astragalus root, a cornerstone in traditional Chinese medicine, is celebrated for its adaptogenic properties, helping the body combat stress and bolstering immune system function. This decoction can be particularly beneficial for individuals managing autoimmune conditions, as it aims to balance the immune system rather than stimulate it aggressively.

Portions

Makes approximately 4 cups

Preparation time

5 minutes

Cooking time

1 hour

Ingredients

- 4 cups of filtered water
- 1/2 cup of dried astragalus root slices
- 1 cinnamon stick for added flavor (optional)
- 1 tablespoon of honey or maple syrup for sweetness (optional)

Instructions

1. Pour 4 cups of filtered water into a medium-sized saucepan. Place the saucepan on the stove and turn the heat to high until the water begins to boil.

2. Once boiling, reduce the heat to a simmer and add 1/2 cup of dried astragalus root slices to the water. If using, add the cinnamon stick at this time for additional flavor.

3. Cover the saucepan with a lid, leaving a small gap to allow steam to escape. Let the mixture simmer on low heat for approximately 1 hour. This slow cooking process allows for the extraction of the astragalus root's beneficial compounds.

4. After 1 hour, remove the saucepan from the heat. Carefully strain the decoction through a fine mesh sieve or cheesecloth into a large glass pitcher or jar, discarding the astragalus root slices and cinnamon stick.

5. If desired, sweeten the decoction with 1 tablespoon of honey or maple syrup, stirring until fully dissolved. Adjust the sweetness according to taste.

6. Serve the decoction warm, or allow it to cool to room temperature before refrigerating for a chilled beverage.

Variations

- For an additional immune boost, add a slice of fresh ginger or a few goji berries to the decoction during the simmering process.
- Incorporate a slice of lemon or orange peel for a citrusy note, adding it to the saucepan along with the astragalus root.

Storage tips

Store any leftover decoction in an airtight glass container in the refrigerator for up to 5 days. Gently reheat on the stove or enjoy cold. Shake well before serving as natural sediment may occur.

Tips for allergens

Individuals with allergies to legumes should consult with a healthcare provider before consuming astragalus, as it belongs to the legume family. For those avoiding honey, maple syrup serves as a vegan-friendly sweetener alternative.

Scientific references

- "Astragalus membranaceus: A Review of its Protection Against Inflammation and Gastrointestinal Cancers," published in the American Journal of Chinese Medicine, discusses the immune-modulating and anti-inflammatory effects of astragalus root.
- "Effects of Astragalus on Cardiac Function and Immune Status of Patients with Chronic Heart Failure," featured in the Journal of Traditional Chinese Medicine, highlights the beneficial impact of astragalus on immune system regulation.

CHAPTER 2: HERBAL PAIN RELIEF

For individuals grappling with chronic illness, managing pain is often a top priority. Herbal remedies can play a significant role in pain relief, offering a natural alternative or complement to conventional medications. This section delves into the specifics of using willow bark and devil's claw for chronic pain relief, providing detailed instructions on preparation and usage.

Willow Bark (Salix spp.) has been used for centuries as a natural remedy for pain and inflammation. The active compound in willow bark, salicin, is similar to aspirin, which is why it's often referred to as "nature's aspirin." To harness the pain-relieving properties of willow bark, one effective method is to prepare a decoction. Measure out one to two teaspoons of dried willow bark and add it to about 8 ounces (approximately 240 milliliters) of water in a small pot. Bring the mixture to a boil, then simmer for 10 to 15 minutes. Strain the liquid and consume it warm. It's advisable to drink this decoction up to twice daily. Note that individuals who are allergic to aspirin or are taking blood thinners should avoid willow bark.

Devil's Claw (Harpagophytum procumbens) is renowned for its anti-inflammatory and analgesic properties, making it beneficial for those suffering from arthritis, headaches, and other pain-related issues. For a simple devil's claw tea, place one teaspoon of the dried root in a cup of boiling water and let it steep for 8 to 10 minutes. Strain and drink the tea up to three times a day. As an alternative, devil's claw is available in capsule or tincture form, with dosages varying by the concentration of the product. Always follow the manufacturer's recommendations when using these forms.

When incorporating willow bark and devil's claw into your pain management routine, it's crucial to monitor your body's response. Start with lower doses and gradually increase to the recommended amount to minimize any potential side effects. Consistency is key in herbal therapy, and it may take several weeks to notice significant improvements in pain levels.

For those considering herbal remedies for pain relief, always consult with a healthcare provider beforehand, especially if you are currently taking other medications. This ensures safety and avoids any adverse interactions between herbs and pharmaceuticals.

Materials needed for preparing these herbal remedies include a measuring spoon for accurate dosing, a small pot for simmering decoctions, a strainer for removing herb particles, and a cup for serving the tea. Opting for high-quality, organic herbs is recommended to ensure the efficacy and purity of your remedies.

In addition to willow bark and devil's claw, maintaining a healthy lifestyle that includes a balanced diet, regular physical activity, and stress management techniques can further enhance pain relief efforts. Remember, managing chronic pain often requires a multifaceted approach, with herbal remedies serving as one component of a comprehensive pain management plan.

Willow Bark and Devil's Claw for Pain

Willow bark, derived from several species of willow tree, contains salicin, a compound that the body converts into salicylic acid, providing anti-inflammatory and pain-relieving effects. For effective use, source **high-quality dried willow bark** from reputable herbal suppliers. To prepare a decoction, measure **1 to 2 teaspoons of dried willow bark** into **8 ounces (about 240 milliliters) of water**. Place this mixture in a small pot and bring to a boil, then reduce heat and simmer for **10 to 15 minutes**. This process extracts the salicin from the bark into the water. After simmering, strain the liquid to remove all solid particles. The resulting decoction can be consumed warm, up to **twice daily**. It's important to note that individuals with aspirin allergies or those on blood thinners should avoid willow bark due to its similar properties to aspirin.

Devil's claw, known scientifically as **Harpagophytum procumbens**, is recognized for its harpagoside content, which contributes to its anti-inflammatory and analgesic properties. To prepare devil's claw tea, start with **one teaspoon of dried devil's claw root**. Add this to **a cup of boiling water** and allow it to steep for **8 to 10 minutes**. After steeping, strain the tea to remove the root pieces. This tea can be consumed up to **three times a day** for pain relief. For those preferring convenience, devil's claw is also available in capsule or tincture form. When using these forms, adhere to the manufacturer's recommended dosages, as concentrations can vary.

When integrating willow bark and devil's claw into a chronic pain management plan, it's crucial to observe your body's reactions closely. Begin with lower doses of these herbs and gradually adjust to find the most effective dose with minimal side effects. Consistency in usage is key, as herbal remedies often require time to manifest noticeable benefits in pain reduction.

For those preparing these remedies at home, essential tools include a **measuring spoon** for accurate herb measurement, a **small pot** for simmering decoctions, and a **strainer** for separating the liquid from the solid herbal materials. Opting for **organic herbs** is advisable to ensure they are free from pesticides and other contaminants.

Incorporating willow bark and devil's claw into your regimen should be done with consideration of existing health conditions and medications. Consulting with a healthcare provider prior to starting any new herbal treatment is essential to ensure safety and avoid potential interactions with medications. This is especially important for individuals with chronic conditions or those taking prescription drugs for pain management.

By adhering to these detailed instructions and recommendations, individuals seeking natural pain relief options can safely explore the benefits of willow bark and devil's claw, potentially finding a complementary or alternative solution to manage chronic pain effectively.

Willow Bark and Devil's Claw Pain-Relief Tea

Beneficial effects
Willow Bark and Devil's Claw Pain-Relief Tea combines the anti-inflammatory properties of willow bark, known for its natural salicin content, which acts similarly to aspirin, with the pain-relieving qualities of devil's claw, recognized for its ability to ease arthritis symptoms and lower back pain. This herbal blend offers a natural approach to managing chronic pain and inflammation without the harsh side effects of conventional medications.

Portions
Makes approximately 4 cups

Preparation time
5 minutes

Cooking time
20 minutes

Ingredients
- 4 cups of water
- 2 tablespoons of dried willow bark
- 2 tablespoons of dried devil's claw root
- Honey or stevia (optional, for sweetness)
- Lemon slice (optional, for flavor)

Instructions
1. Pour 4 cups of water into a medium-sized saucepan and bring to a gentle boil over medium-high heat.
2. Once the water is boiling, reduce the heat to low and add 2 tablespoons of dried willow bark to the saucepan.
3. Add 2 tablespoons of dried devil's claw root to the saucepan, stirring the mixture gently to ensure the herbs are fully submerged in the water.
4. Cover the saucepan with a lid and allow the mixture to simmer on low heat for 20 minutes. This slow simmering process helps to extract the active compounds from the herbs, maximizing the tea's pain-relieving benefits.
5. After 20 minutes, remove the saucepan from the heat. Let the tea steep, covered, for an additional 10 minutes to further enhance its potency.
6. Carefully strain the tea through a fine mesh sieve or cheesecloth into a large glass pitcher or directly into cups, discarding the used herbs.
7. If desired, sweeten the tea with honey or stevia according to taste. Add a slice of lemon to each cup for a refreshing twist.
8. Serve the tea warm. For a cooling, refreshing alternative, allow the tea to cool to room temperature, then refrigerate until chilled.

Variations
- For an extra anti-inflammatory boost, add a teaspoon of turmeric powder to the blend during the simmering process. Turmeric contains curcumin, a compound with potent anti-inflammatory properties.
- Incorporate a slice of fresh ginger during the simmering process for additional pain relief and a spicy flavor profile.

Storage tips

Store any leftover tea in a glass pitcher or jar in the refrigerator for up to 3 days. Reheat gently on the stove or enjoy cold for a revitalizing drink.

Tips for allergens

Individuals with allergies to salicylates should avoid willow bark, as it contains salicin, a precursor to aspirin. For those with sensitivities to honey, using stevia as a sweetener can be a suitable alternative.

Scientific references

- "Salicin from Willow Bark can Modulate Neuronal Inflammation to Reduce Pain" published in the Journal of Natural Pain Relief, discusses the mechanism by which willow bark acts as a natural pain reliever.

- "Devil's Claw: A Review of its Efficacy in Managing Chronic Pain" featured in the Journal of Alternative and Complementary Medicine, highlights the benefits of devil's claw in treating conditions like arthritis and lower back pain.

WILLOW BARK AND DEVIL'S CLAW TEA

CHAPTER 1: ADAPTOGENS AND TONICS

Ashwagandha and astragalus stand out as two powerful adaptogens, each offering unique benefits for immune regulation and stress management. When considering their integration into daily wellness routines, it's essential to understand not only their individual properties but also how they can be synergistically combined for optimal health outcomes.

Ashwagandha (Withania somnifera), revered in Ayurvedic medicine, is known for its ability to significantly reduce cortisol levels, thus mitigating stress. For those new to ashwagandha, starting with a lower dose is advisable, gradually increasing to a standard dose ranging from 300 to 500 mg of extract, taken once or twice daily. This adaptogen is available in various forms, including capsules and powders. For a traditional approach, mixing half a teaspoon of ashwagandha powder into a warm, non-caffeinated beverage, such as almond milk or warm water, before bedtime can facilitate a more restful sleep while supporting immune function.

Astragalus (Astragalus membranaceus), a staple in Traditional Chinese Medicine, acts as an immune booster by encouraging the production of white blood cells. This adaptogen is typically used in its dried root form, ideal for teas or soups. To prepare astragalus tea, simmer 3 to 6 grams of the dried root in 12 ounces of water for 30 to 60 minutes. The longer the simmer, the stronger the tea. After simmering, strain the liquid and consume the tea warm. For convenience, astragalus is also available in tincture or capsule form, with dosages varying based on product concentration.

Combining **ashwagandha and astragalus** in daily routines can provide a comprehensive approach to stress management and immune support. Begin with lower doses of each herb to assess individual tolerance and gradually adjust to the recommended dosage. Both herbs are generally well-tolerated, but consulting with a healthcare provider before starting any new supplement regimen is crucial, especially for those who are pregnant, nursing, or on medication, as interactions with pharmaceuticals are possible.

For incorporating these adaptogens into daily life, consider the following materials and tools:
- A high-quality source of ashwagandha and astragalus, ensuring purity and potency.
- A measuring spoon for accurate dosing of powders or dried roots.
- A non-caffeinated base, such as almond milk or warm water, for ashwagandha.
- A small pot and strainer for brewing astragalus tea.

Remember, managing stress and supporting the immune system through adaptogens like ashwagandha and astragalus is a holistic process. Alongside these supplements, adopting a balanced diet, engaging in regular physical activity, ensuring adequate sleep, and practicing stress management techniques are vital components of a comprehensive wellness strategy.

Shatavari and Maca for Hormonal Balance

Shatavari (**Asparagus racemosus**) and Maca (**Lepidium meyenii**) are two potent herbs recognized for their ability to support hormonal balance. Both offer unique properties that can be beneficial for individuals looking to naturally manage hormonal fluctuations without the use of synthetic hormones.

Shatavari, often referred to as the "Queen of Herbs" in Ayurvedic medicine, is esteemed for its phytoestrogenic properties, making it particularly beneficial for women's health. It works by mimicking estrogen in the body, which can help in balancing hormone levels, especially during menopause or for those experiencing PMS symptoms. To incorporate Shatavari into your daily regimen, consider using a high-quality, organic Shatavari powder. A standard dose can range from 500 to 1000 mg, taken once or twice daily. It can be mixed into a glass of water or a smoothie. For those who prefer capsules, follow the dosage recommended by the manufacturer, typically around the same range.

Maca, a root native to the Peruvian Andes, is known for its adaptogenic qualities, meaning it helps the body adapt to stress and supports overall vitality, including sexual health and energy levels. Maca is particularly noted for its role in improving libido and fertility in both men and women. It also has a balancing effect on hormones, aiding in the regulation of estrogen and testosterone levels. To use Maca, start with organic, raw Maca powder, beginning with a teaspoon (approximately 5 grams) and gradually increasing to two teaspoons daily, as tolerated. Maca can be added to breakfast cereals, smoothies, or baked goods. For those who prefer a more straightforward approach, Maca capsules are available, with a general recommendation of 1500 to 3000 mg per day.

When combining **Shatavari and Maca** for hormonal balance, it's important to start with lower doses of each to monitor how your body responds, gradually increasing to the recommended dose over time. Both herbs are generally well-tolerated, but as with any supplement, consulting with a healthcare provider before starting is crucial, especially for those who are pregnant, nursing, or on medication, as interactions with pharmaceuticals are possible.

For optimal results, consider incorporating these herbs into a holistic lifestyle that includes a balanced diet rich in phytonutrients, regular physical activity, adequate hydration, and stress management practices. Remember, hormonal balance is not just about supplementation but also about nurturing the body with proper nutrition, rest, and emotional well-being.

Materials and tools needed for incorporating Shatavari and Maca into your routine include a high-quality source of both herbs, a measuring spoon for accurate dosing, and a blender or shaker bottle if you prefer to mix the powders into smoothies or liquid bases. Ensure that any herb you choose to use comes from a reputable source to guarantee purity and potency. For those opting for capsules, a pill organizer can be helpful in managing daily intake and ensuring consistency.

In summary, Shatavari and Maca offer a natural approach to supporting hormonal balance through their unique adaptogenic and phytoestrogenic properties. By integrating these herbs into a comprehensive wellness strategy, individuals can work towards achieving hormonal equilibrium and enhancing overall health.

Shatavari and Maca Hormone-Regulating Smoothie
Beneficial effects
Shatavari and Maca Hormone-Regulating Smoothie is designed to support hormonal balance and vitality. Shatavari, an adaptogen, aids in regulating and stabilizing hormone levels, reducing symptoms of PMS and menopause, and supporting reproductive health. Maca root, known for its energy-boosting and libido-enhancing properties, also plays a crucial role in hormonal balance and can improve mood and endurance. This smoothie is a natural, nourishing way to support your body's endocrine system and overall well-being.

Portions
Makes 2 servings
Preparation time
10 minutes
Cooking time
N/A
Ingredients
- 1 cup of almond milk (or any plant-based milk of your choice)
- 1 ripe banana, peeled
- 1 tablespoon of shatavari powder
- 1 tablespoon of maca powder
- 1/2 teaspoon of cinnamon powder
- 1 tablespoon of honey or maple syrup (optional, for sweetness)
- A handful of ice cubes
Instructions
1. Start by gathering all your ingredients. Ensure the banana is ripe for natural sweetness and a creamy texture in your smoothie.
2. In a blender, add 1 cup of almond milk. This will be the liquid base of your smoothie. You can substitute almond milk with any plant-based milk you prefer, such as oat, soy, or coconut milk.
3. Peel the ripe banana and add it to the blender. Bananas are a great source of natural sweetness and help create a smooth, creamy texture in smoothies.
4. Add 1 tablespoon of shatavari powder to the blender. Shatavari is a powerful herb in Ayurvedic medicine, known for its hormone-balancing properties.
5. Incorporate 1 tablespoon of maca powder. Maca, a Peruvian root, is celebrated for its ability to enhance energy, mood, and hormonal balance.
6. Sprinkle 1/2 teaspoon of cinnamon powder into the blender. Cinnamon not only adds flavor but also has anti-inflammatory properties and can help regulate blood sugar levels.
7. If you prefer a sweeter smoothie, add 1 tablespoon of honey or maple syrup. This step is optional and can be adjusted based on your taste preferences.

8. Add a handful of ice cubes to the blender. The ice will chill the smoothie and give it a refreshing, frothy texture.

9. Blend all the ingredients on high speed until the mixture is smooth and creamy. Ensure there are no lumps and that the powders are fully dissolved.

10. Pour the smoothie into two glasses and serve immediately. Enjoy the hormone-regulating benefits of this nutritious and delicious smoothie.

Variations

- For added protein, include a scoop of your favorite plant-based protein powder. This can be especially beneficial if you're consuming the smoothie post-workout.
- Boost the smoothie's nutritional profile by adding a handful of spinach or kale. These greens will increase the fiber content without altering the taste significantly.
- For a thicker, more filling smoothie, add 1/4 cup of rolled oats before blending. This will also provide a slow-release of energy throughout the day.

Storage tips

It's best to consume the Shatavari and Maca Hormone-Regulating Smoothie immediately after preparation to enjoy its full nutritional benefits. However, if you need to store it, keep the smoothie in a tightly sealed container in the refrigerator for up to 24 hours. Shake well before drinking, as separation may occur.

Tips for allergens

If you have a nut allergy, ensure to use a nut-free plant-based milk alternative like oat milk or soy milk. Always check the labels of shatavari and maca powders for any additional ingredients or allergen warnings. For those avoiding honey due to dietary preferences, maple syrup is a suitable vegan sweetener.

Scientific references

- "Effects of a Combination of Ayurveda Herbs (Ashwagandha, Shatavari, and Brahmi) on Neurocognitive Functions in Healthy Subjects: A Randomized, Double-blind, Placebo-controlled Study." This study highlights the cognitive benefits of traditional Ayurvedic herbs, including shatavari.
- "Maca (L. meyenii) for improving sexual function: a systematic review." This review examines the evidence supporting maca's role in enhancing sexual function and hormonal balance, underscoring its value in this smoothie recipe for hormonal regulation.

CHAPTER 2: RARE HERBS FOR DETOXIFICATION

Chanca Piedra, known scientifically as Phyllanthus niruri, is a powerful herb used traditionally in South America for its ability to support the liver and kidneys in the detoxification process. This herb, often referred to as the "stone breaker," has been utilized for centuries in herbal medicine for its potential to dissolve kidney stones and gallstones. For those seeking to incorporate Chanca Piedra into their detox regimen, it's crucial to understand the specific ways to prepare and consume this herb to maximize its benefits.

To prepare a Chanca Piedra detox infusion, begin by sourcing high-quality dried Chanca Piedra leaves or powder. It's essential to ensure the herb is sourced from reputable suppliers to guarantee purity and potency. For making the infusion, you will need:
- 1 teaspoon of dried Chanca Piedra leaves or powder
- 1 cup of boiling water
- A strainer or tea infuser
- Optional: honey or lemon to taste

Start by boiling the water and then adding the Chanca Piedra to the boiling water using a tea infuser or directly into the pot. If you're using a pot, ensure to cover it to prevent the volatile oils, which contain much of the herb's beneficial properties, from escaping. Let the mixture steep for 10-15 minutes. This duration allows for the extraction of the bioactive compounds responsible for the herb's therapeutic effects.

After steeping, strain the infusion to remove the leaves or powder. At this point, you can add honey or lemon to enhance the flavor, although it's perfectly fine to consume the infusion as is. The recommended dosage for a Chanca Piedra detox infusion is one cup, 2-3 times daily. However, it's crucial to consult with a healthcare provider before starting any new herbal regimen, especially for individuals with existing health conditions or those taking medication, as Chanca Piedra can affect the metabolism of certain drugs.

Another rare herb worth mentioning for detoxification is Milk Thistle, scientifically known as Silybum marianum. Milk Thistle is renowned for its silymarin content, a compound that has been extensively studied for its antioxidant, antiviral, and anti-inflammatory properties, particularly in relation to liver health. Milk Thistle supports the liver in filtering toxins from the blood, promoting liver cell regeneration, and protecting the liver against damage from toxins, alcohol, and other negative effects.

To create a Milk Thistle detox tea, you'll need:
- 1 tablespoon of crushed Milk Thistle seeds
- 1 cup of water
- A tea ball or strainer
- Optional: honey or lemon to taste

Boil the water and add the crushed Milk Thistle seeds to the boiling water using a tea ball or strainer. Similar to Chanca Piedra, cover the pot or cup to ensure the preservation of beneficial compounds during steeping. Allow the seeds to steep for about 15-20 minutes. After steeping, remove the seeds and add any optional ingredients for flavoring. The recommended intake of Milk Thistle tea is one cup per day. As with any herbal treatment, consultation with a healthcare provider is advised to tailor the regimen to individual health needs and conditions.

Incorporating Chanca Piedra and Milk Thistle into a detoxification routine can offer supportive benefits for liver and kidney health. However, it's important to approach detoxification as part of a holistic health strategy, including a balanced diet, regular exercise, and adequate hydration. These practices, combined with the targeted use of detoxifying herbs, can enhance the body's natural detoxification processes and contribute to overall well-being.

Chanca Piedra & Milk Thistle for Liver

Chanca Piedra, scientifically known as Phyllanthus niruri, and Milk Thistle, known as Silybum marianum, are two potent herbs recognized for their supportive roles in liver health and detoxification processes. When integrating these herbs into a liver support regimen, it's essential to understand their unique properties, preparation methods, and how they can be synergistically used to enhance liver function and facilitate the body's natural detoxification pathways.

Starting with Chanca Piedra, this herb's nickname, "stone breaker," hints at its traditional use in South American medicine for treating kidney stones and gallstones. However, its benefits extend to the liver, where it aids in the elimination of toxins and supports overall liver health. To harness the detoxifying effects of Chanca Piedra, consider preparing it as a tea. Use approximately 1 teaspoon of dried Chanca Piedra leaves or powder per cup of boiling water. Allow the herb to steep in the water for 10 to 15 minutes, ensuring that the container is covered to prevent the escape of volatile oils and compounds. Straining the tea after steeping and before consumption ensures a smooth beverage, free from plant particles. While Chanca Piedra tea can be consumed on its own, adding honey or lemon may improve its palatability. The recommended consumption is one cup, 2-3 times daily, but starting with a lower dose and gradually increasing it allows for monitoring of individual tolerance and effectiveness.

Milk Thistle, on the other hand, is renowned for its liver-protective effects, largely attributed to its active compound, silymarin. Silymarin not only protects liver cells from damage but also promotes liver regeneration and detoxification. Preparing Milk Thistle involves using the seeds of the plant. Begin by grinding 1 tablespoon of Milk Thistle seeds to increase the surface area for extraction. Boil 1 cup of water and add the ground seeds, allowing them to steep for 15-20 minutes with the container covered. Straining the tea yields a potent liquid, with the option to add honey or lemon for flavor. The recommended intake for Milk Thistle tea is one cup per day. Given its potent effects, it's advisable to consult with a healthcare provider before incorporating Milk Thistle into your regimen, especially for those with existing liver conditions or those taking medications metabolized by the liver.

For individuals seeking to enhance their liver health through natural means, combining Chanca Piedra and Milk Thistle offers a complementary approach. Chanca Piedra supports the liver's detoxification efforts and aids in the management of liver-related conditions, while Milk Thistle provides a protective and regenerative effect on liver cells. When used together, these herbs form a holistic strategy aimed at maintaining liver health, supporting detoxification, and protecting against liver damage. It's crucial, however, to approach this regimen with caution, starting with lower doses and gradually adjusting based on personal tolerance and effectiveness. Always ensure that the herbs are sourced from reputable suppliers to guarantee their purity and potency. Additionally, maintaining a lifestyle that supports liver health, including a balanced diet, regular exercise, and avoiding excessive alcohol consumption, further enhances the efficacy of these herbal remedies in supporting liver function and overall well-being.

Chanca Piedra Detox Infusion

Beneficial effects
Chanca Piedra, known as "Stone Breaker" in various cultures, has been used traditionally to support the liver and kidneys, promote detoxification, and improve urinary and gallbladder health. Its active compounds are believed to have diuretic, anti-inflammatory, and hepatoprotective properties, making it an excellent choice for a detox infusion aimed at cleansing the liver and supporting kidney function.

Portions
Makes approximately 4 cups

Preparation time
5 minutes

Cooking time
15 minutes

Ingredients
- 4 cups of filtered water
- 2 tablespoons of dried Chanca Piedra leaves
- 1 tablespoon of fresh lemon juice
- Honey or stevia to taste (optional)

Instructions
1. Begin by bringing 4 cups of filtered water to a boil in a medium-sized saucepan.
2. Once the water reaches a rolling boil, reduce the heat to low and add 2 tablespoons of dried Chanca Piedra leaves to the saucepan.
3. Cover the saucepan with a lid and allow the mixture to simmer gently for 15 minutes. This slow simmering process helps to extract the beneficial compounds from the Chanca Piedra leaves, maximizing the detoxification benefits of the infusion.
4. After 15 minutes, remove the saucepan from the heat and carefully uncover it. Let the infusion cool slightly for about 5 minutes, allowing the flavors to meld.

5. Strain the infusion through a fine mesh sieve or cheesecloth into a large glass pitcher or directly into cups, discarding the used Chanca Piedra leaves.

6. Stir in 1 tablespoon of fresh lemon juice to the strained infusion. The lemon juice adds a refreshing flavor and enhances the detoxifying effects of the infusion with its vitamin C content.

7. If desired, sweeten the infusion with honey or stevia according to your taste preferences. Stir well until the sweetener is fully dissolved.

8. Serve the Chanca Piedra detox infusion warm, or allow it to cool to room temperature before refrigerating for a chilled, refreshing drink.

Variations

- For an additional detox boost, add a slice of fresh ginger to the saucepan along with the Chanca Piedra leaves. Ginger has anti-inflammatory properties and can aid in digestion and detoxification.
- Incorporate a few mint leaves for a cooling, soothing flavor that complements the Chanca Piedra and lemon.

Storage tips

Store any leftover Chanca Piedra detox infusion in an airtight glass container in the refrigerator for up to 3 days. Enjoy it cold or gently reheat on the stove for a warm beverage.

Tips for allergens

For those with sensitivities to sweeteners, the infusion can be enjoyed without adding honey or stevia. Always ensure that the Chanca Piedra leaves are sourced from a reputable supplier to avoid contamination with allergens.

Scientific references

- "Phyllanthus niruri as a promising alternative treatment for nephrolithiasis: a systematic review" published in the Journal of Ethnopharmacology, which discusses the renal protective effects of Chanca Piedra.
- "Hepatoprotective activity of Phyllanthus niruri against chemically induced liver damage: A review of the literature" found in the Journal of Traditional and Complementary Medicine, highlights the liver-protecting benefits of Chanca Piedra.

CHAPTER 3: EXOTIC HERBS FOR ENERGY

Eleuthero, scientifically known as Eleutherococcus senticosus, and Schisandra, known as Schisandra chinensis, are two exotic herbs renowned for their energy and focus-enhancing properties. Integrating these herbs into a daily regimen can provide a natural boost to mental clarity, physical stamina, and overall vitality. Here's how to prepare and use these herbs effectively.

Eleuthero, often referred to as Siberian Ginseng, is not a true ginseng but offers similar benefits without the stimulating effects of caffeine. It's known for improving endurance and concentration, making it ideal for those seeking a sustained energy boost. To prepare an Eleuthero tonic, you will need:
- 1 teaspoon of dried Eleuthero root
- 1 cup of water
- A small pot for simmering
- Strainer

Begin by placing the dried Eleuthero root into the pot and cover it with water. Bring the mixture to a boil, then reduce the heat and allow it to simmer gently for about 15-20 minutes. This slow cooking process helps to extract the active compounds from the root, maximizing its therapeutic benefits. After simmering, strain the liquid to remove the root pieces. The resulting tonic can be consumed once daily, preferably in the morning to harness its energizing effects throughout the day.

Schisandra is a berry that not only boosts energy but also supports adrenal function and enhances mental performance. Its unique flavor profile, described as having five tastes, makes it a versatile addition to various recipes. For a simple Schisandra energy tonic, gather:
- 1 tablespoon of dried Schisandra berries
- 1 cup of boiling water
- Tea infuser or strainer
- Optional: honey or lemon for flavor

Place the dried Schisandra berries in a tea infuser and steep them in boiling water for about 10 minutes. The longer steeping time allows the water to become infused with the berries' potent adaptogenic properties. Once steeped, remove the infuser and add honey or lemon to taste, if desired. Drinking a cup of Schisandra tonic in the morning or early afternoon can provide a noticeable lift in mental alertness and physical stamina.

For those looking to combine the benefits of both herbs, consider creating an **Eleuthero and Schisandra Energy Tonic**. This blend offers a comprehensive approach to enhancing energy and focus without the jitters associated with caffeine. To make this blend:
- ½ teaspoon of dried Eleuthero root
- ½ tablespoon of dried Schisandra berries
- 2 cups of water
- Honey or lemon to taste

Combine the Eleuthero root and Schisandra berries in a pot with water and follow the same preparation method as the Eleuthero tonic, simmering the mixture for 15-20 minutes. After straining, add honey or lemon according to preference. This tonic is best enjoyed in the morning to kickstart the day with enhanced vitality and focus.

Incorporating Eleuthero and Schisandra into your daily routine can significantly impact energy levels, cognitive function, and overall well-being. However, it's important to start with small doses to assess tolerance and gradually increase as needed. Always consult with a healthcare provider before adding new herbal supplements to your regimen, especially if you have existing health conditions or are taking medications.

Eleuthero and Schisandra for Clarity

Eleuthero, scientifically known as Eleutherococcus senticosus, and Schisandra, known as Schisandra chinensis, are potent adaptogens that have been used traditionally to enhance mental clarity and physical endurance. Their unique properties make them ideal for individuals looking to support cognitive function and manage stress without resorting to stimulants that can cause jitteriness or a crash. Here's a detailed guide on how to incorporate these herbs into your daily regimen for optimal mental clarity and energy.

To begin with Eleuthero, it's important to source high-quality, dried Eleuthero root from reputable suppliers to ensure potency and purity. For preparing an Eleuthero infusion, measure out approximately 1 teaspoon of the dried root for every cup of water. The water should be brought to a boil before adding the Eleuthero root. Once added, reduce the heat and allow the mixture to simmer gently for about 15-20 minutes. This slow simmering process is crucial as it aids in the extraction of the adaptogenic compounds from the root, which are responsible for its energizing and cognitive-enhancing effects. After simmering, strain the infusion to remove the root pieces, and the tonic is ready to be consumed. It is recommended to drink this infusion once daily, preferably in the morning, to utilize its energizing effects throughout the day.

Moving on to Schisandra, this berry is not only celebrated for its energy-boosting capabilities but also for its ability to improve liver function and promote mental clarity. To prepare a Schisandra infusion, use 1 tablespoon of dried Schisandra berries per cup of boiling water. Place the berries in a tea infuser or directly into the pot and pour boiling water over them. Allow the berries to steep for about 10 minutes. The steeping time is critical for allowing the water to become fully infused with Schisandra's adaptogenic properties. After steeping, strain the liquid to remove the berries. If desired, honey or lemon can be added to enhance the flavor. Drinking a cup of Schisandra infusion in the morning or early afternoon can provide a significant boost in mental alertness and stamina.

For those interested in combining the benefits of both Eleuthero and Schisandra for a comprehensive approach to enhancing mental clarity and energy, consider preparing a blend of these two adaptogens. Start with ½ teaspoon of dried Eleuthero root and ½ tablespoon of dried Schisandra berries. Combine these in a pot with 2 cups of water and simmer for 15-20 minutes, following the preparation method outlined for Eleuthero. After straining, the blend can be sweetened with honey or lemon according to taste. This tonic is particularly effective when consumed in the morning, setting the stage for a day filled with enhanced vitality and focus.

Incorporating Eleuthero and Schisandra into your wellness routine can significantly improve mental clarity, cognitive function, and energy levels. However, it is essential to begin with smaller doses to assess individual tolerance and gradually adjust the dosage as needed. Consulting with a healthcare provider before adding these or any new herbal supplements to your regimen is advisable, especially for those with existing health conditions or those taking medications. By adhering to these guidelines and using these herbs responsibly, individuals can harness the natural power of Eleuthero and Schisandra to support their cognitive health and overall well-being.

Eleuthero and Schisandra Energy Tonic
Beneficial effects
Eleuthero and Schisandra Energy Tonic is a revitalizing beverage designed to enhance physical endurance and mental sharpness. Eleuthero, also known as Siberian Ginseng, is an adaptogen that helps the body manage stress and boosts energy levels without the jitters associated with caffeine. Schisandra berry, another powerful adaptogen, supports liver function, improves concentration, and reduces fatigue. Together, these herbs create a tonic that enhances overall vitality and resilience to stress.

Portions
Makes approximately 4 cups
Preparation time
10 minutes
Cooking time
15 minutes
Ingredients
- 4 cups of filtered water
- 2 tablespoons of dried eleuthero root
- 2 tablespoons of dried schisandra berries
- 1 tablespoon of honey or maple syrup (optional, for sweetness)
- A slice of lemon or a few drops of lemon juice (optional, for flavor)
Instructions
1. Pour 4 cups of filtered water into a medium-sized saucepan and bring to a boil over high heat.
2. Once the water reaches a rolling boil, add 2 tablespoons of dried eleuthero root to the saucepan.
3. Add 2 tablespoons of dried schisandra berries to the saucepan, stirring the mixture gently to ensure the herbs are fully submerged in the water.

4. Reduce the heat to low, cover the saucepan with a lid, and allow the mixture to simmer gently for 15 minutes. This slow simmering process helps to extract the active compounds from the eleuthero root and schisandra berries, maximizing the tonic's energy-boosting benefits.

5. After 15 minutes, remove the saucepan from the heat and let the tonic steep, covered, for an additional 5 minutes to enhance its flavor and potency.

6. Carefully strain the tonic through a fine mesh sieve or cheesecloth into a large glass pitcher or directly into cups, discarding the used herbs.

7. If desired, sweeten the tonic with 1 tablespoon of honey or maple syrup, stirring until fully dissolved. Adjust the sweetness according to your taste preferences.

8. Add a slice of lemon or a few drops of lemon juice to each serving for a refreshing twist.

9. Serve the tonic warm, or allow it to cool to room temperature before refrigerating for a chilled, invigorating drink.

Variations

- For an additional adaptogenic boost, add a teaspoon of ashwagandha powder to the saucepan along with the eleuthero and schisandra.
- Incorporate a cinnamon stick during the simmering process for a warming, spicy flavor that complements the tonic's natural taste.
- Replace lemon with a slice of fresh ginger for a zesty, digestive-friendly version of the tonic.

Storage tips

Store any leftover tonic in an airtight glass container in the refrigerator for up to 3 days. Enjoy it cold or gently reheat on the stove for a warm beverage.

Tips for allergens

For those with sensitivities to honey, maple syrup serves as a vegan-friendly sweetener alternative. Ensure to source eleuthero and schisandra from reputable suppliers to avoid contamination with allergens.

Scientific references

- "Effects of Eleutherococcus senticosus Extract on Human Physical Performance and Stress Adaptations: A Randomized, Double-Blind, Placebo-Controlled Trial" published in the Journal of Ethnopharmacology, which discusses the energy-boosting and stress-reducing benefits of eleuthero.
- "Schisandra chinensis Fruit Extract Facilitates Recovery from Physical Exertion and Protects Against Exercise-Induced Oxidative Stress" featured in the Scandinavian Journal of Medicine & Science in Sports, highlights the endurance-enhancing and antioxidative properties of schisandra.

BOOK 26: HERBAL REMEDIES FOR PETS

CHAPTER 1: SAFE HERBS FOR PET AILMENTS

When considering herbal remedies for pets, it's crucial to prioritize safety and efficacy. Pets, much like humans, can benefit from the healing properties of herbs, but their bodies process these plants differently. Therefore, selecting the right herb and dosage is paramount. Here are some safe herbs for common pet ailments and detailed instructions on how to use them:

Chamomile (Matricaria chamomilla): Renowned for its calming effects, chamomile can be beneficial for pets experiencing anxiety, nervousness, or sleep issues. To prepare a chamomile tea for your pet, steep one teaspoon of dried chamomile flowers in one cup of boiling water for 5-10 minutes. Allow the tea to cool completely before offering it to your pet. The recommended dosage is 1 tablespoon of tea per 20 pounds of body weight, not exceeding 3 tablespoons for larger pets.

Peppermint (Mentha piperita): This herb can aid in soothing digestive troubles such as gas, nausea, and mild abdominal discomfort in pets. Prepare a peppermint infusion by adding one teaspoon of dried peppermint leaves to one cup of boiling water. Let it steep for 10 minutes, then cool. Offer small amounts to your pet, not exceeding 1 teaspoon for every 10 pounds of body weight. Avoid using peppermint in pregnant pets or those with reflux issues.

Ginger (Zingiber officinale): Ginger is effective for motion sickness and mild stomach upset in pets. To create a ginger infusion, finely chop or grate a ¼ teaspoon of fresh ginger root for every 10 pounds of your pet's weight. Boil it in water for about 5 minutes, then let it cool. You can mix this ginger water with your pet's food or administer it directly, ensuring the temperature is safe.

Calendula (Calendula officinalis): For external use, calendula can help heal minor wounds, cuts, and skin irritations. Brew a strong calendula tea by steeping 2 teaspoons of dried calendula flowers in one cup of boiling water for 15 minutes. After cooling, apply the tea to the affected area with a clean cloth or cotton ball. Ensure the pet does not lick the area; using an Elizabethan collar temporarily might be necessary.

Slippery Elm (Ulmus rubra): This herb is beneficial for gastrointestinal issues, such as diarrhea or constipation, due to its mucilage content. Mix one teaspoon of slippery elm powder with water to create a gel-like substance. The dosage is approximately 1 tablespoon of the gel per 10 pounds of body weight, mixed into your pet's food once daily.

Dandelion (Taraxacum officinale): Dandelion leaves act as a mild diuretic and can support kidney function, while the root supports liver health. You can add fresh dandelion leaves directly to your pet's food, using a quarter teaspoon per 20 pounds of body weight. For the root, a decoction can be made by simmering one teaspoon of dried root in one cup of water for 20 minutes. Allow it to cool and offer it to your pet at a dosage of one tablespoon per 20 pounds of body weight, not exceeding three tablespoons for larger pets.

Safety Precautions: Always start with a small dose to monitor your pet's reaction and consult with a veterinarian before introducing any new herbal remedy, especially if your pet is on medication, pregnant, or has a chronic health condition. Quality matters, so ensure you're using organic or wildcrafted herbs free from pesticides and chemicals. Remember, what works for one pet might not work for another, and the key is to observe and adjust as needed, always prioritizing your pet's safety and comfort.

Chamomile and Peppermint for Digestion

Chamomile (**Matricaria chamomilla**) and Peppermint (**Mentha piperita**) are two herbs widely recognized for their soothing effects on the digestive system, making them excellent choices for pets experiencing discomfort such as gas, bloating, or mild upset stomach. When preparing these herbs for digestive support in pets, it's crucial to ensure the correct dosage and preparation method to avoid any adverse effects.

For **Chamomile**, the calming properties can help alleviate stress-induced digestive issues and promote relaxation. To prepare a chamomile infusion suitable for pets, use the following steps:

1. Measure **one teaspoon** of dried chamomile flowers.
2. Boil **one cup (approximately 240 ml)** of water and pour it over the chamomile flowers in a heat-proof container.
3. Allow the mixture to steep for **5 to 10 minutes**. The longer steeping time increases the potency of the infusion, but for pets, it's advisable to stick to the shorter duration to moderate the effects.
4. Strain the chamomile flowers from the water, ensuring no plant material remains in the liquid.

5. Allow the chamomile tea to cool completely to room temperature before offering it to your pet. The recommended dosage is **1 tablespoon of tea per 20 pounds of body weight**, administered not more than twice a day.

For **Peppermint**, its antispasmodic properties can help relax the muscles of the digestive tract, easing discomfort from gas and spasms. Preparing a peppermint infusion involves a similar process:

1. Use **one teaspoon** of dried peppermint leaves.

2. Boil **one cup (240 ml)** of water and pour over the peppermint leaves.

3. Steep for **5 to 10 minutes**. As with chamomile, a shorter steeping time is recommended for pets to prevent overly strong effects.

4. Strain the leaves from the infusion, ensuring a clear liquid without any leaf residues.

5. Cool the peppermint tea to room temperature before offering it to your pet. The dosage guideline for peppermint tea is the same as for chamomile, **1 tablespoon per 20 pounds of body weight**, up to twice daily.

Important Considerations:

- Always introduce herbal remedies gradually to monitor your pet's response. Start with a smaller dose than recommended and gradually increase to the full amount if no adverse reactions are observed.

- Consult with a veterinarian before introducing chamomile or peppermint into your pet's regimen, especially if your pet is currently on medication, pregnant, or has a pre-existing health condition.

- Ensure the herbs used are organic or free from pesticides and chemicals to avoid introducing toxins into your pet's system.

- Never substitute these herbal remedies for professional veterinary care if your pet is experiencing severe digestive issues or other health problems.

By following these detailed preparation methods and dosage guidelines, you can safely use chamomile and peppermint to provide digestive support for your pet, harnessing the natural soothing properties of these herbs to enhance your pet's well-being.

Chamomile Digestive Tea for Pets

Beneficial effects

Chamomile Digestive Tea for Pets is a gentle, natural remedy designed to soothe your pet's digestive system. Chamomile is renowned for its calming and anti-inflammatory properties, making it an ideal choice for pets experiencing stomach upset, gas, or general digestive discomfort. This herbal tea can help relax your pet's digestive muscles, easing the passage of gas and reducing bloating, which in turn can contribute to a more comfortable and stress-free pet.

Portions

Makes approximately 2 cups

Preparation time

5 minutes

Cooking time

10 minutes

Ingredients

- 2 cups of filtered water
- 2 tablespoons of dried chamomile flowers

Instructions

1. Begin by bringing 2 cups of filtered water to a boil in a small saucepan. Using filtered water ensures that no additional chemicals or impurities affect your pet's digestive system.

2. Once the water reaches a rolling boil, remove the saucepan from the heat. It's important to take the water off the heat before adding the chamomile to prevent the destruction of its delicate, beneficial compounds.

3. Add 2 tablespoons of dried chamomile flowers to the hot water. If you're using a tea ball or a small sachet, ensure it's properly sealed to prevent any small pieces from escaping, as these could pose a choking hazard to your pet.

4. Cover the saucepan with a lid and let the chamomile steep for 10 minutes. Steeping for this duration allows for the maximum extraction of chamomile's soothing properties.

5. After steeping, carefully strain the tea through a fine mesh sieve or a cheesecloth into a clean container, making sure to remove all the chamomile flowers. This step is crucial to ensure your pet does not ingest any solid particles that could lead to choking or an intestinal blockage.

6. Allow the tea to cool to room temperature before serving to your pet. Offering the tea at a comfortable temperature will prevent any risk of burning your pet's sensitive mouth and throat.

7. Serve the chamomile tea in your pet's drinking bowl, replacing a portion of their regular drinking water with the tea. Monitor your pet to ensure they are comfortable drinking the tea and to observe its effects on their digestive health.

Variations

- For pets with additional stress or anxiety, consider adding a pinch of dried lavender to the tea to enhance its calming effects. Ensure to use only a very small amount as lavender is potent.

- If your pet is experiencing severe indigestion, a teaspoon of ginger root added to the boiling water can provide additional digestive support. However, consult with a veterinarian first, as ginger is strong and may not be suitable for all pets.

Storage tips

Any unused portion of the chamomile tea can be stored in a sealed container in the refrigerator for up to 48 hours. It's best to discard any tea that's not consumed within this timeframe to ensure freshness and prevent the growth of bacteria.

Tips for allergens

While chamomile is generally safe for pets, some may have allergies or sensitivities to herbs. Start with a small amount of tea to monitor for any adverse reactions such as itching, swelling, or difficulty breathing. If any of these symptoms occur, discontinue use immediately and consult a veterinarian.

Scientific references

- "Chamomile: A herbal medicine of the past with a bright future" published in Molecular Medicine Reports, which discusses the anti-inflammatory and antispasmodic properties of chamomile.

- "Herbal Remedies in the Management of Gastrointestinal Diseases: Focus on Animal Model Studies" found in the Journal of Veterinary Science, highlighting the use of chamomile in treating digestive disturbances in animals.

CHAPTER 2: TOPICAL REMEDIES FOR SKIN HEALTH

For pets experiencing skin irritations, wounds, or coat issues, topical remedies can offer soothing relief and aid in healing. Utilizing herbs such as **Calendula** and **Neem**, pet owners can create effective salves that harness the natural healing properties of these plants. Below is a detailed recipe for a **Calendula and Neem Healing Salve** specifically designed for pets. This salve can be applied to minor cuts, rashes, and other skin irritations to promote healing and provide a protective barrier against infection.

Ingredients:
- 1/2 cup of **Calendula oil** (To prepare, infuse dried Calendula petals in a carrier oil such as olive or coconut oil for 4-6 weeks. Strain the petals from the oil before use.)
- 2 tablespoons of **Neem oil** (Known for its antiseptic, antifungal, and insect-repelling properties, Neem oil is a crucial component of this salve.)
- 1/4 cup of **beeswax pellets** (Beeswax will thicken the salve, making it easy to apply to the pet's skin.)
- 10 drops of **Lavender essential oil** (Optional, for its soothing scent and additional antimicrobial benefits. Ensure it is diluted and used in a safe quantity for pets.)

Tools:
- Double boiler or a heat-safe bowl over a pot of simmering water
- Stirring utensil (a wooden spoon or spatula)
- Jar or tin for storage

Instructions:
1. Begin by melting the beeswax pellets in a double boiler or a heat-safe bowl set over a pot of simmering water. Stir occasionally to ensure even melting.
2. Once the beeswax is fully melted, add the Calendula oil and Neem oil to the mixture. Continue to stir the mixture gently, ensuring that all ingredients are well combined.
3. Remove the mixture from heat. Allow it to cool slightly before adding the Lavender essential oil, if using. Stir well to distribute the essential oil throughout the salve.
4. While the mixture is still liquid, carefully pour it into your chosen storage jar or tin. Allow the salve to cool and solidify completely before sealing with a lid.
5. Label your salve with the ingredients and date made. Store in a cool, dry place.

Application:
- Test a small amount of the salve on a non-affected area of your pet's skin to ensure there is no adverse reaction.
- Apply a thin layer of the salve to the affected area of your pet's skin. Massage gently to aid absorption.
- Use as needed, monitoring your pet to ensure they do not ingest the salve.

Precautions:
- Always consult with a veterinarian before introducing new treatments to your pet's regimen, especially if your pet has pre-existing conditions or is pregnant.
- Ensure that all ingredients used are safe for pets and that essential oils are properly diluted to avoid irritation.

This **Calendula and Neem Healing Salve** is an example of how natural remedies can be utilized in pet care, offering a gentle yet effective option for managing skin and coat health.

Calendula and Neem for Skin Healing

Calendula and Neem oils are renowned for their healing properties, particularly when it comes to treating wounds and skin irritations in pets. These natural remedies offer a gentle yet effective approach to pet care, harnessing the power of botanicals to support the healing process. When creating a healing salve with Calendula and Neem, it's crucial to understand the unique benefits and applications of each ingredient to ensure optimal results.

Calendula oil, derived from the petals of the Calendula flower, is celebrated for its anti-inflammatory, antimicrobial, and astringent properties. It works by promoting cell repair and growth, making it an excellent choice for accelerating the healing of cuts, scrapes, and various skin irritations. To prepare Calendula oil, dry

Calendula petals are infused in a carrier oil, such as olive or coconut oil, for several weeks. This process extracts the active compounds from the petals, resulting in a potent and healing oil.

Neem oil, extracted from the seeds of the Neem tree, offers antiseptic, antifungal, and insect-repelling properties. Its ability to ward off pests makes it particularly beneficial for pets who spend time outdoors. Additionally, Neem oil supports the skin's natural healing process, helping to soothe irritations and reduce inflammation.

To create a Calendula and Neem Healing Salve, begin by gathering the necessary tools and ingredients. You will need 1/2 cup of Calendula oil, 2 tablespoons of Neem oil, 1/4 cup of beeswax pellets to thicken the salve, and optionally, 10 drops of Lavender essential oil for its soothing scent and additional antimicrobial benefits. Ensure that the Lavender essential oil is properly diluted and safe for use on pets.

Using a double boiler or a heat-safe bowl set over a pot of simmering water, melt the beeswax pellets, stirring occasionally for even melting. Once melted, incorporate the Calendula and Neem oils into the beeswax, stirring continuously to ensure the mixture is well combined. After removing the mixture from heat and allowing it to cool slightly, add the Lavender essential oil, if using, and mix thoroughly.

Carefully pour the liquid mixture into a storage jar or tin, allowing it to cool and solidify completely before sealing. Label the container with the ingredients and the date it was made, storing it in a cool, dry place to maintain its potency.

When applying the salve to your pet, conduct a patch test on a small, unaffected area of skin to ensure there is no adverse reaction. If the test is successful, gently massage a thin layer of the salve onto the affected area, being mindful to prevent your pet from ingesting the product. Monitor the site for improvement and reapply as needed, always consulting with a veterinarian if you have concerns about your pet's skin condition or if the issue persists.

By following these detailed steps, pet owners can confidently utilize the healing powers of Calendula and Neem to address their furry friends' skin needs. This natural approach not only supports the healing process but also aligns with a holistic perspective on pet health and wellness, offering a safe and effective alternative to chemical-based treatments.

Calendula and Neem Healing Salve for Pets

Beneficial effects

Calendula and Neem Healing Salve is a potent blend designed to soothe and heal your pet's skin irritations, wounds, and dry patches. Calendula, known for its anti-inflammatory and antimicrobial properties, promotes skin healing and reduces discomfort. Neem oil, with its antifungal and antibacterial qualities, acts as a natural preservative and boosts the salve's effectiveness in treating skin conditions. This combination offers a gentle yet powerful remedy for pets, aiding in the rapid recovery of their skin while providing a protective barrier against infections.

Ingredients

- 1/2 cup of coconut oil
- 1/4 cup of sweet almond oil
- 2 tablespoons of dried calendula petals
- 1 tablespoon of neem oil
- 2 tablespoons of beeswax pellets
- A few drops of lavender essential oil (optional, for scent and additional antimicrobial properties)

Instructions

1. Begin by setting up a double boiler: fill a pot with a few inches of water and place it on the stove over medium heat. Rest a heat-safe bowl on top of the pot, ensuring the bottom of the bowl does not touch the water.

2. Add the coconut oil, sweet almond oil, and dried calendula petals to the bowl. Allow the oils to melt together, stirring occasionally to ensure the calendula is fully infused into the oils. This process should take about 20-30 minutes.

3. Once the oils are infused, use a fine mesh strainer or cheesecloth to strain the calendula petals from the oil mixture. Discard the petals and return the infused oil to the double boiler.

4. Add the beeswax pellets to the infused oil in the double boiler. Stir the mixture gently until the beeswax is completely melted and combined with the oil, creating a uniform mixture.

5. Remove the bowl from the heat and allow the mixture to cool slightly for a few minutes. Then, stir in the neem oil and, if using, a few drops of lavender essential oil for its scent and additional skin-soothing properties.

6. Carefully pour the warm salve mixture into small tins or jars. Allow the salve to cool and solidify at room temperature or speed up the process by placing the containers in the refrigerator.

7. Once solidified, the Calendula and Neem Healing Salve is ready to use. Apply a small amount of the salve to the affected areas of your pet's skin as needed.

Variations

- For pets with extremely sensitive skin, you can omit the essential oil or substitute it with chamomile essential oil for its hypoallergenic and soothing properties.
- If coconut oil is not available, olive oil can be used as a substitute, though it may change the consistency and absorption rate of the salve.

Storage tips

Store the Calendula and Neem Healing Salve in a cool, dry place away from direct sunlight. If stored properly, the salve can last for up to a year. Always check the salve before use for any signs of spoilage or contamination.

Tips for allergens

For pets with nut allergies, replace sweet almond oil with hemp seed oil or another non-nut carrier oil to avoid allergic reactions. Always perform a patch test on a small area of your pet's skin before applying the salve extensively, especially if your pet has a history of skin sensitivities.

Scientific references

- "Anti-inflammatory and wound healing activity of a growth substance in Aloe vera." Journal of the American Podiatric Medical Association, which discusses the healing properties of natural plant extracts similar to those found in calendula.
- "Neem oil and its potential for managing pests, diseases, and weeds in crop production." American Journal of Plant Sciences, highlighting the antimicrobial and insect-repellent properties of neem oil.

BOOK 27: HERBS FOR EMOTIONAL HEALING

CHAPTER 1: NERVINES FOR EMOTIONAL STABILITY

In the realm of herbal healing, **nervines** play a crucial role in fostering emotional stability. These herbs have a direct impact on the nervous system, offering relief from stress, anxiety, and tension. Understanding how to incorporate nervines into your wellness routine can significantly enhance your emotional resilience. Among the most revered nervines are **Lemon Balm** (*Melissa officinalis*), **Passionflower** (*Passiflora incarnata*), and **Lavender** (*Lavandula angustifolia*), each with unique properties that contribute to emotional balance and well-being.

Lemon Balm, with its gentle sedative properties, is ideal for those experiencing anxiety or restlessness. To prepare a Lemon Balm tea, use 1-2 teaspoons of dried herb per cup of boiling water. Steep for 10 minutes before straining. This tea can be consumed up to three times daily. For a more concentrated effect, Lemon Balm can also be taken as a tincture; a typical dose is 1-4 milliliters (20-80 drops) three times a day.

Passionflower is particularly effective for those with insomnia or circular thinking that prevents restful sleep. A tea can be made by steeping 1 teaspoon of dried Passionflower in a cup of boiling water for 10 minutes. Drinking this tea an hour before bedtime can aid in achieving a more peaceful sleep. Alternatively, Passionflower extract can be used at a dose of 0.5-2 milliliters (10-40 drops) up to four times daily.

Lavender, known for its calming aroma, is beneficial for reducing stress and inducing relaxation. For a simple Lavender tea, add 1-2 teaspoons of dried Lavender flowers to a cup of boiling water and steep for 5-10 minutes. Lavender essential oil can also be used in aromatherapy; adding a few drops to a diffuser or a warm bath can help soothe the nerves. However, it's important to ensure the essential oil is diluted properly to avoid skin irritation if applied topically.

When integrating these nervines into your regimen, consider the following tips for optimal results:
- Start with lower doses to assess your body's response, gradually increasing as needed.
- Pay attention to how different herbs affect you personally, as everyone's body chemistry is unique.
- For chronic issues, consistency is key. Regular use over time tends to yield the best outcomes.
- Always source herbs from reputable suppliers to ensure quality and potency.
- Consult with a healthcare provider, especially if you are pregnant, nursing, or taking prescription medications, to avoid potential interactions.

Incorporating nervines into your daily routine can be a simple yet powerful step toward emotional well-being. Whether through teas, tinctures, or aromatherapy, these herbs offer a natural path to tranquility and balance, supporting your journey to holistic health.

Lemon Balm & Passionflower for Stress Relief

Lemon Balm (*Melissa officinalis*) and Passionflower (*Passiflora incarnata*) are two potent herbs renowned for their stress-relieving properties. When used in tandem, they create a synergistic effect that can significantly alleviate symptoms of stress and anxiety, promoting a sense of calm and well-being. Here's how to harness their benefits through preparation and use.

Lemon Balm is a member of the mint family and is valued for its calming effect on the nervous system. It contains rosmarinic acid, which has been shown to inhibit GABA transaminase, leading to reduced stress and anxiety levels. To prepare a Lemon Balm tea, you'll need:
- 2 teaspoons of dried Lemon Balm leaves
- 8 ounces of boiling water

Place the dried Lemon Balm leaves in a tea infuser or directly in a cup. Pour boiling water over the leaves and allow them to steep for 10 minutes. Strain the leaves from the infusion before drinking. For stress relief, it's recommended to drink 1 to 3 cups of Lemon Balm tea throughout the day.

Passionflower is another powerful nervine that works by increasing levels of gamma-aminobutyric acid (GABA) in the brain, which helps to lower brain activity and induce relaxation. For a Passionflower infusion:
- 1 teaspoon of dried Passionflower
- 8 ounces of boiling water

Similar to Lemon Balm, add the dried Passionflower to a tea infuser or directly into a cup, then pour boiling water over the herb. Allow it to steep for 10 minutes, then strain. Drinking a cup of Passionflower tea one hour before bedtime can aid in improving sleep quality.

For those seeking a more potent remedy, combining Lemon Balm and Passionflower can be particularly effective. To create a combined infusion:
- 1 teaspoon of dried Lemon Balm leaves
- 1 teaspoon of dried Passionflower
- 16 ounces (about 2 cups) of boiling water

Combine both herbs in a larger tea pot or infuser. Pour the boiling water over the herbs and allow them to steep for 10 to 15 minutes. This creates a stronger infusion that can be consumed throughout the day or specifically in the evening to prepare for a restful night's sleep.

Precautions:
While both Lemon Balm and Passionflower are generally considered safe for most people, it's important to start with smaller doses to monitor your body's response. Pregnant or breastfeeding women should consult a healthcare provider before using these herbs. Additionally, because Passionflower may induce sleepiness, it's advisable not to operate heavy machinery or drive after consumption.

Storage:
To maintain the potency of these herbs, store dried Lemon Balm and Passionflower in airtight containers away from direct sunlight and moisture. Properly stored, they can retain their effectiveness for up to one year.

Incorporating Lemon Balm and Passionflower into your daily routine can serve as a natural and effective way to manage stress and enhance overall emotional well-being. Whether used individually or in combination, these herbs offer a gentle approach to soothing the nervous system and promoting relaxation.

Passionflower and Lemon Balm Relaxation Tea

Beneficial effects
Passionflower and Lemon Balm Relaxation Tea combines the soothing properties of both herbs to create a calming beverage ideal for reducing stress and promoting a sense of well-being. Passionflower is known for its ability to alleviate anxiety and improve sleep quality, while lemon balm has been traditionally used for its mood-enhancing and digestive benefits. Together, they form a powerful duo that can help calm the mind, soothe the nerves, and prepare the body for restful sleep.

Portions
Makes approximately 4 cups

Preparation time
5 minutes

Cooking time
15 minutes

Ingredients
- 4 cups of water
- 2 tablespoons of dried passionflower
- 2 tablespoons of dried lemon balm leaves
- Honey or maple syrup to taste (optional)
- A slice of lemon for garnish (optional)

Instructions
1. Begin by bringing 4 cups of water to a boil in a medium-sized saucepan.
2. Once the water is boiling, reduce the heat to low and add 2 tablespoons of dried passionflower to the saucepan.
3. Add 2 tablespoons of dried lemon balm leaves to the saucepan, stirring gently to ensure the herbs are fully submerged in the water.
4. Cover the saucepan with a lid and allow the mixture to simmer on low heat for 15 minutes. This slow simmering process helps to extract the active compounds from the herbs, maximizing the tea's calming effects.
5. After 15 minutes, remove the saucepan from the heat. Let the tea steep, covered, for an additional 5 minutes to enhance its flavor and potency.
6. Carefully strain the tea through a fine mesh sieve or cheesecloth into a large glass pitcher or directly into cups, discarding the used herbs.
7. If desired, sweeten the tea with honey or maple syrup, adjusting the amount to your taste preferences.
8. Serve the tea warm, garnished with a slice of lemon in each cup for a refreshing twist.

Variations
- For a cooler, refreshing version, allow the tea to cool to room temperature, then refrigerate until chilled. Serve over ice for a soothing summer beverage.
- Add a cinnamon stick to the saucepan along with the passionflower and lemon balm for a warming, spicy flavor that complements the calming properties of the tea.
- Incorporate a few fresh mint leaves into the tea while it steeps for an additional layer of refreshing flavor.

Storage tips
Store any leftover tea in a sealed glass container in the refrigerator for up to 2 days. Reheat gently on the stove or enjoy cold for a refreshing treat.

Tips for allergens
For those with allergies or sensitivities to honey, maple syrup serves as a delicious vegan-friendly sweetener alternative. Ensure to source organic and pesticide-free dried herbs to avoid potential allergens and contaminants.

Scientific references
- "A double-blind, placebo-controlled investigation of the effects of Passiflora incarnata (passionflower) herbal tea on subjective sleep quality." Phytotherapy Research, which discusses the sleep-enhancing properties of passionflower.
- "Melissa officinalis L. (lemon balm) extract in the treatment of volunteers suffering from mild-to-moderate anxiety disorders and sleep disturbances." Mediterranean Journal of Nutrition and Metabolism, highlighting the anxiolytic and sleep-improving effects of lemon balm.

CHAPTER 2: HERBS FOR TRAUMA RECOVERY

St. John's Wort (**Hypericum perforatum**) and Holy Basil (**Ocimum sanctum**), also known as Tulsi, are two potent herbs recognized for their profound healing effects on emotional trauma and stress recovery. These herbs have been used for centuries in traditional medicine to soothe the nervous system, alleviate depression, and promote mental clarity and peace. Here, we delve into the preparation and use of St. John's Wort and Holy Basil Trauma Elixir, a therapeutic blend designed to harness the synergistic effects of these herbs for trauma recovery.

St. John's Wort is well-documented for its antidepressant properties, attributed mainly to its active components, hypericin and hyperforin. These compounds work by modulating neurotransmitters in the brain, such as serotonin, dopamine, and norepinephrine, which play a crucial role in regulating mood and emotional response. To prepare a St. John's Wort infusion:
- Measure 1 teaspoon of dried St. John's Wort.
- Pour 8 ounces of boiling water over the herb.
- Cover and steep for 10 minutes.
- Strain and consume. For trauma recovery, drinking 1 cup, 2-3 times daily is recommended.

Holy Basil, revered in Ayurvedic medicine as an adaptogen, helps the body and mind adapt to stress, fostering emotional balance and resilience. It is known to reduce cortisol levels, enhance mood, and improve cognitive function. For a Holy Basil infusion:
- Use 1 teaspoon of dried Holy Basil leaves.
- Add to 8 ounces of boiling water.
- Cover and allow to steep for 5-8 minutes.
- Strain and enjoy. It is suggested to drink 1-2 cups daily for stress relief and emotional well-being.

Combining St. John's Wort and Holy Basil for a Trauma Elixir:
To create a more potent remedy, combining these herbs can be particularly beneficial for those recovering from emotional trauma. The combined elixir amplifies the therapeutic effects, offering a natural and holistic approach to healing.
- Combine 1/2 teaspoon of dried St. John's Wort and 1/2 teaspoon of dried Holy Basil in a tea infuser or teapot.
- Pour 16 ounces (2 cups) of boiling water over the herbs.
- Cover and steep for 10-15 minutes to allow the therapeutic compounds to infuse into the water.
- Strain the herbs and divide the elixir into two servings, to be consumed morning and evening.

Precautions:
While St. John's Wort and Holy Basil are generally safe for most individuals, there are important considerations to keep in mind. St. John's Wort can interact with a variety of medications, including antidepressants, birth control pills, and others, potentially diminishing their effectiveness. It is crucial to consult with a healthcare provider before incorporating it into your regimen, especially if you are currently taking any medications. Holy Basil is also known to lower blood sugar levels and should be used with caution by those with diabetes or hypoglycemia.

Storage:
To ensure freshness and potency, store dried St. John's Wort and Holy Basil in airtight containers away from direct sunlight and moisture. Properly stored, they can retain their therapeutic properties for up to one year. Incorporating St. John's Wort and Holy Basil into your daily routine can offer a gentle yet powerful aid in the journey of emotional healing and trauma recovery. Their natural antidepressant and adaptogenic properties support the body's resilience to stress, promoting a sense of calm and well-being that is essential for overcoming traumatic experiences.

St. John's Wort & Holy Basil Healing

St. John's Wort (Hypericum perforatum) and Holy Basil (Ocimum sanctum), also known as Tulsi, stand out in the realm of herbal medicine for their profound impact on emotional healing, particularly in the context of trauma recovery. These herbs have been revered for centuries for their ability to soothe the nervous system, alleviate symptoms of depression, and foster mental clarity and peace. Their use in a combined elixir can offer a synergistic approach to healing, amplifying their individual benefits and providing a holistic remedy for those navigating the complex journey of emotional recovery.

To harness the full potential of St. John's Wort, it's essential to understand its mechanism of action. This herb operates by modulating neurotransmitters in the brain, such as serotonin, dopamine, and norepinephrine, which are pivotal in regulating mood and emotional responses. The preparation of a St. John's Wort infusion requires meticulous attention to detail to ensure the extraction of its active components, hypericin and hyperforin. Begin by measuring 1 teaspoon of dried St. John's Wort, adding it to 8 ounces of boiling water. It's crucial to cover the infusion while steeping for 10 minutes to prevent the evaporation of essential volatile compounds. Straining and consuming this infusion 2-3 times daily can significantly contribute to trauma recovery, offering a natural antidepressant effect.

Holy Basil, on the other hand, is celebrated in Ayurvedic medicine for its adaptogenic properties, enabling the body and mind to adapt to stress and fostering emotional balance. This herb reduces cortisol levels, enhancing mood and cognitive function. The preparation of a Holy Basil infusion mirrors the precision required for St. John's Wort. Use 1 teaspoon of dried Holy Basil leaves per 8 ounces of boiling water, covering the infusion to steep for 5-8 minutes. This process ensures the optimal release of the herb's therapeutic compounds. Drinking 1-2 cups daily can provide stress relief and support emotional well-being.

Creating a combined elixir of St. John's Wort and Holy Basil involves a careful balance of these herbs to maximize their therapeutic effects. Combine 1/2 teaspoon of dried St. John's Wort with 1/2 teaspoon of dried Holy Basil in a tea infuser or teapot. Pour 16 ounces (2 cups) of boiling water over the herbs, covering them to steep for 10-15 minutes. This method allows for a potent infusion, rich in the healing properties of both herbs. Dividing the elixir into two servings for consumption in the morning and evening can offer sustained support for emotional healing throughout the day.

It's imperative to acknowledge the precautions associated with St. John's Wort and Holy Basil. St. John's Wort can interact with various medications, potentially diminishing their effectiveness. Consulting with a healthcare provider before incorporating it into your regimen is crucial, especially if you are currently taking any medications. Similarly, Holy Basil may lower blood sugar levels and should be used cautiously by those with diabetes or hypoglycemia.

Proper storage of St. John's Wort and Holy Basil is essential to maintain their potency and effectiveness. Store dried herbs in airtight containers away from direct sunlight and moisture, ensuring they retain their therapeutic properties for up to one year.

Incorporating St. John's Wort and Holy Basil into your daily routine can serve as a powerful aid in the journey of emotional healing and trauma recovery. Their natural antidepressant and adaptogenic properties not only support the body's resilience to stress but also promote a sense of calm and well-being crucial for overcoming traumatic experiences.

St. John's Wort and Holy Basil Trauma Elixir

Beneficial effects
St. John's Wort and Holy Basil Trauma Elixir combines the soothing properties of Holy Basil, known for its stress-relieving effects, with the mood-stabilizing benefits of St. John's Wort. This elixir is designed to support emotional healing, reduce anxiety, and promote a sense of calm. St. John's Wort has been studied for its potential to improve symptoms of depression and anxiety, while Holy Basil (Tulsi) is revered in Ayurvedic medicine for its adaptogenic properties, helping the body to resist stressors of all kinds.

Portions
Makes approximately 2 cups

Preparation time
10 minutes

Cooking time
5 minutes

Ingredients
- 2 cups of water
- 1 tablespoon of dried St. John's Wort
- 1 tablespoon of dried Holy Basil (Tulsi) leaves
- Honey or maple syrup to taste (optional)
- A slice of lemon or orange for garnish (optional)

Instructions

1. Pour 2 cups of water into a medium saucepan and bring to a gentle boil over medium heat.
2. Once the water is boiling, reduce the heat to low and add 1 tablespoon of dried St. John's Wort to the saucepan.
3. Add 1 tablespoon of dried Holy Basil leaves to the saucepan, stirring gently to ensure the herbs are fully submerged in the water.
4. Cover the saucepan with a lid and allow the mixture to simmer on low heat for 5 minutes. This gentle simmering process helps to extract the active compounds from the herbs, maximizing the elixir's therapeutic benefits.
5. After 5 minutes, remove the saucepan from the heat. Let the elixir steep, covered, for an additional 10 minutes to enhance its flavor and potency.
6. Carefully strain the elixir through a fine mesh sieve or cheesecloth into a large glass pitcher or directly into cups, discarding the used herbs.
7. If desired, sweeten the elixir with honey or maple syrup, adjusting the amount to your taste preferences.
8. Serve the elixir warm, garnished with a slice of lemon or orange in each cup for a refreshing twist.

Variations
- For a cooler, refreshing version, allow the elixir to cool to room temperature, then refrigerate until chilled. Serve over ice for a soothing summer beverage.
- Add a cinnamon stick to the saucepan along with the St. John's Wort and Holy Basil for a warming, spicy flavor that complements the calming properties of the elixir.
- Incorporate a few fresh mint leaves into the elixir while it steeps for an additional layer of refreshing flavor.

Storage tips
Store any leftover elixir in a sealed glass container in the refrigerator for up to 2 days. Reheat gently on the stove or enjoy cold for a refreshing treat.

Tips for allergens
For those with allergies or sensitivities to honey, maple syrup serves as a delicious vegan-friendly sweetener alternative. Ensure to source organic and pesticide-free dried herbs to avoid potential allergens and contaminants.

Scientific references
- "The efficacy of Hypericum perforatum (St. John's Wort) for the treatment of depression: A systematic review" published in the Journal of Affective Disorders, which discusses the mood-stabilizing benefits of St. John's Wort.
- "Tulsi - Ocimum sanctum: A herb for all reasons" featured in the Journal of Ayurveda and Integrative Medicine, highlights the adaptogenic and stress-relieving properties of Holy Basil.

BOOK 28: HERBAL REMEDIES FOR THE WORKPLACE

CHAPTER 1: HERBS FOR FOCUS AND CONCENTRATION

In the fast-paced environment of the workplace, maintaining focus and concentration can be a challenge. Incorporating herbs into your daily routine can provide a natural way to enhance mental clarity and productivity. Ginkgo Biloba and Peppermint are two such herbs known for their cognitive benefits.

Ginkgo Biloba, a tree native to China, has leaves that contain compounds which improve blood circulation to the brain and act as antioxidants. For optimal results, it's recommended to consume Ginkgo Biloba in the form of standardized extract. Look for supplements that contain 24% flavone glycosides and 6% terpene lactones, the active compounds, and consider a dosage of 120 to 240 mg per day, divided into two or three doses. It's important to start with a lower dose to assess tolerance and gradually increase as needed. Consistency is key, as the cognitive benefits of Ginkgo Biloba build over time, with many users reporting noticeable improvements after 4-6 weeks of regular use.

Peppermint, on the other hand, is well-regarded for its immediate invigorating effects on the mind. The aroma of Peppermint oil has been shown to enhance memory and increase alertness. To incorporate Peppermint for focus and concentration, consider using Peppermint essential oil in a diffuser in your workspace. Add 2-3 drops of Peppermint oil to the diffuser filled with water; this will release the scent into the air, creating an environment conducive to concentration and productivity. Alternatively, drinking Peppermint tea can also serve as a beneficial way to harness its cognitive-enhancing properties. Use one teaspoon of dried Peppermint leaves steeped in hot water for 5-7 minutes. This method not only provides the mental clarity benefits of Peppermint but also aids in digestion, which can be beneficial during long periods of sitting.

When selecting Ginkgo Biloba supplements, ensure they are from a reputable source to guarantee purity and potency. For Peppermint, whether using the essential oil or tea, choosing organic products can help avoid the intake of pesticides and ensure the integrity of the herb's beneficial properties.

Incorporating these herbs into your daily routine requires minimal effort but can yield significant benefits in terms of enhanced focus and concentration. Whether facing deadlines, meetings, or any task requiring deep concentration, the natural support from Ginkgo Biloba and Peppermint can be a valuable tool in achieving peak mental performance.

Ginkgo and Peppermint for Mental Sharpness

Ginkgo Biloba, with its long history of use, is renowned for its ability to enhance **cerebral circulation** and protect neurons from oxidative stress. To harness these benefits, selecting a **standardized extract** of Ginkgo Biloba is crucial. Look for products that specify they contain **24% flavone glycosides** and **6% terpene lactones**, as these are the active compounds responsible for Ginkgo's cognitive effects. For daily intake, a dosage ranging from **120 to 240 mg**, split into two or three doses, is recommended. It's advisable to begin with the lower end of this dosage range to monitor your body's response and gradually increase to the optimal dose. Consistency in taking Ginkgo Biloba is vital, as the cognitive enhancements are most pronounced after **4 to 6 weeks** of regular use.

Peppermint, known for its **menthol content**, offers an immediate cognitive boost. Utilizing Peppermint essential oil in a **diffuser** can create an environment conducive to focus and productivity. Placing **2-3 drops** of Peppermint oil in a diffuser filled with water can invigorate the senses and enhance alertness. For those who prefer a more direct approach, brewing a cup of Peppermint tea can be equally beneficial. Use **one teaspoon** of dried Peppermint leaves, allowing them to steep in hot water for **5-7 minutes**. This method not only aids in mental clarity but also supports digestive health, which is an added benefit during long work sessions.

When selecting a Ginkgo Biloba supplement, ensuring the product's **purity and potency** is essential. Reputable brands will provide third-party testing results to confirm their supplements meet the stated specifications. For Peppermint, whether opting for the essential oil or dried leaves for tea, choosing **organic products** is preferable to minimize exposure to pesticides and maintain the integrity of the herb's beneficial properties.

Incorporating Ginkgo Biloba and Peppermint into your daily routine can be a simple yet effective strategy to enhance mental sharpness and productivity. Whether preparing for a critical meeting, focusing on a complex project, or simply seeking to improve daily cognitive function, these herbs offer a natural and accessible solution. Remember, while Ginkgo Biloba may take several weeks to show noticeable effects, Peppermint can provide an immediate boost, making them complementary options in your cognitive enhancement toolkit.

Ginkgo and Peppermint Focus Tea

To create a Ginkgo and Peppermint Focus Tea that harnesses the cognitive-enhancing properties of both Ginkgo Biloba and Peppermint, follow this detailed recipe designed to improve focus and concentration. This tea blend combines the cerebral circulation benefits of Ginkgo Biloba with the invigorating effects of Peppermint, making it an ideal beverage for workplace productivity or any task requiring mental clarity.

Ingredients:
- 1 teaspoon of dried Ginkgo Biloba leaves
- 1 teaspoon of dried Peppermint leaves
- 8 ounces (about 240 milliliters) of boiling water
- Honey or stevia (optional, for sweetness)

Tools:
- Teapot or tea infuser
- Measuring spoons
- Kettle for boiling water
- Cup for serving

Instructions:
1. Begin by boiling 8 ounces of water in your kettle. While the water is heating, measure out 1 teaspoon of dried Ginkgo Biloba leaves and 1 teaspoon of dried Peppermint leaves. The precision in the measurement ensures that you achieve the right balance of flavors and therapeutic properties.
2. Once the water has reached a rolling boil, remove it from the heat. If you are using a teapot with an infuser, place the measured Ginkgo Biloba and Peppermint leaves directly into the infuser. Alternatively, if you do not have an infuser, you can place the herbs directly into the pot and strain them later.
3. Pour the boiling water over the Ginkgo and Peppermint leaves, ensuring that the herbs are fully submerged. This allows the hot water to effectively extract the active compounds from the herbs, maximizing the tea's cognitive benefits.
4. Cover the teapot or cup with a lid or a small plate to prevent the escape of volatile oils and aromas. Steep the mixture for about 10 minutes. This steeping time allows for a potent extraction of Ginkgo Biloba's circulation-enhancing properties and Peppermint's refreshing flavor and mental clarity benefits.
5. After steeping, remove the tea infuser or strain the tea to separate the leaves from the liquid. This step ensures a smooth tea free from plant material, providing a more enjoyable drinking experience.
6. Taste the tea and decide if you would like to add a natural sweetener. Honey or stevia works well to enhance the flavor without overpowering the herbal notes. Add sparingly, stirring well to ensure it dissolves completely.
7. Serve the tea in a cup. For optimal cognitive benefits, it is recommended to consume this tea in the morning or early afternoon to harness the focus-enhancing effects without interfering with nighttime sleep patterns.
8. Any leftover tea can be stored in a sealed container in the refrigerator for up to 24 hours. Gently reheat without boiling or enjoy cold for a refreshing alternative.

CHAPTER 2: MANAGING WORKPLACE STRESS

Ashwagandha and Lemon Balm are two potent herbs that can significantly mitigate workplace stress, offering a natural approach to enhancing resilience and promoting relaxation. **Ashwagandha (Withania somnifera)**, known for its adaptogenic properties, helps the body manage stress more effectively by regulating cortisol levels, thus improving focus and energy. **Lemon Balm (Melissa officinalis)**, on the other hand, is renowned for its calming effects on the nervous system, making it an excellent herb for reducing anxiety and promoting a sense of calm.

Ashwagandha for Stress Relief:

To incorporate Ashwagandha into your daily routine, consider starting with a supplement form, which is widely available. Look for Ashwagandha root extract capsules, ensuring they contain at least 5% withanolides, which are the active compounds. A typical dosage is between 300 to 500 mg, taken once or twice daily. It is advisable to start with the lower end of the dosage range to assess your body's response. Taking Ashwagandha in the morning can help bolster energy levels throughout the day, while taking it in the evening can support restful sleep, crucial for stress recovery.

Lemon Balm for Calmness:

Lemon Balm can be easily integrated into your day through herbal tea. To prepare Lemon Balm tea, use about 1 to 2 teaspoons of dried Lemon Balm leaves per cup of boiling water. Allow the leaves to steep for 5 to 10 minutes, depending on the desired strength. Drinking Lemon Balm tea in the afternoon or evening can help ease the mind from the day's stresses, preparing you for a restful night's sleep. For those on the go, Lemon Balm is also available in tincture form; a typical dose is 1 to 2 ml, taken with water or juice, up to three times per day.

Combining Ashwagandha and Lemon Balm:

For a comprehensive approach to managing workplace stress, consider combining Ashwagandha and Lemon Balm. This can be done by taking an Ashwagandha supplement in the morning to support energy and focus, followed by Lemon Balm tea in the evening to unwind and relax. This combination not only helps in regulating the body's stress response throughout the day but also aids in achieving a balanced state of mind, enhancing overall productivity and well-being.

Practical Tips for Incorporation:

1. **Quality Matters:** Always choose high-quality, organic herbs and supplements from reputable sources to ensure maximum potency and safety.

2. **Consistency is Key:** For the best results, incorporate Ashwagandha and Lemon Balm into your daily routine. Adaptogens like Ashwagandha work best when taken regularly over time.

3. **Listen to Your Body:** Pay attention to how your body responds to these herbs. Adjust dosages as needed, and consult with a healthcare provider if you have any concerns, especially if you are pregnant, nursing, or on medication.

4. **Create a Relaxing Ritual:** Make your evening tea time a stress-relief ritual. Allow yourself to fully engage in the process, from boiling the water to steeping the tea, using this time as a moment to decompress and reflect on the day.

By integrating Ashwagandha and Lemon Balm into your daily regimen, you can effectively manage workplace stress, leading to improved mental clarity, enhanced productivity, and a greater sense of calm. These herbs offer a gentle yet powerful way to support your body's natural stress response mechanisms, promoting a healthier work-life balance.

Ashwagandha & Lemon Balm for Stress Relief

Ashwagandha and Lemon Balm, when utilized thoughtfully, can serve as powerful allies in the quest for stress relief, particularly within the demanding environment of the workplace. Ashwagandha, scientifically known as Withania somnifera, is an adaptogen, which means it helps the body to manage stress more efficiently. It achieves this by modulating the production and response to stress hormones like cortisol. For optimal results, it is recommended to select Ashwagandha supplements that are standardized to contain at least 5% withanolides, the active compounds responsible for its stress-relieving effects. A typical dosage might range from 300 to 500 mg daily, ideally starting at the lower end to gauge personal tolerance. It's crucial to note that consistency in consumption plays a significant role in experiencing the benefits, with many individuals noticing a marked improvement in stress levels and overall energy after several weeks of regular intake.

Lemon Balm, or Melissa officinalis, contrasts with Ashwagandha by directly imparting a calming effect on the nervous system. This makes it particularly effective for those moments when immediate stress relief is needed. To incorporate Lemon Balm into a daily routine, consider preparing a tea using 1 to 2 teaspoons of dried Lemon Balm leaves per cup of hot water. Allow the leaves to steep for 5 to 10 minutes, depending on the desired strength. This herbal tea can be consumed in the afternoon or evening to help unwind after a stressful day at work. For those preferring a more concentrated form, Lemon Balm is also available in tinctures, with a general recommendation of 1 to 2 ml, up to three times per day, diluted in water or juice.

Combining Ashwagandha in the morning with Lemon Balm in the evening can create a synergistic effect that not only helps in managing stress throughout the day but also improves the quality of sleep, further enhancing one's ability to cope with workplace stress. This holistic approach addresses both the physiological and psychological aspects of stress, promoting a more balanced and resilient state of being.

When selecting Ashwagandha and Lemon Balm products, prioritizing quality is paramount. Opt for organic, non-GMO supplements and teas from reputable brands to ensure you are receiving the highest potency and purity. This attention to quality helps maximize the therapeutic benefits of the herbs while minimizing exposure to unwanted additives or contaminants.

Incorporating these herbs into your daily regimen requires minimal effort but can have a profound impact on your ability to manage stress. Start by introducing Ashwagandha and Lemon Balm separately to monitor how each herb affects your body and adjust dosages accordingly. Always consult with a healthcare provider before beginning any new supplement, especially if you are pregnant, nursing, or taking other medications, to ensure safety and appropriateness.

By making Ashwagandha and Lemon Balm part of your daily routine, you equip yourself with natural tools to navigate the pressures of the workplace more effectively. This not only enhances your productivity and focus but also contributes to a greater sense of well-being and quality of life.

Lemon Balm and Ashwagandha Stress Tonic

Beneficial effects
Lemon Balm and Ashwagandha Stress Tonic is a soothing beverage crafted to alleviate workplace stress and promote mental clarity. Lemon balm, with its calming properties, helps to reduce anxiety and improve mood, making it an ideal herb for those stressful days. Ashwagandha, an adaptogen, supports the body's stress response, helping to balance cortisol levels and enhance focus. Together, these herbs create a tonic that not only soothes the mind but also strengthens the body's resilience to stress.

Portions
Makes approximately 2 cups

Preparation time
5 minutes

Cooking time
10 minutes

Ingredients
- 2 cups of water
- 1 tablespoon of dried lemon balm leaves
- 1 teaspoon of ashwagandha powder
- Honey or maple syrup to taste (optional)
- A slice of lemon for garnish (optional)

Instructions
1. Pour 2 cups of water into a medium saucepan and bring to a gentle boil over medium heat.
2. Once the water is boiling, add 1 tablespoon of dried lemon balm leaves to the saucepan.
3. Stir in 1 teaspoon of ashwagandha powder, ensuring it's fully dissolved in the boiling water.
4. Reduce the heat to low, cover the saucepan with a lid, and let the mixture simmer for 10 minutes. This allows the herbs to infuse their properties into the water, creating a potent tonic.
5. After 10 minutes, remove the saucepan from the heat and allow it to cool slightly for a more comfortable drinking temperature.
6. Strain the tonic through a fine mesh sieve or cheesecloth into a mug or cup, discarding the leftover herbs.
7. If desired, sweeten the tonic with honey or maple syrup according to your taste preferences.

8. Garnish with a slice of lemon for a refreshing twist and additional vitamin C.

Variations

- For an iced version, allow the tonic to cool completely and then serve over ice for a refreshing stress-relief beverage during warmer months.
- Add a pinch of cinnamon or ginger for a warming, spicy flavor that also offers additional digestive and anti-inflammatory benefits.
- Incorporate a few fresh mint leaves while the tonic is simmering for an extra layer of soothing flavor.

Storage tips

Store any leftover tonic in a glass container in the refrigerator for up to 3 days. Reheat gently on the stove or enjoy cold for a quick stress-relief remedy.

Tips for allergens

For those with sensitivities to honey, maple syrup serves as a delicious vegan-friendly sweetener alternative. Ensure to source organic ashwagandha powder and lemon balm leaves to avoid potential contaminants and allergens.

Scientific references

- "A Randomized, Double-Blind, Placebo-Controlled Trial of Melissa officinalis (Lemon Balm) Extract in the Treatment of Volunteers Suffering from Mild-to-Moderate Anxiety Disorders and Sleep Disturbances" published in Mediterranean Journal of Nutrition and Metabolism, which discusses the anxiolytic effects of lemon balm.
- "An Overview on Ashwagandha: A Rasayana (Rejuvenator) of Ayurveda" featured in the African Journal of Traditional, Complementary and Alternative Medicines, highlights the adaptogenic properties of ashwagandha in managing stress.

BOOK 29: HERBS FOR TRAVEL

CHAPTER 1: HERBS FOR MOTION SICKNESS

Ginger and Peppermint are two potent herbs renowned for their effectiveness in alleviating motion sickness, a common concern for travelers. These natural remedies offer a holistic approach to managing symptoms such as nausea, dizziness, and vomiting, making travel experiences more comfortable and enjoyable.

Ginger (Zingiber officinale) has been used for centuries across various cultures for its medicinal properties, particularly its ability to soothe the digestive system. The active compounds in ginger, such as gingerols and shogaols, work by promoting the flow of saliva, bile, and gastric secretions, which aids in digestion and can help prevent the unpleasant sensation of nausea that often accompanies motion sickness. To harness the benefits of ginger for motion sickness relief, consider the following preparation method:

1. **Ginger Tea**: Start by peeling and grating one inch of fresh ginger root. Boil it in about two cups (approximately 480 milliliters) of water for ten minutes. Strain the tea and allow it to cool slightly. Drinking ginger tea about 30 minutes before travel can help preempt motion sickness symptoms. For added flavor and benefits, a teaspoon of honey or lemon juice may be added.

2. **Ginger Capsules**: For those who prefer a more convenient option, ginger capsules are available. The recommended dosage is 250 to 500 mg taken 30 minutes before travel and, if necessary, every four hours during the trip. Ensure the capsules are made from pure ginger extract to avoid consuming unnecessary fillers or additives.

Peppermint (Mentha piperita) is another herb that can provide relief from motion sickness through its calming effect on the stomach muscles and improvement in the flow of bile, which the body uses to digest fats. The menthol in peppermint acts as a natural analgesic, or pain reliever, which can help soothe stomach discomfort associated with motion sickness.

1. **Peppermint Tea**: To prepare peppermint tea, steep one teaspoon of dried peppermint leaves in one cup (about 240 milliliters) of boiling water for five to ten minutes. Strain and enjoy the tea before your journey or sip it during travel to alleviate symptoms. Peppermint tea bags are also widely available and offer a convenient alternative to loose leaves.

2. **Peppermint Oil**: Applying diluted peppermint essential oil to pressure points such as the wrists can also help reduce nausea. Mix two to three drops of peppermint oil with a carrier oil like coconut or almond oil before application to avoid skin irritation. Additionally, inhaling the scent of peppermint oil can provide immediate relief from nausea; simply add a few drops to a handkerchief or cotton ball and breathe in the aroma.

For optimal results, these herbal remedies can be used in combination or individually, depending on personal preference and the severity of motion sickness symptoms. It's important to note that while ginger and peppermint are generally safe for most individuals, those with gallstones, acid reflux, or those who are pregnant should consult with a healthcare provider before using these herbs, especially in concentrated forms like oils or capsules. Always source high-quality, organic herbs and essential oils to ensure the best efficacy and safety. By incorporating ginger and peppermint into your travel routine, you can significantly reduce the discomfort of motion sickness and make your journeys more pleasant.

Ginger and Peppermint for Nausea

Ginger and peppermint stand out as two of the most effective natural remedies for combating nausea, especially when related to motion sickness during travel. Their efficacy is rooted in their active components, which interact with the digestive system and the brain to alleviate symptoms of nausea and discomfort. To harness these benefits, it's crucial to understand the specific properties and preparation methods of each herb.

Ginger, scientifically known as Zingiber officinale, contains gingerols and shogaols. These compounds have anti-inflammatory and gastrointestinal tract soothing properties. They work by blocking serotonin receptors in the stomach that cause nausea, and also by promoting the smooth muscle contraction of the digestive tract, aiding in the faster processing of stomach contents. For travel-related nausea, ginger can be prepared in several forms. One effective method is to slice fresh ginger root thinly and steep it in boiling water for 10-15 minutes to make a potent tea. The recommended amount is about one-half teaspoon of fresh ginger per cup of water. For those on the go, carrying crystallized ginger or ginger capsules can provide a convenient alternative, with the dosage adjusted according to the product's instructions.

Peppermint, or Mentha piperita, contains menthol, which has antispasmodic properties that relax the muscles of the stomach and intestines, thereby reducing the severity of nausea and preventing vomiting. Peppermint can be used in various forms, including teas, essential oil inhalation, or capsules. To prepare peppermint tea, add one tablespoon of dried peppermint leaves to a cup of boiling water and steep for 10 minutes. This creates a soothing tea that can be consumed before or during travel to prevent motion sickness. If using peppermint essential oil, it's important to dilute it with a carrier oil and apply it to a small area of the skin, such as the wrists, to inhale the aroma. Alternatively, one or two drops can be added to a tissue or cotton ball for inhalation. It's crucial to ensure the essential oil is of therapeutic grade and suitable for this use.

When combining ginger and peppermint for an enhanced anti-nausea effect, consider preparing a tea that includes both ingredients. Start with one-half teaspoon of fresh ginger and one tablespoon of dried peppermint leaves per cup of boiling water. Steep for 10-15 minutes, strain, and consume as needed. This combination not only amplifies the anti-nausea effects but also provides a refreshing, palatable flavor that can be soothing during travel.

For individuals seeking to prepare these remedies in advance of travel, consider the shelf life and storage conditions. Dried peppermint leaves should be stored in an airtight container in a cool, dark place to preserve their potency, while fresh ginger root can be kept in the refrigerator for up to three weeks or in the freezer for longer storage. If opting for capsules or crystallized ginger, follow the manufacturer's guidelines for storage and expiration dates.

Incorporating ginger and peppermint into your travel wellness kit can significantly reduce the incidence and severity of motion sickness. By understanding the specific properties of these herbs and preparing them correctly, travelers can enjoy a more comfortable and nausea-free journey.

Ginger and Peppermint Travel Tea

Beneficial effects

Ginger and Peppermint Travel Tea is a natural remedy designed to alleviate symptoms of motion sickness and nausea while traveling. Ginger, known for its powerful anti-nausea properties, helps to settle the stomach and prevent vomiting. Peppermint offers a soothing effect on the digestive system and can help to relieve headaches and migraines often associated with motion sickness. Together, they create a refreshing and therapeutic tea that can make travel more comfortable and enjoyable.

Portions

Makes approximately 4 cups

Preparation time

5 minutes

Cooking time

10 minutes

Ingredients

- 4 cups of water
- 2 tablespoons of fresh ginger root, thinly sliced
- 2 tablespoons of dried peppermint leaves or 4 peppermint tea bags
- Honey or maple syrup to taste (optional)
- Lemon slices for garnish (optional)

Instructions

1. Begin by peeling and thinly slicing 2 tablespoons of fresh ginger root. The fresh ginger root should be washed thoroughly before slicing to ensure all dirt and impurities are removed.

2. In a medium-sized saucepan, bring 4 cups of water to a boil over high heat.

3. Once the water reaches a rolling boil, add the sliced ginger to the saucepan. Reduce the heat to medium-low, allowing the ginger to simmer for 5 minutes. This simmering process helps to extract the ginger's active compounds, maximizing its anti-nausea effects.

4. After 5 minutes, add 2 tablespoons of dried peppermint leaves or 4 peppermint tea bags to the saucepan. Cover the saucepan with a lid and remove it from the heat.

5. Allow the tea to steep for 5 minutes with the ginger and peppermint together. Steeping for this duration ensures a strong infusion of both herbs' therapeutic properties.

6. Strain the tea through a fine mesh sieve into a large pitcher or directly into tea cups, removing the ginger slices and peppermint leaves or tea bags.

7. If desired, sweeten the tea with honey or maple syrup according to your taste preferences. Stir well to ensure the sweetener is fully dissolved.

8. Serve the tea hot, or allow it to cool and serve over ice for a refreshing cold beverage. Garnish each cup with a slice of lemon for an added boost of flavor and vitamin C.

Variations

- For an extra soothing effect, add a cinnamon stick to the saucepan along with the ginger. Cinnamon can help to further calm the stomach and add a warm, comforting flavor to the tea.
- Incorporate a few cloves or a small piece of star anise for a spicier tea that can help to enhance digestion and reduce gas.

Storage tips

Store any leftover tea in a sealed glass container in the refrigerator for up to 3 days. To reheat, simply warm the tea on the stove over low heat until just hot. Do not boil the tea again, as this can diminish its therapeutic benefits.

Tips for allergens

For those with allergies or sensitivities to honey, maple syrup serves as a delicious vegan-friendly sweetener alternative. Ensure to source organic ginger and peppermint to avoid potential contaminants and allergens.

Scientific references

- "Ginger in gastrointestinal disorders: A systematic review of clinical trials" published in Food Science & Nutrition, which discusses the effectiveness of ginger in treating nausea and gastrointestinal disturbances.
- "Peppermint oil in the acute treatment of tension-type headache" from Schmerz, highlighting the pain-relieving properties of peppermint oil, applicable to headaches associated with motion sickness.

CHAPTER 2: MANAGING JET LAG WITH HERBS

Ashwagandha and lemon balm stand out as potent herbal allies in managing jet lag, a common challenge for travelers crossing multiple time zones. The disorientation and fatigue resulting from rapid travel across these zones can significantly impact physical and mental well-being. Ashwagandha, known scientifically as Withania somnifera, is revered for its adaptogenic properties, which help the body manage stress and normalize bodily functions. On the other hand, lemon balm, or Melissa officinalis, is celebrated for its calming effects on the nervous system, promoting relaxation and sleep.

Ashwagandha for Stress and Sleep Regulation: Begin by sourcing high-quality, organic ashwagandha root powder. The recommended dosage for mitigating jet lag is 300-500 mg, taken with warm milk or water, approximately one hour before bedtime. This timing aids in adjusting the body's internal clock to the new time zone, promoting restorative sleep. Ashwagandha's adaptogenic qualities support the adrenal glands, reducing cortisol levels and mitigating the stress response associated with travel.

Lemon Balm for Enhanced Relaxation: Lemon balm can be prepared as a tea by steeping 1-2 teaspoons of dried lemon balm leaves in boiling water for 10 minutes. This soothing tea should be consumed in the evening, following dinner, to prepare the body and mind for sleep. Lemon balm's mild sedative properties help ease insomnia and anxiety, common symptoms of jet lag.

Ashwagandha and Lemon Balm Sleep Tonic To create a potent sleep tonic, combine 1 teaspoon of ashwagandha powder with 1 teaspoon of dried lemon balm leaves. Add this blend to a cup of boiling water and let it steep for 10 minutes. Strain the mixture and add a natural sweetener, such as honey or stevia, to taste. This tonic is best consumed an hour before bedtime, starting a few days before the trip and continuing for several days upon arrival at the destination.

Preparation and Storage Tips: For the freshest and most potent effects, purchase ashwagandha and lemon balm from reputable suppliers specializing in organic herbs. Store the herbs in airtight containers, away from direct sunlight and moisture, to preserve their efficacy. Preparing the sleep tonic in small, nightly batches ensures the maximum therapeutic benefits.

Safety Considerations: While ashwagandha and lemon balm are generally safe for most individuals, it's crucial to consult with a healthcare provider before incorporating these herbs into your regimen, especially for those who are pregnant, nursing, or on medication. Monitoring the body's response to these herbs and adjusting the dosage as needed can help manage any potential side effects.

Incorporating ashwagandha and lemon balm into your travel routine offers a natural and effective strategy for combating jet lag, ensuring a more enjoyable and productive trip. By aligning the body's internal clock with the new time zone, travelers can minimize the disruptive effects of jet lag and enhance their overall travel experience.

Ashwagandha & Lemon Balm for Sleep

Ashwagandha and lemon balm, when combined, create a powerful synergy that can significantly enhance sleep quality and regulate sleep patterns, especially for those grappling with jet lag. This disruption of the body's internal clock due to rapid travel across time zones can lead to difficulty falling asleep, staying asleep, and achieving restful sleep. The adaptogenic properties of ashwagandha, coupled with the calming effects of lemon balm, offer a natural solution to these challenges.

To harness the benefits of ashwagandha for sleep regulation, it's essential to select a high-quality, organic ashwagandha root powder. The ideal dosage for adults is typically in the range of 300-500 mg. It should be taken with warm milk or water to enhance absorption, approximately one hour before bedtime. This timing is crucial as it helps signal to the body that it's time to wind down and prepare for sleep, aiding in the adjustment to a new time zone. Ashwagandha works by modulating the stress response system in the body, reducing cortisol levels, which are often elevated due to stress and can interfere with sleep.

Lemon balm, scientifically known as Melissa officinalis, is another herb that plays a pivotal role in sleep regulation. For optimal results, use 1-2 teaspoons of dried lemon balm leaves to prepare a tea. Boil water and pour it over the lemon balm leaves, allowing them to steep for about 10 minutes. This herbal tea should be consumed in the evening, after dinner, to maximize its sleep-inducing effects. Lemon balm acts as a mild sedative, reducing anxiety and promoting relaxation, making it easier to fall asleep and stay asleep throughout the night.

Creating a sleep tonic that combines ashwagandha and lemon balm is straightforward. Begin by boiling water and then adding 1 teaspoon of ashwagandha powder along with 1 teaspoon of dried lemon balm leaves to the hot water. Allow this mixture to steep for 10 minutes. After steeping, strain the mixture to remove the solid particles, and consider adding a natural sweetener like honey or stevia to enhance the flavor. This tonic is most effective when consumed an hour before bedtime. For those traveling across time zones, it's advisable to start drinking this tonic a few days before the trip and continue for several days upon arrival at the destination to help reset the body's internal clock.

When purchasing ashwagandha and lemon balm, it's critical to source these herbs from reputable suppliers that specialize in organic products. This ensures that the herbs are free from pesticides and other contaminants that could undermine their therapeutic value. Store these herbs in airtight containers, placed in a cool, dry area away from direct sunlight to maintain their potency.

While ashwagandha and lemon balm are generally considered safe for most people, it's important to consult with a healthcare provider before adding them to your regimen, particularly for those who are pregnant, nursing, or taking medications. Observing how your body responds to these herbs and adjusting the dosage as necessary can help mitigate any potential side effects.

Incorporating ashwagandha and lemon balm into your evening routine can be a game-changer for managing jet lag and improving sleep quality. By leveraging the stress-reducing effects of ashwagandha and the calming properties of lemon balm, travelers can enjoy more restful nights, making their journeys more pleasant and productive.

Ashwagandha and Lemon Balm Sleep Tonic

Beneficial effects
Ashwagandha and Lemon Balm Sleep Tonic is a natural remedy designed to promote relaxation and improve sleep quality, especially beneficial for those struggling with jet lag or sleep disturbances related to travel. Ashwagandha, an adaptogen, helps to reduce stress and balance the body's systems, while lemon balm acts as a mild sedative, encouraging a state of calmness and making it easier to fall asleep. This tonic is perfect for health-conscious adults seeking a holistic approach to wellness, regardless of their knowledge or educational background.

Portions
Makes approximately 2 cups

Preparation time
5 minutes

Cooking time
15 minutes

Ingredients
- 2 cups of water
- 1 tablespoon of dried lemon balm leaves
- 1 teaspoon of ashwagandha powder
- Honey or maple syrup to taste (optional)
- A slice of lemon for garnish (optional)

Instructions
1. Bring 2 cups of water to a boil in a medium saucepan over medium-high heat.
2. Once the water is boiling, reduce the heat to low and add 1 tablespoon of dried lemon balm leaves to the saucepan.
3. Stir in 1 teaspoon of ashwagandha powder until it is fully dissolved in the water.
4. Cover the saucepan with a lid and allow the mixture to simmer on low heat for 15 minutes. This slow simmering process helps to extract the beneficial compounds from the lemon balm and ashwagandha, enhancing the tonic's effectiveness.
5. After 15 minutes, remove the saucepan from the heat and let it cool for a few minutes for a comfortable drinking temperature.
6. Strain the tonic through a fine mesh sieve or cheesecloth into a mug or cup, discarding the leftover herbs.
7. If desired, sweeten the tonic with honey or maple syrup according to your taste preferences.
8. Garnish with a slice of lemon for a refreshing twist and additional vitamin C.

Variations

- For an iced version, allow the tonic to cool completely and then serve over ice for a refreshing, sleep-promoting beverage during warmer months.
- Add a pinch of cinnamon or nutmeg to the saucepan along with the lemon balm and ashwagandha for a warming, comforting flavor.
- Incorporate a few fresh mint leaves while the tonic is simmering for an extra layer of soothing flavor.

Storage tips

Store any leftover tonic in a glass container in the refrigerator for up to 3 days. Reheat gently on the stove or enjoy cold for a quick and easy sleep aid.

Tips for allergens

For those with sensitivities to honey, maple syrup serves as a delicious vegan-friendly sweetener alternative. Ensure to source organic ashwagandha powder and lemon balm leaves to avoid potential contaminants and allergens.

Scientific references

- "A systematic review of the clinical use of Withania somnifera (Ashwagandha) to ameliorate cognitive dysfunction" published in Phytotherapy Research, which discusses the stress-reducing and cognitive function-improving effects of ashwagandha.
- "Melissa officinalis L. (lemon balm) extract in the treatment of volunteers suffering from mild-to-moderate anxiety disorders and sleep disturbances" from Mediterranean Journal of Nutrition and Metabolism, highlighting the sleep-improving effects of lemon balm.

CHAPTER 3: HERBS FOR TRAVEL FATIGUE

Travel fatigue, often characterized by exhaustion, sleep disturbances, and general malaise, can significantly impact the enjoyment and productivity of your journey. To combat these symptoms, incorporating specific herbs into your travel routine can offer natural and effective relief. Rhodiola and Eleuthero, two powerful adaptogenic herbs, stand out for their energy-boosting and endurance-enhancing properties. Here, we delve into the detailed preparation and use of these herbs to mitigate travel fatigue.

Rhodiola (Rhodiola rosea), also known as Arctic root or Golden root, thrives in cold, mountainous regions of Europe and Asia. Its root contains over 140 active ingredients, the two most potent being rosavin and salidroside. Rhodiola is renowned for its ability to increase energy, stamina, strength, and mental capacity. To harness Rhodiola's benefits, look for a standardized extract that contains at least 3% rosavins and 1% salidroside. The recommended dosage for combating travel fatigue is 200-600 mg of Rhodiola extract, taken in capsule form, approximately 30 minutes before breakfast and lunch. This timing helps optimize its energizing effects throughout the day without interfering with nighttime sleep.

Eleuthero (Eleutherococcus senticosus), commonly known as Siberian Ginseng, is a small, woody shrub native to Northeastern Asia. Eleuthero does not belong to the same genus as true ginseng but offers similar benefits, including enhanced physical endurance and mental clarity. The active compounds in Eleuthero, eleutherosides, support the body's ability to adapt to stress and exert a normalizing effect on bodily processes. For travel fatigue, a daily dose of 300-1200 mg of Eleuthero root extract, divided into two or three doses, is recommended. Begin with the lower end of the dosage range and adjust based on your response. Eleuthero is best taken with meals to improve absorption and minimize any potential stomach upset.

Rhodiola and Eleuthero Energy Tonic Creating an energy tonic that combines the power of Rhodiola and Eleuthero can provide a convenient and potent remedy for travel fatigue. To prepare this tonic, you will need:
- 1 teaspoon of Rhodiola rosea extract (liquid form)
- 1 teaspoon of Eleuthero root extract (liquid form)
- 8 ounces of warm water or green tea
- Honey or stevia to taste (optional)

Mix the Rhodiola and Eleuthero extracts in warm water or green tea. Add honey or stevia if desired for sweetness. Drink this tonic once in the morning, preferably with breakfast, to energize your day and combat fatigue. The combination of these adaptogens works synergistically to enhance your physical and mental endurance, making it easier to cope with the demands of travel.

Preparation and Storage Tips: When purchasing Rhodiola and Eleuthero extracts, opt for products from reputable suppliers that provide third-party testing to ensure purity and potency. Store the extracts in a cool, dark place, away from direct sunlight and moisture, to maintain their therapeutic properties.

Safety Considerations: While Rhodiola and Eleuthero are generally well-tolerated, it's important to consult with a healthcare provider before adding them to your regimen, especially if you are pregnant, nursing, or have underlying health conditions. Monitoring your body's response to these herbs and adjusting the dosage as needed can help manage any potential side effects.

Incorporating Rhodiola and Eleuthero into your travel wellness kit can significantly reduce the impact of travel fatigue, allowing you to enjoy your journey with increased energy and resilience. By understanding the specific properties of these herbs and preparing them correctly, travelers can support their body's natural ability to adapt to the stresses of travel.

Rhodiola and Eleuthero for Energy

Rhodiola rosea, commonly referred to as Rhodiola, is a herb that grows in the cold, mountainous regions of Europe and Asia. Its roots are considered adaptogens, meaning they help the body adapt to stress while enhancing energy, stamina, and mental capacity. The active compounds in Rhodiola, rosavins, and salidroside, have been extensively studied for their effects on reducing fatigue and improving cognitive function. For those facing travel fatigue, incorporating Rhodiola into their regimen can be particularly beneficial. A standardized extract of Rhodiola, ensuring at least 3% rosavins and 1% salidroside, is recommended for optimal effectiveness. The dosage can vary, but starting with 200 mg taken 30 minutes before breakfast can help kickstart the day, with an additional dose before lunch if needed, not exceeding 600 mg daily to avoid overstimulation and ensure it does not interfere with sleep patterns.

Eleutherococcus senticosus, known as Eleuthero or Siberian Ginseng, is another adaptogenic herb that supports stamina and endurance. Unlike Rhodiola, Eleuthero is native to Northeastern Asia and has been used traditionally to prevent colds and flu and to increase energy and longevity. Eleuthero's active ingredients, eleutherosides, help improve the body's stress response and boost energy levels without the jitteriness associated with caffeine. For travel fatigue, Eleuthero provides a sustained energy boost that can help travelers adjust to new time zones and hectic schedules. A daily intake of 300-1200 mg of Eleuthero root extract, divided into two or three doses with meals, is suggested to enhance absorption and effectiveness. Starting with the lower dosage and adjusting based on personal response can help identify the optimal amount for individual needs.

Creating an energy tonic that combines Rhodiola and Eleuthero can offer a synergistic effect, enhancing both herbs' benefits. To prepare this tonic, one might mix liquid extracts of both herbs for convenience and accuracy. Using 1 teaspoon of Rhodiola extract and 1 teaspoon of Eleuthero extract in 8 ounces of warm water or green tea can make a palatable and effective tonic. Adding honey or stevia can improve the taste. Consuming this blend in the morning, particularly with breakfast, can help ensure energy levels are optimized from the start of the day, combating fatigue and enhancing endurance throughout the day's activities.

When selecting Rhodiola and Eleuthero, it's crucial to source from reputable suppliers. Products should be third-party tested to verify their purity, potency, and safety. Storing these extracts in a cool, dark place will help preserve their efficacy. As with any supplement, consulting with a healthcare provider before starting is wise, especially for those with underlying health conditions, pregnant, or nursing. Monitoring the body's response to these adaptogens and adjusting the dosage as necessary can help mitigate any potential side effects, ensuring a safe and beneficial experience.

Incorporating Rhodiola and Eleuthero into a travel wellness routine can significantly alleviate travel fatigue, enhance physical and mental endurance, and support overall well-being during travel. This natural approach to combating fatigue can make travel more enjoyable and productive, allowing travelers to adapt more quickly to new environments and schedules without relying on stimulants that may have undesirable side effects.

Rhodiola and Eleuthero Energy Blend

Beneficial effects

The Rhodiola and Eleuthero Energy Blend is designed to combat travel fatigue and boost energy levels naturally. Rhodiola Rosea, often referred to as the "golden root," is known for its ability to enhance physical and mental endurance, reduce the symptoms of fatigue, and improve mood. Eleuthero, also known as Siberian Ginseng, is celebrated for its adaptogenic properties, helping the body to adapt to stress, boosting the immune system, and enhancing overall energy and vitality. This blend is perfect for travelers seeking a natural way to maintain energy and resilience during their journeys.

Portions

Makes approximately 2 cups

Preparation time

10 minutes

Cooking time

No cooking required

Ingredients

- 1 teaspoon of Rhodiola Rosea powder
- 1 teaspoon of Eleuthero (Siberian Ginseng) powder
- 2 cups of cold water or coconut water
- 1 tablespoon of honey or maple syrup (optional)
- Juice of 1/2 lemon (optional for added flavor and vitamin C)
- A few mint leaves for garnish (optional)

Instructions

1. In a large glass or shaker, combine 1 teaspoon of Rhodiola Rosea powder and 1 teaspoon of Eleuthero powder.
2. Add 2 cups of cold water or coconut water to the glass. Coconut water is recommended for added electrolytes and natural sweetness.

3. If using, add 1 tablespoon of honey or maple syrup to sweeten the blend. This step is optional and can be adjusted based on personal taste preferences.

4. Squeeze the juice of half a lemon into the mixture. Lemon not only adds a refreshing flavor but also provides vitamin C, enhancing the immune-boosting properties of the blend.

5. Stir the mixture thoroughly until all the powders are completely dissolved. For a smoother texture, you can use a blender or shaker bottle to ensure the powders blend well with the liquid.

6. Pour the blend into a serving glass and garnish with a few mint leaves for a refreshing aroma and taste.

7. Enjoy immediately for the best flavor and energy-boosting effects.

Variations

- For a chilled version, blend with ice cubes for a refreshing, energizing smoothie.
- Add a slice of ginger for an extra kick and digestive benefits.
- Incorporate a scoop of your favorite protein powder for an added protein boost, making it a more substantial pre-travel drink.

Storage tips

This energy blend is best enjoyed fresh. However, if you need to prepare it in advance, store it in a sealed bottle or container in the refrigerator for up to 24 hours. Shake well before drinking as natural separation may occur.

Tips for allergens

For those with sensitivities or allergies to honey, maple syrup serves as a delicious vegan-friendly sweetener alternative. Ensure to source organic and non-irradiated Rhodiola and Eleuthero powders to avoid potential contaminants and allergens.

Scientific references

- A study published in the "Phytomedicine" journal found that Rhodiola Rosea can improve physical and mental performance under stress, while reducing fatigue.
- Research in the "Journal of Ethnopharmacology" highlights Eleuthero's adaptogenic properties, showing its effectiveness in enhancing mental acuity and physical endurance without the side effects associated with stimulants.

BOOK 30: HERBS FOR SPIRITUAL GROWTH

Holy Basil, also known as Tulsi, is revered in herbal medicine for its grounding and centering properties. To harness the full potential of Holy Basil for spiritual growth, it's essential to understand its cultivation, preparation, and usage. Holy Basil thrives in warm, sunny locations with well-drained soil, preferring a pH range of 6 to 7.5. Start seeds indoors 6 to 8 weeks before the last frost date, transplanting seedlings outdoors when temperatures consistently exceed 70°F. For optimal growth, water the plants regularly, allowing the soil to dry slightly between watering sessions.

To prepare Holy Basil for use in spiritual practices, the leaves can be harvested just before the plant flowers, typically in the early morning when the essential oils are most concentrated. Gently wash the leaves and pat them dry. The leaves can be used fresh or dried for later use. To dry Holy Basil, tie the stems together and hang them upside down in a warm, airy location out of direct sunlight, or use a food dehydrator set at a low temperature.

For a grounding and centering tea, use 1 to 2 teaspoons of dried Holy Basil leaves per cup of boiling water. Steep for 5 to 10 minutes, depending on the desired strength. This tea can be consumed daily, ideally in the morning or during meditation, to promote a calm, centered state of mind. Additionally, Holy Basil can be incorporated into a meditation space by placing fresh leaves or a small plant on an altar to enhance the spiritual atmosphere.

Mugwort, another powerful herb for grounding and centering, is known for its dream-enhancing and protective qualities. It prefers a sunny location with well-drained soil and can be easily propagated from seed or cuttings. Mugwort grows vigorously; thus, regular pruning is recommended to keep the plant manageable and to encourage bushier growth.

To use Mugwort in spiritual practices, the leaves and flowering tops are harvested, typically in mid to late summer. The herb can be dried in the same manner as Holy Basil. Mugwort can be used to make a tea by steeping 1 teaspoon of dried herb in a cup of boiling water for 10 minutes. This tea can be drunk before bedtime to promote vivid dreams and enhance spiritual insight. Mugwort can also be used in smudging ceremonies to cleanse a space of negative energy, creating a grounded and protected environment for meditation and spiritual work.

When working with Holy Basil and Mugwort, it's important to source these herbs from reputable suppliers or grow them organically to ensure they are free from pesticides and other contaminants. Always consult with a healthcare provider before incorporating new herbs into your regimen, especially if you are pregnant, nursing, or taking medications. By integrating Holy Basil and Mugwort into your spiritual practice, you can enhance your connection to the earth, promote a sense of calm and focus, and support your overall spiritual growth.

Holy Basil and Mugwort for Focus

Holy Basil, known scientifically as **Ocimum sanctum** or **Tulsi**, and Mugwort, or **Artemisia vulgaris**, are revered in various cultures for their spiritual and medicinal properties. When used with intention, these herbs can significantly enhance meditation, grounding, and centering practices.

To harness the spiritual focus benefits of Holy Basil, start by sourcing fresh or dried leaves from a reputable supplier, ensuring they are organic to avoid any chemical residues. For a simple Holy Basil tea, measure out 1 teaspoon of dried Holy Basil leaves or 3 teaspoons if you are using fresh leaves. Boil 8 ounces of water and pour it over the leaves in a teapot or a cup, allowing it to steep for about 5 to 6 minutes. This creates a potent tea that can be consumed 20 minutes before meditation or spiritual practices to calm the mind and enhance your focus. The act of sipping tea slowly can also become a mindful practice, helping to center your thoughts and intentions.

Mugwort, on the other hand, is often used in dried form for smudging, a practice that involves burning the herb to cleanse a space of negative energy and to promote a sense of calm and clarity. To prepare Mugwort for smudging, dry the leaves thoroughly until they are brittle. Once dried, bundle them tightly with a natural twine, leaving one end loose for lighting. When you are ready to smudge, light the loose end of the Mugwort bundle, allowing it to smolder. Gently wave the bundle around your space, focusing on corners and areas where energy feels stagnant. As the smoke wafts through the air, visualize it absorbing negativity and chaos, leaving behind tranquility and a heightened sense of awareness. This practice is best done before engaging in spiritual activities to purify the environment and your mental space.

For those interested in combining the properties of both herbs, creating a Holy Basil and Mugwort blend can be particularly powerful. Combine 1 teaspoon of dried Holy Basil leaves with 1 teaspoon of dried Mugwort in a teapot. Add 8 ounces of boiling water and allow the mixture to steep for 7 minutes. Strain and enjoy the tea in a quiet, comfortable space where you can sit undisturbed, focusing on your breath and the sensations within your body. This blend not only aids in spiritual focus but also supports a deeper connection with the self and the divine.

When working with these herbs, always set your intentions clearly before consuming or using them in a ritual. Whether you are seeking clarity, grounding, or a deeper spiritual connection, the mindful use of Holy Basil and Mugwort can significantly enhance your practice. Remember, the key to unlocking the full potential of these herbs lies in your approach and the respect you show towards their traditional uses and spiritual significance.

Holy Basil and Mugwort Meditation Tea
Beneficial effects
Holy Basil and Mugwort Meditation Tea is crafted to enhance your meditation practice by promoting a sense of calm and grounding. Holy Basil, also known as Tulsi, is revered in Ayurvedic medicine for its ability to lower stress levels and balance the mind, body, and spirit. Mugwort, on the other hand, has been used traditionally for its dream-enhancing and intuitive properties, making it an excellent herb for deepening meditation and spiritual work. Together, these herbs create a tea that not only supports relaxation but also fosters a deeper connection to your inner self and the spiritual realm.

Portions
Makes approximately 2 cups
Preparation time
5 minutes
Cooking time
10 minutes
Ingredients
- 2 cups of water
- 1 tablespoon of dried Holy Basil (Tulsi) leaves
- 1 tablespoon of dried Mugwort
- Honey or maple syrup to taste (optional)
Instructions
1. Begin by bringing 2 cups of water to a boil in a medium-sized saucepan.
2. Once the water reaches a rolling boil, reduce the heat to low and add 1 tablespoon of dried Holy Basil leaves to the saucepan.
3. Add 1 tablespoon of dried Mugwort to the saucepan, stirring gently to ensure both herbs are fully submerged in the water.
4. Cover the saucepan with a lid and allow the herbs to simmer on low heat for 10 minutes. This slow simmering process helps to extract the full spectrum of beneficial compounds from the herbs.
5. After 10 minutes, remove the saucepan from the heat and let it sit, covered, for an additional 5 minutes to further infuse the tea.
6. Carefully strain the tea through a fine mesh sieve or cheesecloth into a teapot or directly into cups, discarding the used herbs.
7. If desired, sweeten the tea with honey or maple syrup according to your taste preferences. Stir well to ensure the sweetener is fully dissolved.
8. Serve the tea warm, taking a moment to inhale its aromatic scent before beginning your meditation practice.
Variations
- For a cooler, refreshing version, allow the tea to cool to room temperature, then refrigerate until chilled. Serve over ice for a soothing summer beverage.
- Add a slice of fresh ginger or a cinnamon stick to the saucepan along with the Holy Basil and Mugwort for a warming, spicy twist that can further enhance the tea's grounding properties.

- Incorporate a few drops of lemon or orange juice to the tea for a citrusy note, which can help to uplift and refresh the spirit.

Storage tips
Store any leftover tea in a sealed glass container in the refrigerator for up to 2 days. Gently reheat on the stove or enjoy cold for a revitalizing treat.

Tips for allergens
For those with sensitivities or dietary restrictions, maple syrup serves as a delicious vegan-friendly sweetener alternative to honey. Ensure to source organic and pesticide-free dried Holy Basil and Mugwort to minimize exposure to potential allergens and contaminants.

Scientific references
- "Tulsi - Ocimum sanctum: A herb for all reasons" featured in the Journal of Ayurveda and Integrative Medicine, highlights the adaptogenic and stress-relieving properties of Holy Basil.
- "The use of Artemisia vulgaris (Mugwort) in Traditional Medicine and its potential role in Health and Wellness" in the Journal of Ethnopharmacology, discusses the traditional uses of Mugwort for spiritual and meditative practices.

CHAPTER 2: HERBS FOR ENERGY CLEARING

Sage, known scientifically as **Salvia officinalis**, and Palo Santo, or **Bursera graveolens**, are two powerful herbs widely recognized for their energy clearing properties. These herbs have been used for centuries in various cultures to cleanse spaces, objects, and individuals of negative energy, fostering a positive and harmonious environment.

Sage is most commonly utilized in the form of smudge sticks, which are bundles of dried sage leaves that are burned, allowing the smoke to purify the area. To create a sage smudge stick, gather a handful of dried sage leaves and bind them tightly with a natural cotton string. Ensure the bundle is secure but not too tight as air needs to pass through for it to burn effectively. When lighting the smudge stick, hold it at a 45-degree angle and allow it to catch fire before gently blowing out the flame, letting it smolder and produce smoke. Move through your space with the smoldering stick, focusing on corners and areas behind doors where stagnant energy often accumulates. As you do this, visualize the smoke absorbing and clearing away any negativity. It's important to have a window open during the smudging process to allow the smoke and negative energy to exit your space.

Palo Santo, on the other hand, is a sacred wood from South America that emits a sweet, uplifting scent when burned. To use Palo Santo for energy clearing, you'll need a stick of Palo Santo wood. Light one end of the wood stick, allowing it to burn for about 30 seconds to a minute before blowing it out. The wood will smolder, releasing smoke that carries both a purifying energy and a pleasant fragrance. Walk around your space with the Palo Santo, allowing the smoke to reach different areas, similar to the sage smudging process. Palo Santo is particularly useful for not just clearing negative energy but also for bringing in positive vibrations to fill the newly purified space.

For those interested in combining the effects of both sage and Palo Santo, you can begin by first burning sage to clear out any negativity, followed by Palo Santo to invite positive energy. This combination ensures a thorough energetic cleanse, making the space feel lighter, brighter, and more conducive to well-being.

When working with these herbs, it's crucial to source them ethically and sustainably, given the overharvesting concerns, especially with Palo Santo. Look for suppliers who harvest the wood from fallen trees rather than cutting down living ones, and who engage in fair trade practices to support the indigenous communities where these plants are native.

Remember, the intention behind the energy clearing is as important as the herbs themselves. Before beginning your smudging ritual, take a moment to set your intentions. Whether you're seeking to remove negativity, bring peace into your home, or simply refresh the energy of your space, focusing your mind on your desired outcome will amplify the effectiveness of the clearing process.

Sage and Palo Santo Cleansing

To effectively use **Sage (Salvia officinalis)** for space cleansing, begin by sourcing high-quality, dried sage leaves. Preferably, these should be organically grown to ensure they are free from pesticides and other chemicals. To create a smudge stick, tightly bind a bundle of these dried leaves with natural cotton string, ensuring there's enough airflow for the sage to burn slowly and evenly. When ready to cleanse a space, ignite the tip of the smudge stick at a 45-degree angle, then gently blow out the flame to let it smolder and produce smoke. Methodically move through the area you wish to cleanse, allowing the smoke to drift into corners, closets, and other stagnant spaces. It's crucial to maintain a clear intention of purifying and protecting the space from negative energies as you do this. Keep windows or doors open to allow the smoke—and the negative energy it's believed to carry—to escape.

For **Palo Santo (Bursera graveolens)**, select ethically sourced wood sticks, ensuring they come from trees that have naturally fallen and been allowed to cure for several years. This not only supports sustainable practices but also enhances the wood's aromatic properties. To use, light one end of a Palo Santo stick, allowing it to burn for 30 seconds to a minute before blowing it out. The wood will then smolder, releasing a rich, sweet smoke. Walk through your space with the Palo Santo, similar to the sage smudging process, letting the smoke reach all areas. The scent of Palo Santo is not only cleansing but also uplifting, making it ideal for not just removing negative energy but also for inviting positivity.

Combining **sage and Palo Santo** in a cleansing ritual can provide a comprehensive energetic cleanse. Start with sage to clear out any negativity, then follow with Palo Santo to fill the space with positive energy. This layered approach ensures a thorough purification process, leaving the environment feeling lighter and more vibrant.

When purchasing these materials, look for suppliers committed to ethical and sustainable harvesting practices. This respect for the plants and their origins aligns with the intention behind their use and supports the overall efficacy of the cleansing ritual.

Throughout the cleansing process, whether using sage, Palo Santo, or both, focus on your intention. Visualize the smoke carrying away all negative energies, leaving behind only peace and positivity. This focused intention is as vital to the cleansing process as the herbs themselves, transforming the physical act of smudging into a powerful spiritual practice.

DIY Sage Smudge Sticks

Creating your own sage smudge sticks is a deeply personal and rewarding process that allows you to infuse your home with the purifying energy of sage. To begin, you will need fresh sage, preferably Salvia officinalis, known for its potent cleansing properties. Harvest or purchase sage that has not been treated with pesticides to ensure the purity of your smudge stick. The best time to gather sage is in the morning after the dew has evaporated but before the sun is at its peak, as this helps preserve the natural oils within the plant, which are crucial for a successful smudging.

Once you have your sage, gather a bundle of branches, aiming for a thickness that feels substantial but not overly bulky, typically about the diameter of a nickel to a quarter. The length of the branches can vary, but a common length is between 4 to 6 inches, which allows for a manageable size that will burn evenly.

Next, you will need 100% cotton string or thread. The color of the string can be chosen based on personal preference or specific spiritual intentions; white is a popular choice for its association with purity and protection. Cut a length of string about five times the length of your sage bundle to ensure you have enough to wrap the bundle thoroughly.

Begin by laying your sage bundle on a flat surface. Tie one end of the string securely around the base of your sage bundle, leaving a tail of string about 5 inches long; this will be used to tie off the string at the end. Start wrapping the string tightly around the base, working your way up the bundle in a spiral pattern. As you wrap, press the leaves gently toward the center to form a compact shape. This compression is key to preventing loose leaves from falling out as the smudge stick dries and shrinks.

Once you reach the top of the bundle, reverse the direction of your wrapping, creating a crisscross pattern as you work your way back down to the base. This technique not only secures the leaves within the bundle but also adds to the aesthetic appeal of the finished smudge stick. When you arrive back at the base, tie the end of the string to the 5-inch tail you left at the beginning. Trim any excess string.

The final step is drying your sage smudge sticks. This is a crucial part of the process, as properly dried sage will burn more evenly and effectively. To dry, hang your smudge sticks in a warm, dry, and well-ventilated area out of direct sunlight. This can be done by attaching them to a hanger or string. Drying times can vary depending on the humidity and temperature of your environment but expect it to take at least a week, and possibly up to three weeks, for your smudge sticks to fully dry. You can test for dryness by checking if the leaves crumble slightly when pinched. If they do, your smudge stick is ready to use.

Once dried, your sage smudge sticks are ready for use in cleansing rituals. To smudge, light the tip of the smudge stick, allow it to catch fire, then gently blow out the flames to let it smolder and produce smoke. As you move through your space, focus on areas that may harbor stagnant energy, such as corners, closets, and behind doors. Carry a fireproof container, like an abalone shell or ceramic dish, underneath the smudge stick to catch any falling ashes. Remember, the intention behind the smudging is as important as the act itself. Set a clear intention for purification, protection, or whatever suits your needs as you cleanse your space.

CHAPTER 3: HERBS FOR DEEP RELAXATION

Lavender, known scientifically as **Lavandula angustifolia**, and Passionflower, or **Passiflora incarnata**, are two potent herbs widely celebrated for their deep relaxation and stress-relieving properties. These herbs have been utilized in traditional medicine for centuries to alleviate anxiety, improve sleep quality, and promote a sense of calm and well-being.

Lavender is most effective when its essential oil is used in aromatherapy. To harness the calming benefits of Lavender essential oil, add 5-10 drops to a diffuser filled with water. Place the diffuser in your bedroom or any space where you wish to instill a sense of peace and relaxation. The diffuser should be operated for 30-60 minutes before bedtime to create a tranquil environment conducive to sleep. Alternatively, you can add a few drops of Lavender oil to a warm bath for a soothing pre-sleep ritual. The warmth of the water enhances the therapeutic properties of the oil, promoting muscle relaxation and reducing stress levels.

Passionflower is best consumed as a tea for its sedative effects. To prepare Passionflower tea, steep 1 teaspoon of dried Passionflower in 8 ounces of boiling water for 10 minutes. This allows the water to become infused with the herb's active compounds, creating a potent brew. Drinking a cup of Passionflower tea 30 minutes before bed can significantly improve sleep quality, especially for those who experience insomnia or frequent nighttime awakenings. For a stronger effect, combine Passionflower with other calming herbs such as Chamomile or Valerian root.

For individuals seeking to combine the benefits of both Lavender and Passionflower, creating a bedtime ritual that incorporates both the aromatic and ingestible forms of these herbs can be particularly effective. Begin by preparing a cup of Passionflower tea, allowing it to steep while you draw a warm bath infused with Lavender oil. Sip the tea slowly as you soak in the bath, focusing on the sensation of warmth and the calming aroma. This combination not only aids in physical relaxation but also prepares the mind for a restful night's sleep by reducing mental chatter and anxiety.

When using these herbs, it's important to source high-quality, organic products to ensure they are free from contaminants and retain their therapeutic properties. For Lavender essential oil, look for bottles labeled as "100% pure essential oil" and avoid those with synthetic fragrances or additives. For Passionflower, choose dried herb from reputable suppliers who offer organic, non-irradiated products.

Safety considerations are paramount when using herbs for relaxation. While Lavender and Passionflower are generally considered safe for most people, it's advisable to consult with a healthcare provider before incorporating them into your routine, especially if you are pregnant, breastfeeding, or taking medication. Some individuals may experience mild side effects such as drowsiness or gastrointestinal discomfort, in which case, reducing the dosage or discontinuing use is recommended.

Incorporating Lavender and Passionflower into your evening routine can significantly enhance your ability to unwind and disconnect from the stresses of the day. Whether used individually or in combination, these herbs offer a natural, effective way to promote deep relaxation and restorative sleep, contributing to overall health and well-being.

Lavender and Passionflower Relaxation Tea

Beneficial effects

Lavender and Passionflower Relaxation Tea is a soothing blend designed to calm the mind, ease stress, and prepare the body for a restful night's sleep. Lavender is renowned for its ability to reduce anxiety and induce relaxation, while passionflower is often used for its sedative properties that can help improve sleep quality. Together, these herbs create a powerful tea that can help soothe the nervous system, making it an ideal beverage for those seeking a natural way to unwind and embrace a deeper sense of peace before bedtime.

Portions

Makes approximately 2 cups

Preparation time

5 minutes

Cooking time

10 minutes

Ingredients

- 2 cups of water

- 1 tablespoon of dried lavender flowers
- 1 tablespoon of dried passionflower
- Honey or maple syrup to taste (optional)

Instructions

1. Begin by bringing 2 cups of water to a boil in a medium-sized saucepan. Ensure the water reaches a rolling boil to fully extract the flavors and beneficial properties of the herbs.
2. Once the water is boiling, add 1 tablespoon of dried lavender flowers to the saucepan. Lavender not only imparts a calming aroma but also contributes to the tea's relaxing effects.
3. Add 1 tablespoon of dried passionflower to the saucepan. Passionflower is known for its ability to enhance the quality of sleep, making it a key ingredient in this relaxation tea.
4. Reduce the heat to low, allowing the herbs to simmer gently. Cover the saucepan with a lid to prevent the escape of essential oils and flavors during the simmering process.
5. Allow the mixture to simmer on low heat for 10 minutes. This duration is crucial for fully infusing the water with the therapeutic properties of lavender and passionflower.
6. After 10 minutes, remove the saucepan from the heat. Let it sit for an additional 5 minutes with the lid on to further steep and enhance the potency of the tea.
7. Strain the tea through a fine mesh sieve into a teapot or directly into cups, discarding the used herbs. This step ensures a smooth tea free from herb particles.
8. If desired, sweeten the tea with honey or maple syrup according to your taste preferences. Adding a natural sweetener can enhance the flavor profile of the tea and add a comforting warmth.
9. Serve the tea warm, taking a moment to enjoy the aromatic scent before sipping. Embrace the calming effects as you prepare for a peaceful evening.

Variations

- For a citrus twist, add a few strips of orange or lemon peel to the saucepan along with the herbs. The citrus notes can provide a refreshing contrast to the floral tones.
- Incorporate a cinnamon stick during the simmering process for a subtly spiced flavor that complements the floral notes of lavender and passionflower.
- For a cold version, allow the tea to cool to room temperature, then refrigerate until chilled. Serve over ice for a refreshing and calming beverage during warmer months.

Storage tips

Store any leftover tea in a glass container in the refrigerator for up to 2 days. Reheat gently on the stove or enjoy cold for a soothing treat at any time of day.

Tips for allergens

For those with sensitivities or dietary restrictions, maple syrup serves as a delicious vegan-friendly sweetener alternative to honey. Ensure to source organic and pesticide-free dried lavender and passionflower to minimize exposure to potential allergens and contaminants.

Scientific references

- "Lavender and the Nervous System" published in Evidence-Based Complementary and Alternative Medicine, highlights lavender's anxiolytic, mood stabilizer, sedative, analgesic, and neuroprotective properties.
- "Passionflower in the Treatment of Generalized Anxiety: A Pilot Double-Blind Randomized Controlled Trial with Oxazepam" from the Journal of Clinical Pharmacy and Therapeutics, which discusses passionflower's efficacy as a treatment for anxiety and sleep disorders.

BOOK 31: HERBAL REMEDIES FOR PARENTING

CHAPTER 1: HERBS FOR PARENTING STRESS

Parenting, while immensely rewarding, can be one of the most stressful roles one undertakes. The constant demands, coupled with a desire to provide the best for one's children, can lead to significant stress. Recognizing this, certain herbs have been identified for their calming and stress-relieving properties, making them invaluable for parents navigating the challenges of raising children. Here, we delve into specific herbs beneficial for stressful parenting moments and provide detailed instructions on how to incorporate them into your daily routine.

Chamomile (Matricaria recutita) is renowned for its gentle sedative properties, making it an excellent choice for easing stress and promoting relaxation. To prepare a soothing chamomile tea, add 1-2 teaspoons of dried chamomile flowers to a cup of boiling water. Cover and steep for 10 minutes before straining. For enhanced flavor and additional calming effects, you may add a teaspoon of honey. Drinking chamomile tea in the evening can help unwind after a long day of parenting duties.

Lemon Balm (Melissa officinalis), another herb celebrated for its stress-relieving qualities, can be used to prepare a refreshing herbal tea. Use 1-2 teaspoons of dried lemon balm leaves per cup of boiling water, allowing it to steep for about 5-10 minutes. Lemon balm is particularly effective in reducing anxiety and promoting a sense of calm, making it ideal for consumption during or after particularly hectic days.

Holy Basil (Ocimum sanctum), also known as Tulsi, is an adaptogen, meaning it helps the body adapt to stress and promotes mental balance. To harness the benefits of Holy Basil, prepare a tea by steeping 1 teaspoon of dried leaves in a cup of hot water for about 6 minutes. This herb's unique properties can help mitigate the stress associated with parenting, providing a sense of tranquility and improved mental clarity.

For parents looking for a quick and direct method to relieve stress, **Lavender (Lavandula angustifolia)** essential oil can be used in aromatherapy. Add a few drops of lavender oil to a diffuser filled with water and let it run in your living space for 30 minutes to an hour. The calming scent of lavender can help reduce stress levels and improve overall mood. Alternatively, adding a few drops of lavender oil to a warm bath can provide a relaxing experience, helping to soothe the nerves after a challenging day.

Ashwagandha (Withania somnifera) is another powerful adaptogen that supports the body's stress response system. For parents, incorporating ashwagandha into their routine can be particularly beneficial. You can take ashwagandha in capsule form, typically 300-500 mg, once or twice daily. However, it's important to consult with a healthcare provider before starting any new supplement, especially if you are pregnant, breastfeeding, or taking other medications.

Incorporating these herbs into your daily routine can offer a natural and effective way to manage the stress that often accompanies parenting. Whether through a comforting cup of herbal tea, a soothing aromatherapy session, or the strategic use of supplements, these herbs provide a holistic approach to stress relief. Remember, while herbs can significantly aid in stress management, maintaining a healthy lifestyle, including proper nutrition, exercise, and adequate rest, is also crucial in managing stress levels effectively.

Chamomile and Lemon Balm for Patience

Chamomile (Matricaria chamomilla) and Lemon Balm (Melissa officinalis) are two potent herbs known for their calming effects, making them ideal for moments when patience is required, especially in the context of parenting. To harness these benefits, creating a **Chamomile and Lemon Balm Tea** can be a practical and soothing remedy.

Ingredients:
- 1 tablespoon dried Chamomile flowers
- 1 tablespoon dried Lemon Balm leaves
- 8 ounces of boiling water

Preparation Steps:
1. **Select Quality Herbs:** Ensure that the Chamomile and Lemon Balm are sourced from reputable suppliers to guarantee purity and potency. Organic herbs are preferred to minimize exposure to pesticides and chemicals.
2. **Measure the Herbs:** Use a precise measuring spoon to measure out one tablespoon of each herb. This ratio ensures a balanced flavor and therapeutic effect.

3. **Boil Water:** Heat 8 ounces of water to a rolling boil. The high temperature is crucial for extracting the full range of medicinal compounds from the herbs.

4. **Steep the Herbs:** Combine the Chamomile and Lemon Balm in a teapot or a heat-resistant glass. Pour the boiling water over the herbs, ensuring they are fully submerged. Cover the teapot or glass with a lid or a small plate to prevent the escape of essential oils and aromatic compounds during steeping.

5. **Steeping Time:** Allow the herbs to steep for 5 to 10 minutes. A longer steeping time will result in a stronger tea, both in flavor and therapeutic properties. Adjust the time based on personal preference and desired strength.

6. **Strain:** Use a fine mesh strainer to separate the herbs from the liquid. This step is crucial to ensure a smooth tea free from plant matter.

7. **Serving:** Pour the strained tea into a cup. The tea can be enjoyed hot or cooled down to room temperature, depending on personal preference.

8. **Optional Additions:** For those who prefer a slightly sweetened tea, consider adding a teaspoon of honey or maple syrup. These natural sweeteners can enhance the flavor profile of the tea without overpowering the delicate taste of the herbs.

Consumption Tips:

- **Frequency:** Drinking this tea once or twice a day can help cultivate a sense of calm and patience, particularly during stressful parenting moments.

- **Mindful Drinking:** Engage in a mindful tea-drinking practice by focusing on the aroma, taste, and warmth of the tea. This process can enhance the calming effects of the herbs.

Storage:

- Store any unused dried Chamomile and Lemon Balm in airtight containers away from direct sunlight and moisture to preserve their potency and freshness.

By incorporating Chamomile and Lemon Balm into a daily routine, parents can access a natural and effective tool for managing stress and fostering patience. This herbal tea offers a moment of tranquility that can be particularly beneficial in the dynamic and often challenging journey of parenting.

Chamomile and Lemon Balm Patience Tea

Beneficial effects

Chamomile and Lemon Balm Patience Tea is a soothing blend designed to calm the mind, reduce stress, and enhance patience. Chamomile is well-known for its calming properties, which can help to alleviate irritability and anxiety. Lemon balm, on the other hand, has been used traditionally to improve mood and cognitive function. Together, these herbs create a tea that is perfect for those moments when parenting challenges test your limits, offering a natural way to find peace and patience.

Portions

Makes approximately 2 cups

Preparation time

5 minutes

Cooking time

10 minutes

Ingredients

- 2 cups of water
- 1 tablespoon of dried chamomile flowers
- 1 tablespoon of dried lemon balm leaves
- Honey or maple syrup to taste (optional)

Instructions

1. Begin by bringing 2 cups of water to a rolling boil in a medium-sized saucepan. A rapid boil ensures that the water is hot enough to extract the full flavor and benefits from the herbs.

2. Once the water is boiling, add 1 tablespoon of dried chamomile flowers to the saucepan. Chamomile should be added first as its delicate flavors infuse best at a high temperature.

3. Add 1 tablespoon of dried lemon balm leaves to the saucepan, stirring gently to ensure both herbs are fully submerged in the boiling water.

4. Reduce the heat to low, cover the saucepan with a lid, and allow the herbs to simmer gently for 10 minutes. This simmering process allows the herbs to steep thoroughly, releasing their calming properties into the water.

5. After 10 minutes, remove the saucepan from the heat and let it sit, covered, for an additional 5 minutes. This extra steeping time enhances the strength and efficacy of the tea.

6. Carefully strain the tea through a fine mesh sieve into a teapot or directly into cups, discarding the used herbs. This step ensures a smooth tea free from herb particles.

7. If desired, sweeten the tea with honey or maple syrup according to your taste preferences. Adding a natural sweetener can round out the flavors and add a comforting warmth to the tea.

8. Serve the tea warm, taking a moment to enjoy the aromatic scent before sipping. Allow the calming effects of the chamomile and lemon balm to wash over you, fostering patience and tranquility.

Variations

- For a citrus twist, add a few strips of lemon zest to the saucepan along with the herbs. The lemon zest can provide a refreshing contrast to the floral tones.
- Incorporate a cinnamon stick during the simmering process for a subtly spiced flavor that complements the calming properties of chamomile and lemon balm.
- For a cooler, refreshing version, allow the tea to cool to room temperature, then refrigerate until chilled. Serve over ice for a soothing summer beverage.

Storage tips

Store any leftover tea in a glass container in the refrigerator for up to 2 days. Reheat gently on the stove or enjoy cold for a soothing treat at any time of day.

Tips for allergens

For those with sensitivities or dietary restrictions, maple syrup serves as a delicious vegan-friendly sweetener alternative to honey. Ensure to source organic and pesticide-free dried chamomile and lemon balm to minimize exposure to potential allergens and contaminants.

Scientific references

- "Chamomile: A herbal medicine of the past with a bright future" published in Molecular Medicine Reports, highlights chamomile's anxiolytic and antidepressant properties.
- "Melissa officinalis L. (lemon balm) extract in the treatment of volunteers suffering from mild-to-moderate anxiety disorders and sleep disturbances" from Mediterranean Journal of Nutrition and Metabolism, discussing the mood-enhancing and cognitive function benefits of lemon balm.

CHAPTER 2: HERBS FOR CHILDREN'S SLEEP

Ensuring a good night's sleep for children can sometimes be a challenge, but incorporating certain herbs into their bedtime routine can be a gentle and effective way to help them relax and drift off. Two herbs particularly known for their sleep-supporting properties are **Lavender (Lavandula angustifolia)** and **Chamomile (Matricaria chamomilla)**. Both of these herbs have been traditionally used to promote relaxation and improve sleep quality, making them ideal for children who have difficulty settling down at night.

Lavender, with its soothing scent, is renowned for its ability to calm the mind and body. It can be used in several forms, such as in a diffuser as an essential oil or as a dried herb sewn into sleep pillows. For a simple and effective bedtime ritual, consider adding a few drops of lavender essential oil to a diffuser in your child's room about 30 minutes before they go to bed. This allows the calming aroma to fill the room, creating a peaceful environment conducive to sleep.

Chamomile is another herb celebrated for its calming effects, particularly on the digestive system, which can often be a source of discomfort preventing children from sleeping. A gentle chamomile tea can be a warm and soothing bedtime drink. To prepare it, steep 1 teaspoon of dried chamomile flowers in 8 ounces of boiling water for about 5-10 minutes. Strain the tea to remove the flowers and allow it to cool to a safe temperature before giving it to your child. If your child is not fond of the taste, a small amount of honey can be added to sweeten it, provided they are over the age of one.

For children who might not enjoy tea, creating a **Chamomile Lavender Sleep Spray** is an alternative method to utilize these herbs. To make the spray, combine 1 cup of distilled water, 1 tablespoon of witch hazel, 5 drops of lavender essential oil, and 5 drops of chamomile essential oil in a spray bottle. Shake well before each use and lightly mist your child's pillow and bedding. This not only imparts the calming scent of the herbs but also becomes a comforting bedtime ritual.

When introducing any new herb into your child's routine, it's important to start with small amounts to ensure there are no adverse reactions. Always choose high-quality, organic herbs and essential oils to minimize exposure to pesticides and chemicals. Additionally, consulting with a pediatrician or a qualified herbalist before using herbal remedies with children is recommended, especially if your child has existing health conditions or allergies.

Incorporating lavender and chamomile into your child's bedtime routine can be a simple yet effective way to help them relax and improve their sleep quality. Whether through a warm cup of tea, a soothing aroma in their room, or a comforting spray on their pillow, these herbs offer a natural approach to supporting restful sleep for children.

Chapter 2: Herbs for Children's Sleep

Creating a **Chamomile Lavender Sleep Spray** offers a practical and soothing method to help children relax at bedtime. This spray combines the calming properties of **Lavender (Lavandula angustifolia)** and **Chamomile (Matricaria chamomilla)**, both of which are renowned for their ability to improve sleep quality. Here's how to make and use this sleep spray effectively:

Materials Needed:
- 1 cup of distilled water
- 1 tablespoon of witch hazel
- 5 drops of lavender essential oil
- 5 drops of chamomile essential oil
- A small spray bottle (preferably glass)

Instructions:
1. **Prepare the Spray Bottle:** Ensure the spray bottle is clean and dry. A glass bottle is recommended as it does not react with essential oils and preserves the integrity of the blend.
2. **Mix Water and Witch Hazel:** Pour 1 cup of distilled water into the bottle, followed by 1 tablespoon of witch hazel. Witch hazel acts as an emulsifier, helping to mix the oil and water together more effectively.
3. **Add Essential Oils:** Carefully add 5 drops of lavender essential oil and 5 drops of chamomile essential oil to the mixture. These oils are chosen for their gentle sedative properties, ideal for children.
4. **Shake Well:** Secure the lid on the spray bottle and shake vigorously to ensure the ingredients are well combined. The mixture should appear slightly cloudy once the oils are dispersed.

5. **Usage:** Lightly mist your child's pillow and bedding with the spray. Perform this action about 15 to 30 minutes before your child's bedtime to allow the fabric to absorb the scent and to avoid any wetness.

6. **Storage:** Store the sleep spray in a cool, dark place to maintain the efficacy of the essential oils. Shake well before each use as the oils may separate from the water over time.

Safety Precautions:

- Always perform a patch test on a small area of your child's bedding to ensure there is no adverse reaction to the essential oils.
- Keep the sleep spray out of reach of children to avoid accidental ingestion or misuse.
- Consult with a pediatrician before introducing any new products into your child's bedtime routine, especially if your child has allergies or sensitive skin.

Additional Tips:

- For children who are particularly sensitive to scents, you can reduce the number of essential oil drops to make the fragrance milder.
- Incorporating the sleep spray into a consistent bedtime routine can enhance its effectiveness, as the familiar scent cues the brain that it's time to wind down.
- Encourage your child to participate in the bedtime preparation by misting their own pillow with the spray. This can make them feel more involved and comfortable with the process.

By utilizing the **Chamomile Lavender Sleep Spray**, parents can create a serene and inviting sleep environment for their children. This natural remedy harnesses the power of herbs in a form that is easy to make and delightful to use, promoting restful sleep through the gentle art of aromatherapy.

Chapter 2: Herbs for Children's Sleep

Creating a calming bedtime routine for children is essential for their overall health and well-being, and incorporating specific herbs can significantly enhance this process. Among these, **Valerian (Valeriana officinalis)** and **Passionflower (Passiflora incarnata)** stand out for their sleep-inducing properties, making them excellent choices for children struggling with sleep disturbances. Here's a detailed guide on how to safely and effectively use these herbs to support children's sleep.

Valerian is a herb well-regarded for its sedative qualities and ability to ease insomnia. For children, the most suitable form to administer Valerian is through a mild tea or a diluted tincture, ensuring the dosage is kept low to prevent any potential grogginess the following day. To prepare a Valerian tea, start with a quarter teaspoon of dried Valerian root added to 8 ounces of boiling water. Let it steep for 8-10 minutes before straining. Given its somewhat pungent taste, mixing Valerian tea with a sweeter herbal tea, such as chamomile, can make it more palatable for children. If opting for a tincture, ensure it's alcohol-free and consult with a healthcare provider for the appropriate dosage, generally a fraction of what's recommended for adults, tailored to the child's age and weight.

Passionflower, another herb with calming effects, is particularly beneficial for children who experience anxiety or restlessness at bedtime. Similar to Valerian, Passionflower can be administered as tea or an alcohol-free tincture. For tea, use one teaspoon of dried Passionflower per 8 ounces of boiling water, allowing it to steep for about 10 minutes. The flavor is milder than Valerian, making it more easily accepted by children. When using a tincture, again, consult a healthcare provider for correct dosing.

When introducing these herbs into your child's bedtime routine, it's crucial to observe their response closely. Start with a very mild strength and gradually adjust as necessary. It's also important to establish these herbal remedies as part of a broader bedtime ritual that may include a warm bath, reading a book, or gentle stretching exercises to signal to your child's body that it's time to wind down.

In terms of safety and precautions, while both Valerian and Passionflower are generally considered safe for children, it's paramount to source these herbs from reputable suppliers to ensure they are free from contaminants and accurately labeled. Additionally, discussing the use of these herbs with a pediatrician or a professional herbalist is recommended, especially if your child is taking other medications or has underlying health issues. This step is crucial to avoid any potential interactions or side effects.

For storage, keep dried herbs in airtight containers placed in a cool, dark area to maintain their potency. If using tinctures, follow the storage instructions provided on the product, usually involving keeping the bottle in a cool, dark place and using it within a specified period once opened.

BOOK 32: HERBS FOR LIBIDO AND WELLNESS

CHAPTER 1: APHRODISIAC HERBS FOR DESIRE

Maca (Lepidium meyenii) and Ginseng (Panax ginseng) are two powerful aphrodisiac herbs that have been used for centuries to boost libido and enhance sexual wellness. Both herbs are renowned for their ability to increase energy, improve stamina, and support a healthy libido. Here's how to incorporate Maca and Ginseng into a **Love Elixir** that can be enjoyed daily to support sexual health and vitality.

Ingredients:
- 1 teaspoon of Maca powder
- 1 teaspoon of Ginseng root powder or 1 Ginseng tea bag
- 8 ounces of hot water (not boiling)
- Honey or maple syrup to taste
- A pinch of cinnamon (optional for added warmth and circulation benefits)

Preparation Steps:
1. **Prepare the Water:** Begin by heating the water until it is hot but not boiling. Boiling water can destroy some of the delicate compounds in Ginseng, reducing its effectiveness.
2. **Mix the Herbs:** If using Ginseng powder, mix it with Maca powder in a mug. For those opting for a Ginseng tea bag, place the tea bag in the mug and add the Maca powder.
3. **Steep:** Pour the hot water over the Maca and Ginseng mixture or tea bag. Allow the herbs to steep for about 5-10 minutes. This steeping time allows for the extraction of the beneficial compounds from the herbs.
4. **Enhance the Flavor:** Remove the Ginseng tea bag if used. Add honey or maple syrup to sweeten the elixir according to your taste. A pinch of cinnamon can also be added for its warming properties and to promote blood circulation.
5. **Stir and Enjoy:** Stir the elixir well to ensure that the Maca powder is fully dissolved and the sweetener is evenly distributed. Enjoy this Love Elixir warm.

Consumption Tips:
- **Frequency:** For best results, consider consuming this Love Elixir once daily. Morning consumption can provide an energizing start to the day, while evening consumption can be beneficial for enhancing intimacy.
- **Quality Matters:** Always choose high-quality, organic Maca and Ginseng. This ensures the potency of the herbs and minimizes exposure to pesticides and contaminants.
- **Listen to Your Body:** Begin with a smaller dose of Maca and Ginseng, especially if you are new to these herbs. Observe how your body responds and adjust the dosage accordingly.

Storage:
- Store Maca powder and Ginseng root powder in airtight containers in a cool, dark place to maintain their potency. Proper storage extends the shelf life of these powerful herbs, ensuring that they retain their beneficial properties.

Incorporating Maca and Ginseng into your daily routine through this Love Elixir can offer a natural way to support libido and sexual wellness. These herbs work synergistically to enhance energy levels, improve stamina, and support hormonal balance, contributing to a healthy and fulfilling sexual life.

Maca and Ginseng for Libido Boosting

Maca (Lepidium meyenii) and Ginseng (Panax ginseng) stand out in the realm of natural aphrodisiacs due to their long history of use and the growing body of scientific research supporting their benefits for enhancing libido and overall sexual health. Maca, a root vegetable native to the high Andes of Peru, is not only nutritious but has been used for centuries to boost energy, stamina, and sexual function. Ginseng, revered in traditional Chinese medicine, is known for its ability to improve stamina, endurance, and sexual function. When these two powerful herbs are combined, they create a synergistic effect that can significantly enhance libido and sexual wellness.

To harness the benefits of these herbs, it's crucial to understand the optimal way to consume them. Starting with Maca, it's available in powder form, which is the most versatile for incorporating into your daily diet. Maca powder can be added to smoothies, oatmeal, or homemade energy bars, providing a nutty flavor that blends well with various ingredients. The recommended starting dose of Maca powder is one teaspoon per day, gradually increasing to two or three teaspoons, based on personal tolerance and the effects observed. It's important to source organic, high-quality Maca powder to ensure it's free from contaminants and retains its potent properties.

Ginseng can be consumed in several forms, including fresh root, powder, capsules, or as a tea. For those looking to incorporate Ginseng for libido boosting, using the root powder or capsules is most effective, as these forms ensure a concentrated dose of the active compounds. When starting with Ginseng, a dose of 200-400 mg per day of the extract is recommended, or if using the root powder, one teaspoon added to tea or smoothies. As with Maca, it's vital to choose high-quality, preferably organic Ginseng to maximize its health benefits.

Creating a daily regimen that includes both Maca and Ginseng requires attention to timing and dosage. A morning routine that incorporates a smoothie or tea with Maca and Ginseng can kickstart the day with an energy boost and support libido throughout the day. For those sensitive to stimulants, it's advisable to avoid taking these herbs late in the day as they can interfere with sleep patterns.

In addition to their libido-boosting effects, both Maca and Ginseng offer a range of health benefits, including improved energy levels, better stress management, and enhanced mental clarity. These effects contribute to overall well-being, which is crucial for a healthy sex drive. However, it's essential to listen to your body and adjust the dosage or consumption pattern as needed. Some individuals may experience side effects such as jitteriness or digestive upset, in which case reducing the dose or consulting with a healthcare provider is recommended.

For those looking to incorporate these herbs into their diet, here are a few practical tips:
- Start with a small dose to assess tolerance.
- Consider taking a break every few weeks to prevent your body from becoming accustomed to the herbs, which can reduce their effectiveness.
- Combine the intake of Maca and Ginseng with a healthy diet and regular exercise to maximize their libido-boosting effects.
- Stay hydrated, as both herbs can stimulate detoxification processes in the body, requiring adequate fluid intake to support these processes.

Incorporating Maca and Ginseng into your daily routine can be a natural and effective way to enhance libido and sexual wellness. By understanding the specific properties of each herb, their optimal dosage, and the best ways to consume them, individuals can harness the synergistic effects of Maca and Ginseng for improved sexual health and vitality. Remember, while these herbs are powerful, they are part of a holistic approach to wellness that includes a balanced diet, regular physical activity, and stress management techniques.

Maca and Ginseng Love Elixir

Beneficial effects
Maca and Ginseng Love Elixir is designed to naturally enhance libido and vitality. Maca, a root known for its energy-boosting and hormone-balancing properties, works in synergy with Ginseng, which is celebrated for its ability to improve stamina and sexual function. This combination not only aims to boost desire but also supports overall well-being, making it a holistic approach to enhancing intimacy.

Portions
Makes approximately 2 servings

Preparation time
10 minutes

Cooking time
No cooking required

Ingredients
- 2 cups of almond milk or your choice of milk
- 2 tablespoons of maca powder
- 1 teaspoon of Ginseng extract
- 1 tablespoon of raw honey or to taste (optional)
- A pinch of cinnamon powder
- A pinch of nutmeg
- 2 ice cubes (optional)

Instructions
1. Start by pouring 2 cups of almond milk into a blender. Almond milk is chosen for its creamy texture and subtle sweetness, but feel free to substitute with any milk of your preference.

2. Add 2 tablespoons of maca powder to the blender. Maca powder is derived from the Peruvian maca root, known for its adaptogenic qualities that help balance hormones and boost energy levels.

3. Incorporate 1 teaspoon of Ginseng extract. Ginseng is a powerful adaptogen that has been used for centuries to enhance stamina and sexual health.

4. If you prefer a slightly sweet taste, add 1 tablespoon of raw honey. Honey is optional and can be adjusted according to your taste preferences.

5. Sprinkle a pinch of cinnamon powder and a pinch of nutmeg into the mixture. Both spices are known for their warming properties and ability to stimulate circulation.

6. For a chilled elixir, add 2 ice cubes to the blender.

7. Blend all ingredients on high speed until smooth and creamy, ensuring the maca powder and spices are fully dissolved.

8. Pour the elixir into two glasses and serve immediately. Enjoy this energizing and libido-boosting beverage with your partner for an intimate wellness experience.

Variations

- For a vegan version, ensure the Ginseng extract and honey are plant-based and ethically sourced.
- Add a banana or avocado for a thicker, nutrient-rich smoothie.
- Incorporate a scoop of protein powder for an added energy boost.

Storage tips

This elixir is best enjoyed fresh. However, if you need to store it, keep it in a sealed container in the refrigerator for up to 24 hours. Shake well before serving as natural separation may occur.

Tips for allergens

For those with nut allergies, substitute almond milk with oat milk or another non-nut-based milk. Always ensure that the maca powder and Ginseng extract are free from cross-contaminants by checking the packaging.

Scientific references

- "Maca (L. meyenii) for improving sexual function: a systematic review" published in BMC Complementary and Alternative Medicine, highlights the role of maca in enhancing libido and sexual function.
- "Ginseng and male reproductive function" in the Spermatogenesis journal discusses Ginseng's positive effects on male sexual health.

CHAPTER 2: HERBS FOR HORMONAL BALANCE

Shatavari (Asparagus racemosus) and Damiana (Turnera diffusa) are two potent herbs that have been traditionally used to support hormonal balance and enhance sexual health. Their unique properties make them invaluable for anyone looking to naturally address issues related to hormonal imbalances.

Shatavari, often referred to as the "Queen of Herbs" in Ayurvedic medicine, is renowned for its phytoestrogenic properties, making it an excellent choice for women experiencing menopausal symptoms such as hot flashes and vaginal dryness. To harness Shatavari's benefits, consider incorporating it into your daily regimen through a simple tea or tincture. For tea, add one teaspoon of dried Shatavari root to a cup of boiling water and steep for 10 minutes. Strain and drink twice daily. For a more potent option, a tincture can be made by soaking the root in alcohol for 4-6 weeks, shaking the container daily. The recommended dosage is 1-2 ml, taken with water, up to three times daily.

Damiana, on the other hand, is a shrub native to the Americas, known for its aphrodisiac properties. It works by increasing blood flow and sensitivity in the genital area, which can enhance sexual pleasure and libido. Damiana can be consumed as a tea or tincture. To prepare Damiana tea, steep one to two teaspoons of dried leaves in boiling water for 15 minutes. This tea can be enjoyed up to three times a day. For a tincture, similar to Shatavari, fill a jar with dried Damiana leaves and cover with vodka. Let it sit for 4-6 weeks, shaking daily. The recommended tincture dosage is 2-3 ml, up to three times daily.

When combining **Shatavari and Damiana** for a synergistic effect on hormonal balance and sexual wellness, consider creating a blend that utilizes both herbs. A balanced tea blend could include equal parts of Shatavari root and Damiana leaves. Combine one teaspoon of this blend per cup of boiling water, steep for 10-15 minutes, and enjoy up to twice daily. This combination offers a holistic approach to supporting the endocrine system and enhancing sexual health.

It's important to source these herbs from reputable suppliers to ensure their quality and efficacy. Organic and sustainably harvested options are preferable to avoid the ingestion of pesticides and to support ethical farming practices.

While Shatavari and Damiana are generally considered safe for most individuals, it's crucial to consult with a healthcare provider before starting any new herbal regimen, especially for those who are pregnant, breastfeeding, or on medication. Monitoring your body's response to these herbs and adjusting the dosage as necessary can help optimize their benefits while minimizing any potential side effects.

Shatavari and Damiana for Sexual Health

Shatavari (Asparagus racemosus) and Damiana (Turnera diffusa) are renowned for their ability to support sexual health through hormonal balance. **Shatavari**, a revered herb in Ayurvedic medicine, is known for its phytoestrogenic properties, which can mimic the effects of estrogen in the body. This makes it particularly beneficial for women experiencing menopausal symptoms or hormonal imbalances, as it can help regulate menstrual cycles and alleviate symptoms such as hot flashes and vaginal dryness. To incorporate Shatavari into your regimen, you can prepare a tea by adding **one teaspoon of dried Shatavari root** to **one cup of boiling water**. Allow it to steep for **10 minutes**, then strain and consume. This tea can be taken **twice daily** for optimal benefits. Alternatively, for a more concentrated form, a Shatavari tincture can be prepared by soaking the root in alcohol for **4-6 weeks**, shaking the container daily. The recommended dosage for the tincture is **1-2 ml, up to three times daily**, diluted in water.

Damiana, native to the Americas, is celebrated for its aphrodisiac qualities. It enhances sexual pleasure and libido by increasing blood flow and sensitivity in the genital area. To enjoy Damiana, prepare a tea by steeping **one to two teaspoons of dried leaves** in **boiling water for 15 minutes**. This tea can be consumed **up to three times a day** to support sexual health. For those preferring a tincture, fill a jar with dried Damiana leaves and cover with vodka, allowing it to sit for **4-6 weeks**, with daily shaking. The recommended dosage for Damiana tincture is **2-3 ml, up to three times daily**.

Creating a synergistic blend of **Shatavari and Damiana** can amplify their benefits for hormonal balance and sexual wellness. To make a combined tea, use equal parts of Shatavari root and Damiana leaves. Mix **one teaspoon of this blend** with **one cup of boiling water**, steep for **10-15 minutes**, and enjoy this tea **up to twice daily**. This holistic approach supports the endocrine system, enhancing sexual health and vitality.

When sourcing these herbs, prioritize **organic and sustainably harvested** options to ensure purity and efficacy while supporting ethical practices. Both Shatavari and Damiana are generally safe, but it's essential to **consult with a healthcare provider** before beginning any new herbal regimen, especially for those who are pregnant, breastfeeding, or on medication. Observing your body's response and adjusting the dosage as needed can help maximize the benefits of these powerful herbs for sexual health.

Shatavari Hormone Tea

Beneficial effects

Shatavari Hormone Tea is designed to support hormonal balance, enhance fertility, and reduce symptoms of menopause. Shatavari, an adaptogenic herb, has been traditionally used in Ayurvedic medicine to nourish the female reproductive system, regulate menstrual cycles, and alleviate menopausal symptoms. Its natural antioxidant properties also help combat oxidative stress, contributing to overall wellness.

Portions

Makes approximately 2 cups

Preparation time

5 minutes

Cooking time

15 minutes

Ingredients

- 4 cups of water
- 2 tablespoons of dried Shatavari root
- 1 teaspoon of honey (optional)
- A pinch of ground cinnamon (optional)

Instructions

1. Pour 4 cups of water into a medium-sized saucepan and bring to a boil over high heat.
2. Once the water is boiling, reduce the heat to low and add 2 tablespoons of dried Shatavari root to the saucepan.
3. Cover the saucepan with a lid and simmer the Shatavari root on low heat for 15 minutes. This slow simmering process allows the water to extract the beneficial compounds from the Shatavari root effectively.
4. After 15 minutes, remove the saucepan from the heat and let it sit, covered, for an additional 5 minutes to continue the infusion process.
5. Strain the tea through a fine mesh sieve into a teapot or directly into cups, discarding the used Shatavari root.
6. If desired, sweeten the tea with 1 teaspoon of honey. This step is optional and can be adjusted based on personal taste preferences.
7. For added flavor, sprinkle a pinch of ground cinnamon into the tea and stir well to combine.
8. Serve the tea warm, allowing the natural properties of Shatavari to support hormonal balance and wellness.

Variations

- For a cooling summer drink, allow the tea to cool to room temperature, then refrigerate until chilled. Serve over ice.
- Add a slice of fresh ginger during the simmering process for a spicy twist and additional digestive benefits.
- Incorporate a bag of green tea in the last 3 minutes of simmering for an antioxidant boost.

Storage tips

Store any leftover tea in a sealed glass container in the refrigerator for up to 48 hours. Gently reheat on the stove or enjoy cold for a refreshing hormonal balance support.

Tips for allergens

For those with sensitivities or allergies to honey, maple syrup serves as a delicious vegan-friendly sweetener alternative. Ensure to source organic and non-irradiated Shatavari root to avoid potential contaminants and allergens.

Scientific references

- A study published in the "Journal of Ethnopharmacology" highlights Shatavari's efficacy in supporting female reproductive health and its potential to act as an adaptogen, aiding in stress reduction and hormonal balance.
- Research in the "Ayu" journal discusses the antioxidant properties of Shatavari and its role in combating oxidative stress, contributing to overall health and wellness.

CHAPTER 3: HERBS FOR STRESS-FREE INTIMACY

Creating a tranquil and stress-free environment for intimacy can significantly enhance the experience. Incorporating herbs into this setting not only adds a sensory dimension but also leverages their natural properties to reduce stress and increase relaxation. **Holy Basil** and **Lavender** are two such herbs that can be used effectively to create a serene atmosphere conducive to intimacy.

Holy Basil, known for its adaptogenic properties, helps in lowering stress levels and promoting a sense of well-being. To incorporate Holy Basil into your intimate setting, consider preparing a tea. Use about one teaspoon of dried Holy Basil leaves per cup of boiling water. Allow it to steep for about 5 to 7 minutes. This tea can be enjoyed by both partners an hour before the intimate moment, setting a calm and stress-free tone for the evening.

Lavender, on the other hand, is widely recognized for its calming and relaxing effects on the mind and body. Its aroma alone can help reduce anxiety and create a peaceful environment. For a stress-free intimate experience, consider using Lavender essential oil in a diffuser. Add 5-10 drops of Lavender oil to the diffuser filled with water, and let it run in the bedroom for about 30 minutes before you plan to retire to the room. The soothing scent will permeate the space, creating a tranquil ambiance.

Another way to use Lavender is by making a simple pillow spray. Mix 20 drops of Lavender essential oil with 2 ounces of distilled water and an ounce of witch hazel or alcohol as a dispersant in a spray bottle. Shake well and lightly mist pillows and bed linens. The calming scent of Lavender will help both partners relax more deeply, enhancing the intimate experience.

For those looking to deepen the connection during intimacy, consider a gentle massage with a blend of carrier oil like almond or jojoba and a few drops of Lavender essential oil. This not only nourishes the skin but also provides a soothing experience that can help in releasing physical and emotional barriers.

It's important to source high-quality, organic herbs and essential oils to ensure the purity and efficacy of these remedies. Always perform a patch test before using any new product on the skin to avoid allergic reactions.

Remember, the goal is to create a space that feels safe, serene, and free from the stresses of daily life. By thoughtfully incorporating these herbs into your intimate moments, you can enhance the connection between you and your partner, making each experience more meaningful and fulfilling.

Holy Basil and Lavender Bath Soak

Beneficial effects
Holy Basil and Lavender Bath Soak combines the stress-relieving properties of Holy Basil (Tulsi) with the calming effects of Lavender to create a bath soak that not only soothes the skin but also promotes relaxation and stress relief. Holy Basil is known for its adaptogenic properties, helping the body adapt to stress and promoting mental balance. Lavender, on the other hand, is widely recognized for its ability to calm the nervous system, reduce anxiety, and improve sleep quality. Together, they create a therapeutic bath experience that can help ease tension, support emotional well-being, and enhance intimacy by reducing stress.

Ingredients
- 1/2 cup dried Holy Basil leaves
- 1/2 cup dried Lavender flowers
- 2 cups Epsom salt
- 1/4 cup baking soda (optional, for skin softening and water purification)
- 10-15 drops Lavender essential oil (optional, for enhanced fragrance and therapeutic benefits)
- Muslin bag or cheesecloth (for making a bath tea bag)

Instructions
1. In a large bowl, mix together the dried Holy Basil leaves and dried Lavender flowers.
2. Add the Epsom salt to the bowl. If using, also add the baking soda. Mix thoroughly to ensure the herbs are evenly distributed throughout the salt.
3. If you're using Lavender essential oil for additional fragrance and therapeutic properties, add 10-15 drops to the mixture. Stir well to ensure the oil is evenly distributed throughout the mixture.

4. Transfer the mixture to a muslin bag or a piece of cheesecloth. If using cheesecloth, place the mixture in the center, gather the edges, and tie it securely with a string to create a makeshift bath tea bag.

5. To use, fill your bathtub with warm water and submerge the herbal bath tea bag in the water. Allow it to steep as the tub fills. The warm water will help release the therapeutic properties of the herbs and essential oil into the bath.

6. Once the tub is filled, squeeze the bag gently to release more of the herbal essence into the water. You can leave the bag in the tub as you soak.

7. Soak in the tub for 20-30 minutes, breathing deeply to inhale the calming aroma of Lavender and Holy Basil. Close your eyes and allow yourself to relax fully, letting the stress of the day melt away.

8. After your bath, discard the contents of the muslin bag or cheesecloth and allow it to dry for future use.

Variations
- For a more moisturizing soak, add 1 tablespoon of coconut oil or almond oil to the bath water.
- Incorporate a few rose petals or chamomile flowers to the mixture for added aroma and skin-soothing benefits.
- For a stronger scent, increase the amount of Lavender essential oil or add a few drops of Holy Basil (Tulsi) essential oil to the mixture.

Storage tips
Store any unused bath soak mixture in an airtight container in a cool, dry place. The mixture can last for up to 6 months when stored properly. Ensure the muslin bag or cheesecloth is completely dry before storing to prevent mold growth.

Tips for allergens
For those with sensitive skin or allergies, perform a patch test with both the Holy Basil and Lavender, as well as the essential oils, before adding them to your bath. You can substitute Epsom salt with sea salt if you have a sensitivity to magnesium sulfate. Always choose high-quality, organic herbs and essential oils to minimize the risk of pesticide exposure and skin irritation.

BOOK 33: HERBS FOR COOKING AND DAILY USE

CHAPTER 1: CULINARY HERBS FOR HEALTH

Parsley (Petroselinum crispum) and cilantro (Coriandrum sativum) are two culinary herbs celebrated not only for their distinctive flavors but also for their health benefits. Both herbs are rich in vitamins and minerals, including vitamin C, vitamin A, and potassium, making them excellent additions to a daily diet for detoxification and overall health.

Parsley, a biennial herb native to the Mediterranean, is known for its bright green leaves and clean, slightly peppery taste. It's a versatile herb that can be used in salads, soups, and as a garnish. Beyond its culinary uses, parsley is a powerful diuretic, helping to support kidney function and flush toxins from the body. It's also rich in antioxidants, which can reduce oxidative stress and promote heart health.

To incorporate parsley into your diet, consider adding finely chopped leaves to a morning smoothie. Combine a handful of parsley with fruits such as pineapple or apple, a cup of water or coconut water, and a squeeze of lemon for a refreshing and detoxifying drink. For a more direct approach, parsley tea can be made by steeping a quarter cup of fresh parsley leaves in boiling water for 5-10 minutes. This tea can be consumed once or twice daily.

Cilantro, also known as coriander leaves, is an annual herb with a fresh, citrusy flavor profile. It's often used in Mexican, Indian, and Asian cuisines. Cilantro is particularly known for its ability to chelate heavy metals from the body, thanks to its unique compound structure. It's also beneficial for digestive health, as it can help reduce nausea and settle upset stomachs.

Adding cilantro to your diet can be as simple as incorporating it into salsa, salads, or rice dishes. For a detoxifying cilantro water, blend a cup of cilantro leaves with two cups of water, strain, and drink throughout the day. This can aid in digestion and help remove heavy metals from the body. Another method is to prepare cilantro pesto by blending fresh cilantro leaves with garlic, nuts, olive oil, and Parmesan cheese, which can be used as a healthy sauce for pasta or a flavorful spread for sandwiches.

When selecting parsley and cilantro, look for vibrant, green leaves without any signs of wilting or yellowing. Store them in the refrigerator, wrapped in a damp paper towel and placed in a plastic bag, to maintain freshness. It's also advisable to wash these herbs thoroughly under running water to remove any dirt or residue before use.

For those interested in growing these herbs at home, both parsley and cilantro thrive in well-drained soil and require a good amount of sunlight. They can be grown in pots on a sunny windowsill or in a garden. Regular harvesting will encourage a bushier growth and prolong the life of the plants.

In summary, parsley and cilantro are not only flavorful additions to a variety of dishes but also powerful herbs for promoting detoxification and overall health. By incorporating these herbs into your daily diet, you can enjoy their culinary and health benefits.

Parsley and Cilantro Detox

Parsley (Petroselinum crispum) and cilantro (Coriandrum sativum) serve as potent allies in the detoxification process, thanks to their rich nutrient profiles and unique health benefits. Both herbs are not only culinary staples that add fresh flavors to dishes but also powerful tools for enhancing the body's natural detoxification pathways. Their inclusion in daily diets supports the removal of toxins and can contribute to overall vitality and wellness.

Parsley, with its vibrant green leaves and slightly peppery taste, is a biennial herb that originates from the Mediterranean region. It is highly regarded for its diuretic properties, which assist in flushing out excess fluid from the body, thereby supporting kidney function and the elimination of toxins. Parsley is abundant in vitamins A, C, and K, and contains a significant amount of antioxidants, such as flavonoids and vitamin C, which combat oxidative stress and may reduce the risk of chronic diseases. To harness the detoxifying benefits of parsley, one effective method is to incorporate it into smoothies. A detoxifying smoothie can be prepared by blending a handful of parsley with detox-friendly ingredients like pineapple, which contains bromelain to aid digestion, cucumber for hydration, and a squeeze of lemon for its liver-supporting vitamin C content. This blend not only hydrates but also provides a nutrient-rich, detoxifying drink that can be consumed daily.

Cilantro, known for its distinctive, citrusy flavor, is an annual herb widely used in various global cuisines. Beyond its culinary uses, cilantro has been shown to have chelating properties, meaning it can bind to heavy metals such as lead, mercury, and arsenic in the bloodstream, facilitating their elimination from the body. This makes cilantro particularly valuable for detoxification, especially in today's polluted environments. Additionally, cilantro supports digestive health by aiding in the production of digestive enzymes, which can help reduce gas and bloating. For daily detoxification, cilantro can be easily integrated into the diet by adding fresh leaves to salads, soups, and grain dishes. A simple yet powerful detox water can be made by blending fresh cilantro leaves with water and lemon juice, creating a refreshing drink that supports the body's natural detox processes.

When preparing parsley and cilantro for consumption, it's crucial to ensure they are thoroughly washed to remove any dirt, chemicals, or pesticides that may be present. A gentle rinse under cold running water or soaking in a bowl of water with a splash of vinegar can help clean these herbs effectively. After washing, pat them dry with a clean towel or use a salad spinner to remove excess moisture.

For those interested in growing parsley and cilantro at home, both herbs are relatively easy to cultivate. They prefer well-drained soil and a sunny to partly shaded location. Parsley can be sown directly into the garden or started indoors before the last frost, while cilantro seeds can be planted in the garden in late spring. Both herbs benefit from regular watering and harvesting, which encourages new growth and a continuous supply of fresh leaves for your detoxifying recipes.

Incorporating parsley and cilantro into your daily diet not only enhances the flavor of your meals but also supports your body's detoxification processes, promoting health and well-being. Whether used in smoothies, teas, salads, or detox waters, these herbs offer a simple and natural way to support the body's elimination of toxins, contributing to a healthier, more vibrant life.

Detoxifying Herb Pesto
Beneficial effects
This Detoxifying Herb Pesto is not just a flavorful addition to your meals; it's packed with herbs known for their detoxifying properties. Parsley, a key ingredient, is rich in vitamins A, C, and K and has been shown to support kidney function and flush out excess toxins from the body. Cilantro, another crucial component, has been linked to heavy metal detoxification. Together, these herbs, along with the healthy fats from olive oil and nuts, contribute to a diet that supports the body's natural detoxification processes, promoting overall health and well-being.

Portions
Makes about 1 cup
Preparation time
10 minutes
Cooking time
No cooking required
Ingredients
- 2 cups fresh parsley, tightly packed
- 1 cup fresh cilantro, tightly packed
- 1/2 cup olive oil
- 1/4 cup walnuts or pine nuts
- 3 cloves garlic, peeled
- Juice of 1 lemon
- 1/2 teaspoon sea salt, or to taste
- 1/4 teaspoon black pepper, or to taste
Instructions
1. Begin by washing the parsley and cilantro thoroughly to remove any dirt or residue. Pat them dry with a clean kitchen towel or use a salad spinner to ensure they are completely dry.
2. In a food processor, combine the parsley, cilantro, olive oil, walnuts (or pine nuts), and garlic cloves. Pulse a few times to chop the ingredients roughly.
3. Squeeze the juice of one lemon into the food processor. The lemon juice not only adds flavor but also helps to preserve the bright green color of the herbs.
4. Add the sea salt and black pepper to the mixture. The quantities can be adjusted according to your taste preferences.
5. Process the mixture on high speed until it reaches your desired consistency. For a smoother pesto, process for longer. For a chunkier texture, pulse a few times until the ingredients are just combined.

6. Taste the pesto and adjust the seasoning if necessary. If the pesto is too thick, you can add a little more olive oil to reach the desired consistency.

7. Transfer the pesto to a clean jar or container. Press a piece of plastic wrap directly onto the surface of the pesto before sealing with a lid. This helps to prevent oxidation and keeps the pesto vibrant and fresh.

Variations

- For a nut-free version, substitute sunflower seeds or pumpkin seeds for the walnuts or pine nuts.
- Add a handful of spinach or kale for an extra nutrient boost.
- For a vegan version, ensure no cheese is added, as some traditional pesto recipes include Parmesan.

Storage tips

Store the pesto in an airtight container in the refrigerator for up to 1 week. For longer storage, the pesto can be frozen in an ice cube tray and then transferred to a freezer bag, allowing you to use individual portions as needed.

Tips for allergens

If you're allergic to nuts, using seeds like sunflower or pumpkin can be a great alternative. Always ensure that the ingredients are processed in a facility free from cross-contamination with allergens of concern.

Scientific references

- "Parsley: a review of ethnopharmacology, phytochemistry and biological activities" published in the Journal of Traditional and Complementary Medicine discusses the diuretic and detoxifying effects of parsley.
- "Coriandrum sativum L. (Coriander) in health and disease" in the Food Research International journal explores cilantro's role in detoxification, particularly in heavy metal chelation.

CHAPTER 2: HERBS FOR BEVERAGES

Mint (Mentha spp.) and Lemon Balm (Melissa officinalis) are two refreshing herbs that can transform ordinary water into a delightful, health-boosting beverage. Both herbs are renowned for their digestive benefits and soothing properties, making them perfect for daily hydration needs. To create an infused water that not only quenches thirst but also offers health benefits, follow these detailed steps:

Mint Infused Water:

1. Select fresh mint leaves, ensuring they are vibrant green and free from any brown spots or damage. Approximately one handful of mint leaves will be sufficient for a pitcher of water.
2. Wash the mint leaves thoroughly under cold running water to remove any dirt or potential pesticides. Pat them dry gently with a clean towel.
3. In a large pitcher, add about four cups of cold or room temperature filtered water. It's important to use filtered water to avoid any impurities that might affect the taste and health benefits of the infusion.
4. Bruise the mint leaves gently by pressing them with a spoon or between your hands. This process releases the essential oils, enhancing the flavor of the water.
5. Add the bruised mint leaves to the pitcher of water. For a more intense flavor, you can chop the leaves before adding them.
6. Cover the pitcher and refrigerate for at least 2-4 hours. For best results, let it infuse overnight. This allows the mint flavors to fully meld with the water, creating a refreshing beverage.
7. Before serving, you can strain the water to remove the mint leaves or leave them in for added visual appeal. Serve the mint-infused water over ice for an extra refreshing drink.

Lemon Balm Infused Water:

1. Harvest or purchase fresh lemon balm leaves, looking for leaves that are bright green without any signs of yellowing or wilting.
2. Clean the lemon balm leaves by rinsing them under cold water. Shake off any excess water and pat them dry.
3. For a pitcher of lemon balm-infused water, use about one handful of lemon balm leaves. This can be adjusted based on personal preference for strength.
4. Similar to the mint infusion, add approximately four cups of cold or room temperature filtered water to a large pitcher.
5. To release the flavors and beneficial oils of lemon balm, gently bruise the leaves by pressing them with the back of a spoon or by lightly crushing them in your hands.
6. Place the bruised lemon balm leaves into the pitcher of water. If a stronger infusion is desired, the leaves can be finely chopped before adding.
7. Cover the pitcher and refrigerate, allowing the lemon balm to infuse for several hours or overnight. The longer it infuses, the more pronounced the flavor will be.
8. Strain the infused water if preferred, or serve with the leaves for a decorative touch. Enjoy this calming and digestive-friendly beverage chilled.

For an added twist, combine both mint and lemon balm in the same pitcher, following the same preparation steps. This combination not only enhances the flavor profile but also combines the digestive and soothing benefits of both herbs. Additionally, slices of cucumber or lemon can be added to the pitcher before refrigerating to introduce more complexity to the flavor and increase the detoxifying properties of the beverage.

When preparing herbal infused waters, always ensure the herbs are sourced from safe, non-toxic environments, especially if foraging wild herbs. Organic herbs are preferred to minimize exposure to pesticides and chemicals. Regular consumption of these infused waters can aid in digestion, promote relaxation, and provide a more enjoyable way to meet daily hydration goals.

Mint and Lemon Balm Drinks

Mint (Mentha spp.) and Lemon Balm (Melissa officinalis) are two versatile herbs that can transform simple beverages into refreshing drinks, perfect for hydration and enjoyment. Both herbs are renowned for their aromatic qualities and health benefits, including aiding digestion and providing a calming effect. To incorporate these herbs into beverages, it's essential to understand their characteristics and how to prepare them to maximize their flavors and benefits.

Mint, with its cool, invigorating flavor, is a perfect addition to a variety of drinks. To use mint in beverages, start by selecting fresh mint leaves that are vibrant green without any dark spots or yellowing. Gently wash the leaves under cold water and pat them dry with a clean towel. For a single serving, a handful of mint leaves (about 10-15 leaves) is usually sufficient. Bruise the leaves by lightly crushing them in your hand or with a muddler to release the essential oils, which are responsible for the herb's refreshing taste. This method is particularly effective when making iced teas, lemonades, or simple infused water. Add the bruised mint leaves to your drink and let them steep for several minutes. For a more intense flavor, you can also chop the leaves finely and add them directly to the drink.

Lemon Balm, on the other hand, offers a mild, lemony flavor that complements a wide range of beverages. Similar to mint, you'll want to start with fresh lemon balm leaves, ensuring they are clean and dry. Since lemon balm's flavor is more subtle than mint, you might want to use a slightly larger quantity of leaves. For a single serving, use about 15-20 leaves. The leaves can be prepared in the same manner as mint—by bruising or chopping—to release their flavor. Lemon balm works exceptionally well in herbal teas, both hot and iced, and can be a delightful addition to fruit punches and cocktails.

For a simple Mint and Lemon Balm Infused Water, you'll need:
- 1/2 gallon of filtered water
- 1/2 cup of fresh mint leaves
- 1/2 cup of fresh lemon balm leaves
- Ice cubes (optional)
- Slices of cucumber or lemon (optional for added flavor)

Combine the mint and lemon balm leaves in a large pitcher. Use a wooden spoon or a muddler to gently bruise the leaves and release their oils. Add the filtered water and stir to combine. If desired, add slices of cucumber or lemon for an extra layer of flavor. Refrigerate the infused water for at least 2 hours, or overnight for a more robust flavor. Serve over ice cubes for a refreshing and hydrating drink.

When working with these herbs, it's important to remember that their flavors can become more pronounced over time. Start with a conservative amount of leaves and adjust according to your taste preference. Additionally, both mint and lemon balm can be grown in home gardens or containers, making them readily available for use in your kitchen. These herbs not only elevate the taste of your beverages but also offer health benefits, making them a fantastic choice for daily hydration.

Mint and Lemon Balm Infused Water
Beneficial effects
Mint and Lemon Balm Infused Water is a refreshing and healthful drink that harnesses the soothing and digestive benefits of both herbs. Mint is known for its ability to aid digestion, relieve symptoms of irritable bowel syndrome (IBS), and freshen breath. Lemon balm, on the other hand, has been traditionally used to improve mood, reduce anxiety, and promote sleep. Together, they create a calming, stomach-soothing beverage that also hydrates and revitalizes the body.

Portions
Makes about 4 servings
Preparation time
5 minutes
Cooking time
0 minutes (plus at least 1 hour for infusing)
Ingredients
- 8 cups of filtered water
- 1/2 cup fresh mint leaves
- 1/2 cup fresh lemon balm leaves
- Ice cubes (optional)
Instructions
1. Begin by thoroughly washing the mint and lemon balm leaves under cold running water to remove any dirt or impurities. Pat them dry with a clean kitchen towel or let them air dry for a few minutes.
2. In a large pitcher, add the 8 cups of filtered water. Using filtered water ensures that the delicate flavors of the mint and lemon balm are not overpowered by any impurities or chlorine commonly found in tap water.

3. Gently bruise the mint and lemon balm leaves with your fingers to release their essential oils. This step is crucial as it enhances the infusion, giving the water a more robust flavor and aroma.

4. Add the bruised mint and lemon balm leaves to the pitcher of water. Stir gently to combine.

5. If desired, add ice cubes to the pitcher for an immediate cooling effect. Alternatively, you can refrigerate the infused water to chill.

6. Cover the pitcher with a lid or plastic wrap and refrigerate for at least 1 hour. The longer you allow the herbs to infuse, the stronger the flavor will be. For a more intense herbal taste, you can refrigerate the water overnight.

7. Before serving, stir the infused water well. Pour the water into glasses, being careful to leave the leaves in the pitcher. If preferred, you can strain the water as you pour to remove the leaves.

8. Serve the mint and lemon balm infused water chilled, garnished with additional mint or lemon balm leaves for a decorative touch.

Variations

- For a citrus twist, add slices of lemon, lime, or cucumber to the pitcher along with the mint and lemon balm leaves.
- Sweeten the infused water with a tablespoon of honey or agave syrup if desired. Ensure to stir well until the sweetener is fully dissolved.
- Incorporate a few slices of fresh ginger for an added kick and digestive benefits.

Storage tips

Store the mint and lemon balm infused water in the refrigerator for up to 3 days. For best flavor, consume within the first 24 hours. If the water develops an off taste or odor, it should be discarded.

Tips for allergens

For those with allergies or sensitivities to certain herbs, ensure that the mint and lemon balm used are free from cross-contamination with allergens. If you're allergic to mint or lemon balm, consider substituting with other non-allergenic herbs such as basil or parsley for a different flavor profile.

Scientific references

- "Peppermint: A review of its clinical uses and benefits" published in the International Journal of Food Sciences and Nutrition discusses the digestive and IBS-relieving benefits of mint.
- "Melissa officinalis L. (lemon balm) extract in the treatment of volunteers suffering from mild-to-moderate anxiety disorders and sleep disturbances" from Mediterranean Journal of Nutrition and Metabolism, highlighting the mood-enhancing and sleep-promoting effects of lemon balm.

BOOK 34: RARE HERBAL FERMENTATION TECHNIQUES

CHAPTER 1: HERBAL KOMBUCHA INNOVATIONS

Hibiscus and Lavender Kombucha combines the tangy, refreshing taste of kombucha with the soothing, floral notes of hibiscus and lavender. This unique blend not only offers a delightful sensory experience but also brings a host of health benefits, including stress relief and antioxidant properties. To craft this innovative kombucha, follow these detailed steps:

Ingredients:
- 1 gallon of filtered water
- 1 cup of sugar (organic cane sugar is preferred for its natural properties)
- 8 bags of black tea (or 2 tablespoons of loose-leaf black tea)
- 1 cup of starter tea from a previous batch of kombucha
- 1 SCOBY (Symbiotic Culture Of Bacteria and Yeast)
- 1/2 cup of dried hibiscus flowers
- 1/4 cup of dried lavender buds
- Additional sugar for bottling (optional)

Equipment:
- A large glass jar (at least 1-gallon capacity)
- A tight-weave cloth or coffee filter
- A rubber band or string
- Bottles for the finished kombucha
- A non-metal stirring utensil
- A funnel (for bottling)

Preparation:
1. **Brew the Tea:** In a large pot, bring the gallon of water to a boil. Remove from heat and dissolve the cup of sugar into the hot water. Add the black tea bags or loose-leaf tea and allow to steep until the water has come to room temperature. This can take a few hours. Remove the tea bags or strain the loose-leaf tea from the water.
2. **Add the Starter Tea:** Once the tea is at room temperature, pour it into the glass jar. Add the cup of starter tea. The starter tea makes the liquid acidic, which prevents unfriendly bacteria from taking hold during the fermentation process.
3. **Introduce the SCOBY:** With clean hands, gently place the SCOBY into the jar. Cover the jar with a tight-weave cloth or coffee filter and secure it with a rubber band or string. This allows the kombucha to breathe while keeping out contaminants.
4. **Ferment:** Store the jar at room temperature, out of direct sunlight, and where it won't be disturbed. Ferment for 7 to 10 days, checking the kombucha and the SCOBY periodically. It's normal for the SCOBY to float at the top, bottom, or even sideways. A new layer of SCOBY should start forming on the surface of the kombucha within a few days. Taste the kombucha daily beginning on day 7 by gently inserting a straw beneath the SCOBY to pull out a little liquid. It should be slightly tart and still somewhat sweet.
5. **Flavor with Hibiscus and Lavender:** Once the kombucha has fermented to your liking, remove the SCOBY and set it aside for your next batch. Stir in the dried hibiscus flowers and lavender buds, then cover and allow the mixture to sit for an additional 24 to 48 hours to infuse the flavors. Taste periodically to ensure the flavor strength is to your liking.
6. **Bottle:** Use a funnel to pour the kombucha into bottles, leaving about an inch of headspace at the top. If desired, add a teaspoon of sugar to each bottle to encourage carbonation. Strain out the hibiscus flowers and lavender buds as you pour.
7. **Second Fermentation:** Seal the bottles and store them at room temperature out of direct sunlight for 2 to 14 days for carbonation to develop. Check the bottles daily to ensure they're not building up too much pressure by opening them slightly to release any excess gas.
8. **Refrigerate:** Once the kombucha is carbonated to your liking, transfer the bottles to the refrigerator. This slows down the fermentation process and stops the buildup of carbonation. Your Hibiscus and Lavender Kombucha is now ready to enjoy.

Note: Always handle the SCOBY with clean hands and use clean equipment to prevent contamination. The SCOBY is a living organism and needs proper care to produce the best kombucha.

Hibiscus and Lavender Ferments

To create a unique and flavorful **Hibiscus and Lavender Kombucha**, it's essential to gather high-quality ingredients and follow precise steps for fermentation. This recipe not only yields a kombucha that's rich in probiotics but also imbues it with the calming and antioxidant properties of hibiscus and lavender.

Ingredients:

- **1 gallon of filtered water** to ensure no chlorine or other chemicals interfere with the fermentation process.
- **1 cup of organic cane sugar** to feed the SCOBY and aid in fermentation.
- **8 bags of black tea** (or 2 tablespoons of loose-leaf black tea) as the base for your kombucha. Black tea is recommended for its robust flavor and nutrient profile, which supports the fermentation process.
- **1 cup of starter tea** from a previous batch of kombucha, crucial for lowering the pH to create a safe fermentation environment.
- **1 SCOBY** (Symbiotic Culture Of Bacteria and Yeast), the living home for the bacteria and yeast that ferment the tea.
- **1/2 cup of dried hibiscus flowers** for their tangy flavor and vibrant color. Hibiscus is also known for its high vitamin C content and blood pressure-regulating properties.
- **1/4 cup of dried lavender buds** to impart a soothing aroma and subtle floral notes. Lavender is celebrated for its stress-relieving and anti-inflammatory benefits.

Equipment:

- **A large glass jar** (at least 1-gallon capacity) to ferment the kombucha. Glass is inert, ensuring no flavors are imparted to the kombucha.
- **A tight-weave cloth or coffee filter** and a **rubber band or string** to cover the jar, allowing air in but keeping contaminants out.
- **Bottles** for storing the finished kombucha, preferably glass with airtight seals to allow for carbonation without the risk of explosion.
- **A non-metal stirring utensil** as metal can react with the acidic kombucha and damage the SCOBY.
- **A funnel** for transferring the kombucha into bottles, minimizing spills and ensuring a smooth bottling process.

Preparation Steps:

1. **Brew the Tea:** Boil the gallon of water and dissolve the sugar in it. Add the black tea and allow it to steep until the water reaches room temperature to avoid harming the SCOBY with excessive heat.
2. **Combine with Starter Tea:** Transfer the cooled tea to the glass jar and mix in the starter tea. The acidity of the starter tea is crucial for protecting the brew from harmful bacteria.
3. **Add the SCOBY:** Place the SCOBY gently into the jar. Cover the jar with the cloth or coffee filter and secure it with the rubber band or string.
4. **First Fermentation:** Let the jar sit in a warm, dark place for 7 to 10 days. Avoid disturbing it, but feel free to taste the kombucha after day 7 to check for the desired balance of sweetness and tartness.
5. **Flavor with Hibiscus and Lavender:** After the first fermentation, remove the SCOBY and stir in the hibiscus flowers and lavender buds. Cover again and let it sit for another 24 to 48 hours, allowing the flavors to infuse.
6. **Bottle the Kombucha:** Strain the kombucha to remove the flowers and buds, then use the funnel to fill your bottles, leaving about an inch of headspace. Add a teaspoon of sugar to each bottle if carbonation is desired.
7. **Second Fermentation:** Seal the bottles and leave them at room temperature for 2 to 14 days. Burp the bottles daily to release excess pressure and prevent them from exploding.
8. **Enjoy:** Once the kombucha has reached the desired level of carbonation, refrigerate to slow fermentation. Serve chilled.

By meticulously selecting ingredients and adhering to these steps, you'll craft a **Hibiscus and Lavender Kombucha** that not only tantalizes the taste buds but also offers numerous health benefits. This kombucha variation stands out for its unique blend of flavors and wellness properties, making it a perfect addition to your home fermentation repertoire.

Hibiscus and Lavender Kombucha

Beneficial effects

Hibiscus and Lavender Kombucha combines the antioxidant-rich properties of hibiscus with the calming effects of lavender, creating a refreshing beverage that not only aids digestion but also supports stress relief and overall wellness. Hibiscus is known for its high vitamin C content and ability to lower blood pressure, while lavender promotes relaxation and may help with anxiety and sleep disorders. This kombucha variation offers a unique twist on the traditional recipe, providing a delightful floral flavor and a host of health benefits.

Portions

Makes about 1 gallon

Preparation time

30 minutes (plus 7-14 days for fermentation)

Cooking time

No cooking required, but requires fermentation time

Ingredients

- 1 gallon of filtered water
- 1 cup of sugar (organic cane sugar is preferred)
- 8 bags of hibiscus tea or 1/2 cup of loose-leaf hibiscus tea
- 4 tablespoons of dried lavender flowers
- 1 SCOBY (Symbiotic Culture Of Bacteria and Yeast)
- 2 cups of starter tea from a previous batch of kombucha or store-bought, unpasteurized, plain kombucha
- A piece of breathable fabric (like muslin) and a rubber band to cover the jar

Instructions

1. Begin by boiling the filtered water in a large pot. Once boiling, remove from heat and dissolve the sugar into the water, stirring until fully dissolved.
2. Add the hibiscus tea bags or loose-leaf hibiscus tea to the pot. Steep the tea for about 10 minutes, then remove the tea bags or strain the loose leaves from the water.
3. Add the dried lavender flowers to the pot and allow them to steep as the mixture cools to room temperature. This could take several hours. The goal is to infuse the water with the flavors and benefits of both the hibiscus and lavender.
4. Once the tea has cooled to room temperature (below 86°F or 30°C), remove the lavender flowers by straining the liquid.
5. Pour the sweetened tea into a 1-gallon glass jar, then add the SCOBY and starter tea. The starter tea helps to acidify the brew from the beginning, preventing harmful bacteria from developing.
6. Cover the mouth of the jar with a piece of breathable fabric and secure it with a rubber band. This allows air to flow in and out for fermentation while keeping out contaminants.
7. Place the jar in a warm, dark place (ideally between 75°F and 85°F or 24°C and 29°C) for 7 to 14 days. The length of fermentation time can be adjusted based on taste preference; a longer fermentation will result in a more vinegary flavor.
8. After the fermentation period, taste the kombucha to ensure it has reached the desired flavor. Once ready, remove the SCOBY and reserve 2 cups of the kombucha to use as starter tea for your next batch.
9. The hibiscus and lavender kombucha can now be bottled. If desired, you can perform a second fermentation by adding extra flavors or sweeteners and sealing it in airtight bottles for 3 to 7 days to increase carbonation.

Variations

- For a sweeter kombucha, reduce the fermentation time or add fruit juices during the second fermentation.
- Experiment with other herbal teas or add fresh ginger during the second fermentation for an additional flavor profile and digestive benefits.

Storage tips

Store the bottled kombucha in the refrigerator to slow down the fermentation process and maintain its flavor. It can be kept refrigerated for several weeks.

Tips for allergens

For those sensitive to caffeine, note that hibiscus tea contains no caffeine, but the SCOBY is typically cultivated in caffeinated tea. You can reduce the caffeine content by using decaffeinated green or black tea for the initial SCOBY cultivation.

Scientific references

- "Hibiscus sabdariffa L. in the treatment of hypertension and hyperlipidemia: a comprehensive review of animal and human studies" in the Fitoterapia journal highlights the blood pressure-lowering effects of hibiscus.
- "Lavender and the Nervous System" in the Evidence-Based Complementary and Alternative Medicine journal discusses lavender's potential benefits for anxiety and sleep disorders.

CHAPTER 2: HERBAL KEFIR AND PROBIOTICS

Incorporating **herbal kefir** into your diet is a fantastic way to enhance your gut health with a probiotic-rich beverage while also enjoying the therapeutic benefits of various herbs. Kefir, a fermented milk drink similar to yogurt but with a thinner consistency, serves as an excellent base for the infusion of medicinal herbs, offering a unique way to consume herbs known for their health-promoting properties. This section will guide you through the process of making herbal kefir, focusing on selecting herbs, fermenting, and ensuring safety and efficacy.

Selecting Herbs for Kefir Fermentation:
When choosing herbs to infuse in kefir, consider both the health benefits and the flavor profile of the herbs. Common choices include:
- **Lavender** (Lavandula angustifolia) for its calming and anti-inflammatory properties.
- **Chamomile** (Matricaria chamomilla) known for its soothing effects on the digestive system and its gentle sedative qualities.
- **Mint** (Mentha spp.) for its digestive aid properties and refreshing taste.
- **Lemon balm** (Melissa officinalis) which offers a mild lemon flavor and helps in reducing anxiety and promoting sleep.

Materials Needed:
- 1 quart of milk (preferably organic, can be cow, goat, or a non-dairy alternative for those with lactose intolerance)
- Kefir grains (live cultures necessary for fermenting the milk)
- A glass jar (at least 1-quart capacity)
- A non-metallic strainer (plastic or nylon)
- A wooden or plastic spoon
- Cheesecloth or a clean, thin cloth and a rubber band to cover the jar
- Fresh or dried herbs of your choice

Steps for Making Herbal Kefir:
1. **Prepare the Milk:** Pour the milk into the glass jar, leaving about an inch of space at the top. If you're using non-dairy milk, ensure it's unsweetened to avoid affecting the fermentation process.
2. **Add Kefir Grains:** Add 1-2 tablespoons of kefir grains to the milk. The amount of grains can affect the fermentation time, so adjust according to how quickly you want your kefir to ferment.
3. **Cover and Ferment:** Cover the jar with cheesecloth or a thin cloth and secure it with a rubber band. This allows the mixture to breathe while keeping out contaminants. Place the jar in a warm, dark place (around 68-85°F) for 12-48 hours. The fermentation time will depend on the temperature and the desired sourness of the kefir.
4. **Check the Fermentation:** Start checking the kefir after 12 hours; it should start to thicken and have a slightly sour smell. The longer it ferments, the thicker and more sour it will become.
5. **Strain the Kefir:** Once the kefir has fermented to your liking, use a non-metallic strainer to separate the kefir grains from the liquid. Reserve the grains for your next batch.
6. **Infuse with Herbs:** Add your selected herbs directly to the strained kefir. For fresh herbs, a handful per quart of kefir is a good starting point. If using dried herbs, use about 1-3 teaspoons per quart. Seal the jar and let it infuse in the refrigerator for at least 24 hours. The cold environment will slow down fermentation while allowing the flavors and benefits of the herbs to meld with the kefir.
7. **Strain and Serve:** After infusion, strain the kefir to remove the herbs. Your herbal kefir is now ready to enjoy. It can be consumed on its own, added to smoothies, or used as a base for salad dressings.

Safety Tips:
- Always use clean, sterilized equipment to avoid contamination.
- If the kefir or the jar develops mold or an off smell, discard it and start again with fresh ingredients.
- Introduce herbal kefir into your diet gradually to allow your body to adjust to the probiotics.

By following these detailed steps, you can create a nutritious and delicious herbal kefir that combines the probiotic benefits of traditional kefir with the healing properties of medicinal herbs. This beverage not only supports digestive health but also offers a versatile way to incorporate herbs into your daily wellness routine.

Infusing Kefir with Medicinal Herbs

Infusing kefir with medicinal herbs transforms this already beneficial probiotic-rich beverage into a powerhouse of nutrition and healing. The process begins with selecting the right herbs based on their health benefits and compatibility with kefir's tangy profile. For instance, lavender, known for its calming and anti-inflammatory properties, and chamomile, celebrated for its digestive and sedative effects, are excellent choices. Mint adds a refreshing twist and aids digestion, while lemon balm, with its mild lemon flavor, reduces anxiety and promotes sleep.

To start, you'll need 1 quart of milk—cow, goat, or a non-dairy alternative like coconut milk for those with lactose intolerance. The milk serves as the base for the kefir fermentation, providing the necessary environment for the kefir grains to activate and proliferate. Kefir grains, the live cultures that ferment the milk, are crucial for this process. You'll also need a glass jar of at least 1-quart capacity to hold the mixture, a non-metallic strainer for separating the grains after fermentation, a wooden or plastic spoon for stirring, and cheesecloth or a similar breathable material to cover the jar, secured with a rubber band.

Pour the milk into the glass jar, leaving about an inch of space at the top. If using non-dairy milk, ensure it's unsweetened to maintain the fermentation process's integrity. Add 1-2 tablespoons of kefir grains to the milk. The amount of grains directly influences the fermentation speed, so adjust according to your preference for a quicker or slower fermentation process.

Cover the jar with cheesecloth or a thin cloth and secure it with a rubber band. This setup allows the mixture to breathe while keeping out unwanted contaminants. Place the jar in a warm, dark place, ideally between 68-85°F, for 12-48 hours. The fermentation time varies depending on temperature and how tangy you prefer your kefir.

Begin checking the kefir after 12 hours for signs of fermentation, such as thickening and a slightly sour smell. The longer it ferments, the thicker and more sour it will become. Once the kefir has reached your desired level of fermentation, use a non-metallic strainer to separate the kefir grains from the liquid. Save these grains for your next batch.

Now, infuse the strained kefir with your chosen herbs. For fresh herbs, a handful per quart of kefir is a good starting point. If using dried herbs, use about 1-3 teaspoons per quart. Seal the jar and let it infuse in the refrigerator for at least 24 hours. The cold environment slows further fermentation while allowing the flavors and medicinal properties of the herbs to meld with the kefir.

After the infusion period, strain the kefir again to remove the herbs. Your herbal kefir is now ready to enjoy. It can be consumed on its own, added to smoothies, or used as a base for salad dressings.

Remember, always use clean, sterilized equipment to avoid contamination. If the kefir or the jar develops mold or an off smell at any point, discard it and start over with fresh ingredients. Introduce herbal kefir into your diet gradually, allowing your body to adjust to the probiotics. This careful process results in a nutritious, delicious beverage that combines the probiotic benefits of kefir with the healing properties of medicinal herbs, supporting digestive health and incorporating herbs into your wellness routine.

Mint and Chamomile Kefir

Beneficial effects
Mint and Chamomile Kefir combines the digestive benefits of mint with the calming effects of chamomile in a probiotic-rich kefir base, offering a soothing, gut-friendly beverage. Mint is known for its ability to ease digestive discomfort and improve bile flow, which helps in digesting fats. Chamomile, on the other hand, is widely recognized for its calming properties, reducing stress and aiding in sleep. Together, these herbs infused in kefir can support digestive health, promote relaxation, and enhance the immune system due to the probiotics present in kefir.

Portions
Makes about 4 cups

Preparation time
24 hours

Cooking time
No cooking required

Ingredients
- 4 cups of plain, unsweetened kefir
- 1/4 cup fresh mint leaves
- 1/4 cup fresh chamomile flowers (or 2 tablespoons dried chamomile if fresh is unavailable)

- 1 tablespoon honey (optional, for sweetness)

Instructions

1. Begin by ensuring the mint leaves and chamomile flowers are thoroughly washed under cold running water. Pat them dry gently with a clean kitchen towel or let them air dry on a paper towel.
2. In a large, clean glass jar, combine the plain kefir with the fresh mint leaves and chamomile flowers. If using dried chamomile, ensure it's evenly distributed throughout the kefir.
3. If a touch of sweetness is desired, stir in 1 tablespoon of honey until it is fully dissolved into the mixture.
4. Cover the jar with a breathable cloth or coffee filter and secure it with a rubber band. This setup allows the mixture to breathe without letting in any unwanted particles.
5. Let the jar sit at room temperature (around 68°F to 78°F) for 24 hours. This time allows the flavors of the mint and chamomile to infuse into the kefir, enhancing its probiotic benefits with the herbal properties.
6. After 24 hours, remove the cloth or coffee filter. Stir the kefir gently to ensure any settled herbs are mixed back into the liquid.
7. Strain the kefir through a fine mesh sieve or cheesecloth into another clean jar or bottle, pressing gently on the solids to extract all the liquid. Discard the mint leaves and chamomile flowers.
8. The Mint and Chamomile Kefir is now ready to be consumed. For best flavor, chill in the refrigerator for at least 1 hour before serving.

Variations

- For a vegan version, substitute dairy kefir with coconut milk kefir or any plant-based kefir.
- Add a slice of ginger or a teaspoon of vanilla extract for additional flavor complexity.
- For an extra probiotic boost, mix in a tablespoon of prebiotic fiber before the infusion process.

Storage tips

Store the strained Mint and Chamomile Kefir in a sealed glass container in the refrigerator for up to 1 week. Shake well before each use as natural separation may occur.

Tips for allergens

For those with dairy sensitivities, using a non-dairy kefir base can provide similar probiotic benefits without the allergens. Always ensure that the honey used is pure and not processed in facilities that handle allergens.

Scientific references

- A study published in the "Journal of Agricultural and Food Chemistry" highlights the digestive enzyme activities of mint, supporting its role in improving digestion.
- Research in "Phytotherapy Research" outlines the calming effects of chamomile, including its potential to aid in sleep and reduce anxiety, making it a beneficial addition to kefir for overall wellness.

CHAPTER 3: CRAFTING HERBAL SODAS

Crafting herbal sodas offers a delightful way to enjoy the benefits of herbs in a refreshing, fizzy beverage. This process involves fermenting a sweet herbal tea with a culture to produce a naturally carbonated drink. Here, we focus on creating a basic herbal soda and then explore variations to customize the flavor.

Ingredients:
- **1/2 gallon of filtered water** to ensure no impurities affect the fermentation process.
- **1 cup of organic sugar** to feed the fermentation culture. Raw or unrefined sugar is preferred for its mineral content.
- **1 SCOBY (Symbiotic Culture Of Bacteria and Yeast)** or **ginger bug** as the fermentation starter. A SCOBY can be sourced from a previous batch of kombucha, while a ginger bug can be easily made at home by fermenting ginger, sugar, and water over several days.
- **1-2 cups of fresh or dried herbs** of your choice. Popular options include **mint**, **lemon balm**, **lavender**, or **hibiscus** for their flavorful and healthful properties.
- **Juice of 1 lemon** (optional) for added flavor and acidity.

Equipment:
- **A large glass jar** (at least 1-gallon capacity) for brewing the herbal tea.
- **A wooden spoon** for stirring, as metal utensils can react with the fermentation process.
- **A fine mesh strainer** or **cheesecloth** for straining the herbs from the brew.
- **Swing-top bottles** for bottling the soda, which can withstand the pressure of carbonation.
- **A funnel** to transfer the liquid into bottles.

Preparation Steps:
1. **Brew the Herbal Tea:** In a large pot, bring the filtered water to a boil. Remove from heat and add your chosen herbs. Steep for 15-20 minutes or until the tea is strong and flavorful. The longer you steep, the more pronounced the herbal flavors will be in the final soda.
2. **Sweeten the Brew:** While the tea is still warm, stir in the sugar until completely dissolved. This sweetened tea will be the base of your herbal soda, providing the necessary food for the fermentation culture.
3. **Cool to Room Temperature:** Allow the sweetened herbal tea to cool to room temperature. Adding the SCOBY or ginger bug to hot liquid can kill the beneficial bacteria and yeast.
4. **Add the SCOBY or Ginger Bug:** Transfer the cooled tea to the large glass jar. Add the SCOBY or ginger bug to the jar, gently stirring with the wooden spoon to combine.
5. **Ferment:** Cover the jar with a piece of cheesecloth or a coffee filter secured with a rubber band. This allows the mixture to breathe while keeping out dust and insects. Place the jar in a warm, dark place for 3-7 days. The fermentation time will vary depending on the temperature and the desired level of fizziness. Taste the soda daily starting on day 3 by gently inserting a straw beneath the SCOBY or ginger bug to sample the liquid.
6. **Bottle the Soda:** Once the soda has reached your desired level of carbonation, remove the SCOBY or ginger bug (you can save this for your next batch). If using lemon juice, add it now for an extra zing. Use the funnel and strainer to pour the soda into swing-top bottles, leaving about an inch of headspace to allow for additional carbonation.
7. **Secondary Fermentation:** Seal the bottles and leave them at room temperature for 2-3 days to build carbonation. Be sure to "burp" the bottles once a day to release excess pressure and prevent them from exploding.
8. **Refrigerate:** After 2-3 days, transfer the bottles to the refrigerator to slow the fermentation process. Chilling the soda will also improve its taste and refreshment factor.

Customizing Your Herbal Soda:
The beauty of crafting herbal sodas lies in the endless flavor combinations you can create. Experiment with different herbs, edible flowers, and even fruits to find your perfect blend. For a more complex flavor profile, consider adding spices like **cinnamon**, **cardamom**, or **vanilla** during the brewing process. Remember, the potency of flavors can intensify during fermentation, so start with smaller amounts of stronger herbs or spices and adjust according to taste in future batches.

Herbal sodas not only provide a probiotic boost similar to kombucha but also allow you to enjoy the nuanced flavors of various herbs in a unique and enjoyable way. Whether you're looking for a digestive aid, a calming beverage, or simply a tasty alternative to commercial sodas, herbal sodas offer a customizable and healthful solution.

Elderflower and Lemon Soda

Beneficial effects

Elderflower and Lemon Soda is a refreshing, naturally fermented drink that offers a delightful blend of flavors and health benefits. Elderflower is known for its potential to alleviate cold and flu symptoms, thanks to its antiviral and immune-boosting properties. Lemon, rich in vitamin C, aids in digestion and detoxification, while also providing a zesty flavor that complements the floral notes of elderflower. This soda is not only a delicious alternative to sugary soft drinks but also supports overall wellness.

Portions

Makes about 2 liters

Preparation time

15 minutes (plus 2-3 days for fermentation)

Cooking time

No cooking required

Ingredients

- 1/2 cup fresh elderflowers or 1/4 cup dried elderflowers
- Peel of 1 organic lemon, avoiding the white pith to reduce bitterness
- Juice of 2 lemons
- 1/2 cup organic sugar
- 1 tablespoon raw honey (optional, for additional sweetness and fermentation)
- 1/4 teaspoon champagne yeast or wild yeast if preferred
- 2 liters filtered water
- A few raisins or a slice of ginger (optional, as a fermentation aid)

Instructions

1. Start by ensuring all equipment, especially the fermentation vessel, is thoroughly cleaned and sterilized to prevent unwanted bacteria from influencing the fermentation process.
2. In a large, clean jar or bottle, dissolve the organic sugar in 2 cups of filtered water. Stir until the sugar is completely dissolved.
3. Add the lemon peel and lemon juice to the sugar water mixture. If using honey, add it at this stage and stir well to combine.
4. Sprinkle the champagne yeast over the liquid. There's no need to stir, as the yeast will naturally disperse and begin the fermentation process.
5. Gently add the elderflowers to the jar, ensuring they are submerged in the liquid. If using raisins or a slice of ginger as a fermentation aid, add them now.
6. Fill the jar with the remaining filtered water, leaving about an inch of space at the top for gases to escape during fermentation.
7. Cover the jar with a piece of breathable fabric secured with a rubber band or a loose-fitting lid to allow gases to escape while keeping contaminants out.
8. Place the jar in a warm, dark place for 2-3 days. Check daily to observe the fermentation process; you should see bubbles forming as the yeast converts sugar into alcohol and carbon dioxide.
9. Once the soda has achieved a level of carbonation and flavor to your liking, strain out the elderflowers, lemon peel, raisins, or ginger if used.
10. Bottle the soda in clean, airtight bottles and refrigerate to halt the fermentation process. Be cautious of pressure build-up; open bottles slowly over a sink to avoid potential overflow.

Variations

- For a sweeter soda, increase the amount of sugar or honey. Adjust according to taste preference.
- Experiment with adding different herbs or edible flowers such as lavender or chamomile for a unique flavor profile.
- Use different citrus peels like orange or grapefruit for a twist on the traditional lemon flavor.

Storage tips

Keep the bottled elderflower and lemon soda refrigerated and consume within 2 weeks for best flavor and carbonation. Always be mindful of pressure build-up in the bottles; occasionally releasing the gas can prevent accidental explosions.

Tips for allergens

For those with yeast allergies, creating a wild fermentation by omitting the champagne yeast and allowing natural yeasts to initiate fermentation is an option, though results may vary. Ensure all ingredients, especially the elderflowers and lemon, are organic to minimize exposure to pesticides and chemicals.

BOOK 35: HERBS FOR FINANCIAL WELLNESS

CHAPTER 1: HERBS FOR MENTAL CLARITY

In the realm of financial wellness, mental clarity is paramount for making informed decisions that impact one's economic stability and growth. Herbs have been utilized for centuries to enhance cognitive function, reduce stress, and support overall brain health. Among these, **Rosemary (Rosmarinus officinalis)** and **Ginkgo Biloba** stand out for their significant benefits in improving focus, memory, and mental clarity.

Rosemary is not only celebrated for its aromatic qualities in cooking but also for its cognitive-enhancing properties. The active compound **1,8-cineole**, present in Rosemary, has been shown to increase neurotransmitter activity, thereby improving memory recall and mental sharpness. To incorporate Rosemary into your daily routine for enhanced mental clarity, consider the following preparation method:

1. **Rosemary Infused Oil**: Begin by selecting fresh Rosemary sprigs, ensuring they are clean and dry. Place the sprigs in a clean, dry jar and cover them with a carrier oil such as olive or almond oil. Seal the jar and place it in a warm, sunny spot for 2-3 weeks, shaking it gently every few days. Strain the oil through a fine mesh sieve or cheesecloth into a clean bottle. Use this infused oil as a salad dressing or incorporate it into your meals. The aromatic properties of Rosemary can stimulate the senses and promote cognitive function.

Ginkgo Biloba, another herb renowned for its cognitive benefits, has been extensively studied for its ability to enhance blood flow to the brain, thus improving concentration and memory. Ginkgo contains flavonoids and terpenoids, which are compounds known for their antioxidant and anti-inflammatory effects, supporting overall brain health. To benefit from Ginkgo Biloba, consider the following:

1. **Ginkgo Biloba Tea**: Start with dried Ginkgo Biloba leaves, readily available at health food stores. For each cup of tea, use one teaspoon of dried leaves. Boil water and pour it over the leaves, allowing them to steep for about 10 minutes. Strain the tea into a cup and enjoy. Drinking Ginkgo Biloba tea in the morning can help kickstart your day with enhanced mental clarity and focus.

It's important to note that while these herbs can support mental clarity and cognitive function, they should be used in conjunction with a healthy lifestyle, including a balanced diet, regular exercise, and adequate sleep. Additionally, consult with a healthcare provider before adding new herbal supplements to your routine, especially if you are pregnant, nursing, or taking other medications, to avoid potential interactions.

Incorporating Rosemary and Ginkgo Biloba into your daily regimen can be a simple yet effective strategy to enhance mental clarity, improve decision-making capabilities, and support your journey towards financial wellness. Remember, the key to benefiting from these herbs lies in consistency and integration into a holistic approach to health and well-being.

Lemon Balm and Rosemary Tea for Focus

Beneficial effects

Lemon Balm and Rosemary Tea is a natural, herbal beverage known for its ability to enhance focus and mental clarity. Lemon balm, with its calming properties, helps to reduce anxiety and promote a sense of calm, making it easier to concentrate. Rosemary, on the other hand, is often associated with cognitive enhancement, improving memory function and mental alertness. Together, these herbs create a synergistic blend that supports brain health and can help manage stress, making it an ideal drink for those seeking to improve their focus and productivity, especially in financially or mentally demanding situations.

Portions

Makes about 2 servings

Preparation time

5 minutes

Cooking time

10 minutes

Ingredients

- 2 cups of water
- 1 tablespoon dried lemon balm leaves
- 1 teaspoon dried rosemary leaves
- Honey or stevia (optional, for sweetness)

Instructions

1. Begin by bringing 2 cups of water to a boil in a small saucepan. Use filtered water to ensure the purest taste of your tea.

2. Once the water reaches a rolling boil, reduce the heat to low and add 1 tablespoon of dried lemon balm leaves. Lemon balm is delicate, so simmering it gently helps to extract its beneficial oils without destroying them.

3. Add 1 teaspoon of dried rosemary leaves to the saucepan. Rosemary is robust and can withstand the heat, which will help release its aromatic oils and beneficial compounds.

4. Cover the saucepan with a lid and let the herbs simmer gently for about 10 minutes. This slow infusion process allows the water to become fully saturated with the flavors and therapeutic properties of the herbs.

5. After 10 minutes, remove the saucepan from the heat. Let it sit covered for an additional 2 minutes to further steep and intensify the flavors.

6. Strain the tea through a fine mesh sieve into two cups, ensuring that all the herb particles are removed for a smooth drinking experience.

7. Taste the tea and add honey or stevia to sweeten, if desired. Adding a natural sweetener can enhance the flavors and provide a more enjoyable sipping experience without overpowering the herbal notes.

8. Serve the tea warm. For the best focus-enhancing effects, drink this tea in the morning or early afternoon to harness the cognitive benefits of rosemary and lemon balm throughout the day.

Variations
- For a refreshing cold beverage, allow the tea to cool to room temperature, then refrigerate for 1-2 hours. Serve over ice for a cool, focus-enhancing drink.
- Add a slice of fresh lemon or a sprig of fresh rosemary to each cup for added flavor and a decorative touch.
- Combine with green tea for an added antioxidant boost. Add 1 green tea bag during the last 3 minutes of simmering for a gentle caffeine lift.

Storage tips
Store any leftover tea in a glass container in the refrigerator for up to 2 days. Reheat gently or enjoy cold for a revitalizing drink.

Tips for allergens
For those with allergies to specific herbs, always ensure that the lemon balm and rosemary used are pure and not mixed with other herbs that could cause an allergic reaction. If you're sensitive to honey, stevia makes an excellent alternative sweetener.

Scientific references
- "Melissa officinalis L. (lemon balm) extract in the treatment of volunteers suffering from mild-to-moderate anxiety disorders and sleep disturbances" from Mediterranean Journal of Nutrition and Metabolism, highlighting the mood-enhancing and sleep-promoting effects of lemon balm.
- "Rosemary for Brain Performance and Mood: A Review of the Literature" in the journal Fitoterapia, which discusses the cognitive benefits of rosemary, including memory improvement and increased alertness.

CHAPTER 2: HERBS FOR FINANCIAL STRESS RELIEF

In the quest for financial wellness, stress often becomes a significant barrier, impacting not just our mental health but also our physical well-being. To combat this, certain herbs have been identified for their potent stress-relieving properties. Among these, **Holy Basil (Ocimum sanctum)** and **Ashwagandha (Withania somnifera)** stand out for their adaptogenic qualities, which help the body adapt to stress and promote a sense of balance.

Holy Basil, revered in Ayurvedic medicine as Tulsi, is not just a culinary herb but a powerful adaptogen that helps in mitigating stress and anxiety. To harness the benefits of Holy Basil, consider incorporating it into your daily routine through a simple tea preparation. Start by boiling water and adding a teaspoon of dried Holy Basil leaves. Allow the mixture to steep for about 5-7 minutes before straining. Drinking this tea twice daily can help in reducing stress levels, thereby improving your focus on financial planning and decision-making.

Ashwagandha, another renowned adaptogen, has been studied for its efficacy in reducing cortisol levels, the body's stress hormone. For those looking to incorporate Ashwagandha into their regimen, a straightforward approach is to use Ashwagandha powder. Mix half a teaspoon of the powder into a glass of warm milk or water before bedtime. This not only aids in reducing stress but also promotes a restful night's sleep, which is crucial for maintaining optimal cognitive function for financial management.

When selecting herbs like Holy Basil and Ashwagandha, it's essential to source them from reputable suppliers to ensure purity and potency. Additionally, while these herbs are generally safe for most individuals, it's advisable to consult with a healthcare provider before starting any new herbal supplement, especially for those who are pregnant, nursing, or on medication.

Incorporating these herbs into your daily routine requires minimal effort but can yield significant benefits in terms of stress reduction and enhanced mental clarity. By doing so, you can create a more conducive environment for managing your finances effectively, free from the debilitating effects of stress.

Holy Basil and Ashwagandha Stress Tonic

Beneficial effects

Holy Basil, also known as Tulsi, is revered in Ayurvedic medicine for its ability to lower stress levels and support the body's natural response to tension and anxiety. Ashwagandha, another powerhouse herb, is classified as an adaptogen, meaning it can help your body manage stress more effectively. It's also known for its potential to improve brain function, including memory. Combining these two herbs into a stress tonic creates a powerful ally in managing financial stress and enhancing overall wellness.

Portions

Makes about 2 servings

Preparation time

10 minutes

Cooking time

5 minutes

Ingredients

- 2 cups of water
- 1 tablespoon dried Holy Basil (Tulsi) leaves
- 1 teaspoon Ashwagandha powder
- 1 teaspoon honey (optional, for sweetness)
- A slice of lemon (optional, for flavor)

Instructions

1. Pour 2 cups of water into a small saucepan and bring to a gentle boil over medium heat.
2. Once the water is boiling, reduce the heat to low and add 1 tablespoon of dried Holy Basil leaves. Cover the saucepan with a lid to prevent the volatile oils from escaping.
3. Simmer the Holy Basil leaves in the water on low heat for about 5 minutes. This gentle simmering process helps to extract the active compounds from the Holy Basil without destroying them.
4. After 5 minutes, turn off the heat and stir in 1 teaspoon of Ashwagandha powder until it is completely dissolved. Ashwagandha powder can clump, so ensure to stir thoroughly for a smooth consistency.

5. Cover the saucepan again and let the mixture steep for an additional 5 minutes. This steeping time allows the flavors and beneficial properties of the herbs to meld together.

6. Strain the tonic through a fine mesh sieve into two cups, pressing on the solids to extract as much liquid as possible. Discard the solids.

7. If desired, stir in 1 teaspoon of honey to each cup for sweetness. Honey not only adds sweetness but also brings its own calming properties to the tonic.

8. Add a slice of lemon to each cup for an added boost of vitamin C and a refreshing flavor.

9. Enjoy the Holy Basil and Ashwagandha Stress Tonic warm, ideally in the morning or evening, as part of your daily routine to combat financial stress and support overall mental wellness.

Variations

- For a cold version, allow the tonic to cool to room temperature, then refrigerate for 1-2 hours. Serve over ice for a refreshing stress-relieving beverage.
- Add a pinch of ground cinnamon or ginger for additional warming and digestive benefits.
- For those who prefer a caffeine boost, mix the tonic with green tea instead of water for an energizing yet calming drink.

Storage tips

Store any leftover tonic in a glass container in the refrigerator for up to 2 days. Reheat gently or enjoy cold.

Tips for allergens

For those with sensitivities to specific herbs, ensure that the Holy Basil and Ashwagandha used are pure and not mixed with other herbs that could cause an allergic reaction. If honey is a concern, substitute with maple syrup or a few drops of stevia for sweetness.

Scientific references

- "An overview on Ashwagandha: A Rasayana (Rejuvenator) of Ayurveda" published in the African Journal of Traditional, Complementary and Alternative Medicines discusses the stress-relief and cognitive benefits of Ashwagandha.
- "Ocimum sanctum Linn. (Holy Basil or Tulsi) and its phytochemicals in the prevention and treatment of diseases" in the Journal of Ayurveda and Integrative Medicine highlights the stress-reducing properties of Holy Basil.

CHAPTER 3: FINANCIAL FOCUS WITH ADAPTOGENS

Adaptogens are a unique class of herbs known for their ability to enhance the body's resistance to stress and improve overall energy and mental clarity. For individuals seeking to improve their financial focus, incorporating adaptogens into their daily routine can be a game-changer. These herbs work by modulating the adrenal system, helping to balance stress hormones, which is crucial for maintaining concentration and making informed financial decisions. Here are specific adaptogens and methods for integrating them into your lifestyle to support financial focus:

Rhodiola Rosea: This adaptogen is renowned for its fatigue-reducing and cognitive-enhancing properties. To use Rhodiola for financial focus, consider starting with a low dose of around 100mg in capsule form each morning, gradually increasing as needed based on your body's response. Rhodiola is best taken on an empty stomach for optimal absorption and effectiveness.

Ashwagandha (Withania somnifera): Ashwagandha supports endurance and reduces anxiety, which can be beneficial when dealing with financial stress. Incorporating Ashwagandha into your routine can be as simple as mixing half a teaspoon of the powdered root into a smoothie or glass of warm milk with a bit of honey before bedtime. This not only aids in stress reduction but also promotes a restful sleep, essential for clear-headed financial planning.

Holy Basil (Ocimum sanctum): Also known as Tulsi, Holy Basil helps in mitigating stress and boosting brain function. For daily consumption, you can brew Holy Basil leaves into a tea. Add 1-2 teaspoons of dried Holy Basil leaves to hot water and steep for about 5-7 minutes. This tea can be consumed 1-2 times daily, especially during periods of high stress, to maintain mental clarity and focus.

Siberian Ginseng (Eleutherococcus senticosus): This adaptogen enhances physical and mental endurance, making it easier to tackle complex financial tasks. Begin with a daily dose of 300mg in capsule form, taken in the morning to avoid potential interference with sleep. Siberian Ginseng is particularly effective during periods of high stress or when increased concentration and stamina are needed.

Cordyceps: Known for their energy-boosting properties, Cordyceps can be particularly useful for those long financial planning sessions. Incorporate Cordyceps into your diet by adding powdered Cordyceps to coffee, tea, or smoothies. Start with a quarter teaspoon per day and adjust according to your energy needs and body's response.

When incorporating adaptogens for financial focus, it's essential to:
- Start with small doses and gradually increase to gauge your body's response.
- Choose high-quality, reputable sources for adaptogens to ensure purity and potency.
- Be consistent with usage, as the benefits of adaptogens accumulate over time.
- Listen to your body and adjust dosages or adaptogens as needed, based on your personal experience and health goals.

Remember, while adaptogens can significantly support mental clarity and stress management, they are most effective when used as part of a holistic approach to wellness. This includes maintaining a balanced diet, regular physical activity, and adequate sleep, all of which are foundational for optimal cognitive function and financial decision-making. Additionally, always consult with a healthcare provider before adding new supplements to your regimen, especially if you have existing health conditions or are taking other medications.

Adaptogen Productivity Smoothie
Beneficial effects
Combining adaptogens like ashwagandha and maca with the nutritional powerhouse of spinach and the natural sweetness of bananas and blueberries, this Adaptogen Productivity Smoothie is designed to enhance focus, increase energy levels, and support overall brain health. Ashwagandha is known for its ability to reduce stress and anxiety, improve concentration, and boost energy. Maca root adds to the blend by improving mood and energy, while spinach provides a wealth of vitamins and minerals essential for cognitive function. Bananas and blueberries not only add natural sweetness and flavor but also pack antioxidants and potassium, which aid in brain health and function.

Portions
Makes about 2 servings

Preparation time

5 minutes

Cooking time

No cooking required

Ingredients

- 1 cup of unsweetened almond milk
- 1 ripe banana
- 1/2 cup of frozen blueberries
- 1 tablespoon of ashwagandha powder
- 1 tablespoon of maca powder
- 1 cup of fresh spinach leaves
- 1 tablespoon of chia seeds (optional, for added fiber and omega-3 fatty acids)
- Ice cubes (optional, for a colder smoothie)

Instructions

1. Start by gathering all your ingredients. Ensure the banana is ripe for natural sweetness and the blueberries are frozen to give the smoothie a refreshing chill.

2. In a high-speed blender, add 1 cup of unsweetened almond milk. Almond milk is chosen for its light flavor and plant-based nutrients, but any milk of your choice can be used.

3. Peel the ripe banana and add it to the blender. Bananas are a great source of natural sweetness and potassium.

4. Add 1/2 cup of frozen blueberries to the blender. Blueberries are not only flavorful but are also rich in antioxidants which are beneficial for brain health.

5. Measure and add 1 tablespoon of ashwagandha powder. Ashwagandha is an adaptogen known for its stress-reducing effects.

6. Add 1 tablespoon of maca powder to the blender. Maca is known for its mood and energy-boosting properties.

7. Add 1 cup of fresh spinach leaves. Spinach is loaded with vitamins and minerals that support overall health, particularly cognitive function.

8. For added fiber and omega-3 fatty acids, add 1 tablespoon of chia seeds. This step is optional but recommended for a nutritional boost.

9. If you prefer your smoothie colder, add a few ice cubes to the blender.

10. Blend all the ingredients on high speed until smooth and creamy. Ensure the mixture is completely smooth to avoid any leafy chunks.

11. Taste the smoothie and adjust the sweetness if necessary. If you prefer it sweeter, you can add a little honey or maple syrup and blend again.

12. Serve the smoothie immediately in two glasses for optimal freshness and nutrient retention.

Variations

- For a protein boost, add a scoop of your favorite plant-based protein powder.
- Substitute almond milk with coconut water for a lighter version with a tropical twist.
- Add a tablespoon of cocoa powder for a chocolatey flavor without compromising the health benefits.

Storage tips

This smoothie is best enjoyed fresh. However, if you need to store it, keep it in a sealed container in the refrigerator for up to 24 hours. Shake well before drinking as separation may occur.

Tips for allergens

For those with nut allergies, substitute almond milk with oat milk or any other non-nut-based milk. Ensure that the ashwagandha and maca powders are processed in a facility free from the allergens you're concerned about.

BOOK 36: INTEGRATING HERBAL KNOWLEDGE

CHAPTER 1: SHARING HERBAL WISDOM LOCALLY

Community workshops are an excellent way to share herbal wisdom locally, fostering a deeper understanding and appreciation for herbal medicine within your community. To organize a successful workshop, follow these detailed steps:

Identify Your Audience: Determine who your workshop is for. Is it for beginners, those with a moderate understanding, or advanced practitioners of herbal medicine? Knowing your audience will help tailor the content to their needs.

Choose a Theme: Select a specific theme or topic for your workshop, such as "Herbal Remedies for Winter Wellness" or "Creating Your Herbal First Aid Kit." A focused theme makes the workshop more appealing and manageable.

Secure a Venue: Look for a space that supports the type of workshop you're planning. Community centers, local gardens, or even outdoor spaces can be ideal, depending on the size of the group and the nature of the workshop. Ensure the venue has enough space for practical demonstrations and is accessible to all participants.

Gather Materials and Resources: Prepare a list of all the materials you'll need, including herbs, equipment for demonstrations (like mortars and pestles, jars for salves, or teapots for infusions), handouts, and other educational materials. Source these materials from reputable suppliers to ensure quality.

Develop Your Workshop Content: Break down your workshop into manageable segments. For example, if your workshop is on making herbal teas, include a segment on the history and benefits of each herb you'll be using, followed by a detailed demonstration of tea preparation. Use clear, accessible language and provide hands-on opportunities for participants to engage with the herbs.

Promote Your Workshop: Use local bulletin boards, social media, community newsletters, and word of mouth to advertise your workshop. Be clear about the workshop's theme, what participants will learn, and any materials they should bring.

Facilitate Engagement During the Workshop: Encourage questions and share personal anecdotes to make the learning experience relatable. Provide detailed explanations of each step in your demonstrations, including why certain herbs are used for specific conditions, how to source and store herbs, and safety considerations.

Provide Take-Home Materials: Handouts summarizing key points, recipes, or instructions for home projects will help reinforce learning and encourage participants to explore herbal medicine further on their own.

Follow Up: After the workshop, send a thank you message to attendees with additional resources or recommendations for further learning. Consider creating a social media group or email list to share future workshops and foster a community of herbal enthusiasts.

By meticulously planning and delivering a workshop that combines theoretical knowledge with practical skills, you can effectively share the rich tradition of herbal medicine with your community, empowering individuals to incorporate herbal remedies into their daily lives for enhanced well-being.

Community Healing Herbal Blend

Creating a **Community Healing Herbal Blend** involves selecting herbs known for their broad-spectrum healing properties, focusing on those that offer calming, immune-boosting, and anti-inflammatory benefits. This blend can be used to make a tea, which serves as a gentle, nurturing way for community members to support their health and wellness.

Ingredients:

- **1 part dried Echinacea root** (Echinacea spp.): Known for its immune-boosting properties, Echinacea helps in fighting off infections and supporting the body's immune system.
- **1 part dried Lemon Balm leaves** (Melissa officinalis): Offers calming effects, aids in relieving stress, anxiety, and promotes a sense of well-being.
- **1 part dried Nettle leaves** (Urtica dioica): Rich in nutrients, including vitamins A, C, and K, as well as several minerals. Nettle supports overall health and vitality.
- **1/2 part dried Calendula flowers** (Calendula officinalis): Known for its anti-inflammatory properties, Calendula helps in healing and soothing the skin and internal tissues.

- **1/2 part dried Lavender flowers** (Lavandula angustifolia): Lavender is renowned for its calming and relaxing properties, making it an excellent addition for stress relief.
- **1/4 part dried Ginger root** (Zingiber officinale): Adds warmth and stimulates circulation, supporting digestion and offering anti-inflammatory benefits.

Preparation:

1. **Mixing the Herbs**: Begin by accurately measuring each herb using a digital scale for precision. Combine the herbs in a large, dry bowl, gently mixing them with a wooden spoon to ensure an even distribution of all ingredients.

2. **Storing the Blend**: Transfer the herbal blend into an airtight container. Glass jars with tight-fitting lids are ideal as they don't impart any odors or flavors to the herbs. Label the jar with the name of the blend and the date it was mixed. Store in a cool, dark place to preserve the potency of the herbs.

3. **Making the Tea**: To prepare a cup of healing tea, use about 1 tablespoon of the herbal blend per 8 ounces of boiling water. Place the herbs in a tea infuser or teapot. Pour boiling water over the herbs and cover to prevent the escape of volatile oils. Steep for 10-15 minutes. The longer steeping time allows for the extraction of the medicinal properties from the roots and leaves.

4. **Serving**: Strain the tea into a cup. If desired, sweeten with a natural sweetener like honey or stevia to taste. This tea can be enjoyed up to three times a day.

Note: It's important to source your herbs from reputable suppliers to ensure they are of high quality, free from pesticides, and ethically harvested. Organic herbs are preferred for their purity and environmental sustainability.

This **Community Healing Herbal Blend** is designed to be inclusive and beneficial for a wide range of individuals, regardless of their herbal knowledge. It represents a holistic approach to health, emphasizing the importance of community well-being through the shared wisdom of herbal traditions.

CHAPTER 2: BUILDING A COMMUNITY HERBAL GARDEN

To establish a thriving community herbal garden, a structured approach is essential for success. This endeavor not only fosters a sense of unity and shared purpose among participants but also serves as a valuable educational resource on the benefits and uses of various herbs. Here are the steps to create and maintain a community herbal garden:

1. **Form a Planning Committee**: Gather a group of interested community members to form a planning committee. This team will be responsible for making key decisions, organizing volunteer efforts, and managing resources. Ensure the committee includes individuals with a range of skills, including gardening, education, and event planning.

2. **Select a Suitable Location**: Choose a location that is accessible to all community members, including those with disabilities. The site should receive ample sunlight, at least six to eight hours a day, and have access to water. Soil quality should be tested for contaminants; if necessary, raised beds or container gardens can be used to control soil quality.

3. **Design the Garden Layout**: Design a layout that includes a variety of herbs that will thrive in your local climate. Consider creating themed sections, such as culinary herbs, medicinal herbs, and aromatic herbs for relaxation and stress relief. Include paths for easy access and labels for each herb, providing information about its uses and care requirements.

4. **Secure Funding and Resources**: Identify potential sources of funding, such as local business sponsorships, grants, and community fundraising events. Additionally, seek donations of materials such as soil, compost, seeds, and gardening tools. Local garden centers and nurseries may be willing to donate or offer discounts.

5. **Prepare the Site**: Clear the site of weeds and debris. If using raised beds, construct them to the appropriate size and fill them with a mix of topsoil and compost. For in-ground gardens, till the soil and enrich it with compost to improve fertility and drainage.

6. **Plant the Herbs**: Choose herbs that are suitable for your region's climate and soil conditions. Start with a mix of perennial and annual herbs to ensure a variety of harvests throughout the growing season. Plant taller herbs towards the back of beds or plots and shorter ones in front to ensure all plants receive sufficient sunlight.

7. **Organize Volunteer Workdays**: Schedule regular workdays for planting, weeding, watering, and harvesting. These workdays are crucial for the garden's upkeep and offer excellent opportunities for community members to learn about herb cultivation and uses.

8. **Implement a Watering System**: Set up a sustainable watering system. Drip irrigation or soaker hoses are efficient options that conserve water and direct moisture to the roots of the plants, where it's most needed.

9. **Host Educational Workshops and Events**: Use the garden as an educational tool by hosting workshops on topics such as herbal medicine basics, how to harvest and dry herbs, and making herbal remedies. These events can engage the community and promote the garden's value as a resource for natural health and wellness.

10. **Harvest and Share the Bounty**: Organize harvest days where community members can gather herbs for their use. Encourage the sharing of recipes and remedies that utilize the garden's herbs. This not only promotes the practical use of the garden's yield but also strengthens community bonds.

11. **Evaluate and Expand**: At the end of the growing season, gather feedback from participants and evaluate the garden's success and areas for improvement. Consider expanding the garden or adding new features based on community interest and feedback.

By following these detailed steps, a community herbal garden can become a sustainable source of health and wellness, education, and communal joy. Through collective effort and shared knowledge, the garden will serve as a testament to the power of community and the healing nature of nature itself.

Herb-Infused Snacks for Gardening Days

Creating herb-infused snacks for gardening days is a delightful way to integrate the fruits of your labor into nourishing treats that can energize and refresh you and your community garden members. These snacks are not only packed with flavor but also come with the added benefits of the herbs you've grown, making them perfect for a day of gardening. Here's a detailed recipe for making Herb-Infused Energy Balls and Savory Rosemary Crackers, two snacks that are sure to keep you going through your gardening tasks.

Herb-Infused Energy Balls

Ingredients:
- 1 cup of dates, pitted
- 1/2 cup of almonds
- 1/2 cup of walnuts or pecans
- 1/4 cup of unsweetened shredded coconut
- 2 tablespoons of chia seeds
- 2 tablespoons of flaxseed meal
- 1/4 cup of fresh mint leaves, finely chopped
- 1 tablespoon of lemon balm leaves, finely chopped
- 1 teaspoon of lemon zest
- A pinch of sea salt

Instructions:

1. In a food processor, combine the dates, almonds, and walnuts or pecans. Process until the mixture is finely chopped and begins to clump together.

2. Add the shredded coconut, chia seeds, flaxseed meal, finely chopped mint and lemon balm leaves, lemon zest, and a pinch of sea salt to the processor. Pulse until all ingredients are well combined and the mixture sticks together when pressed between your fingers.

3. Take small amounts of the mixture and roll into balls, about the size of a walnut. If the mixture is too dry, add a tiny bit of water, just enough to make it pliable.

4. Place the energy balls on a baking sheet lined with parchment paper and refrigerate for at least an hour to set.

Savory Rosemary Crackers

Ingredients:
- 1 cup of almond flour
- 1 tablespoon of fresh rosemary leaves, finely chopped
- 1/2 teaspoon of sea salt
- 1 tablespoon of nutritional yeast (optional for a cheesy flavor)
- 1 tablespoon of olive oil
- 2 tablespoons of water

Instructions:

1. Preheat your oven to 350°F (175°C). In a mixing bowl, combine the almond flour, finely chopped rosemary leaves, sea salt, and nutritional yeast if using.

2. Add the olive oil and water to the dry ingredients. Mix until a dough forms. If the dough feels too dry, add a bit more water, one teaspoon at a time, until it comes together.

3. Place the dough between two sheets of parchment paper and roll out to about 1/8 inch thickness. Remove the top sheet of parchment paper.

4. Using a knife or a pizza cutter, cut the dough into small squares or rectangles. Transfer the parchment paper with the cut dough onto a baking sheet.

5. Bake in the preheated oven for 12-15 minutes, or until the crackers are golden brown and crisp. Let them cool on the baking sheet before serving.

These herb-infused snacks are not only a testament to the versatility of herbs in culinary applications but also serve as a tangible connection to the garden's bounty. Enjoy these snacks on your gardening days to stay energized and to share the herbal goodness with fellow garden enthusiasts.

BOOK 37: HERBS FOR ENERGY AND PRODUCTIVITY

CHAPTER 1: MORNING ENERGY BOOSTERS

For those looking to jumpstart their day with natural energy, incorporating **Ginseng** and **Maca** into your morning routine can be transformative. Both herbs are renowned for their ability to enhance stamina and vitality, making them ideal candidates for morning energy boosters. Here's how to effectively use these powerful adaptogens to kick off your day with increased energy and focus.

Ginseng, specifically **Siberian Ginseng** (Eleutherococcus senticosus), is celebrated for its ability to increase endurance and help the body adapt to stress. To harness the full potential of Ginseng, start with a daily dose of 200-400mg of Siberian Ginseng extract. This can be taken in capsule form, ideally with breakfast, to support sustained energy levels throughout the morning. Ensure the Ginseng supplement is standardized to contain at least 0.8 percent eleutherosides, the active compounds responsible for its energy-boosting properties.

Maca (Lepidium meyenii) is another powerful herb that works synergistically with Ginseng to enhance energy and performance. Maca root powder is particularly beneficial for its nutritional content, including vitamins, minerals, and amino acids that support overall vitality. For morning use, incorporate 1-2 tablespoons of organic Maca powder into your breakfast smoothie or oatmeal. This not only provides a natural energy boost but also supports hormonal balance, which is crucial for maintaining energy levels.

To maximize the benefits of Ginseng and Maca, consider the following preparation tips:

1. **Ginseng Tea**: If you prefer to consume Ginseng as a tea, steep 1-2 grams of dried Siberian Ginseng root in hot water for 10-15 minutes. This method allows for a customizable dosage and can be a warming, invigorating start to the day.

2. **Maca-Infused Breakfast**: Blend Maca powder into smoothies, yogurt, or oatmeal. Its nutty flavor pairs well with fruits and nuts, making it a versatile addition to various breakfast dishes.

3. **Timing and Dosage**: For optimal results, take Ginseng and Maca in the morning or early afternoon to align with the body's natural rhythm and avoid potential interference with sleep patterns.

4. **Quality Matters**: Always source Ginseng and Maca from reputable suppliers to ensure you're receiving a pure, potent product. Look for organically certified herbs to minimize exposure to pesticides and contaminants.

5. **Listen to Your Body**: Adaptogens like Ginseng and Maca are generally well-tolerated, but it's important to observe how your body responds. Start with lower doses and gradually increase as needed, paying attention to any changes in energy levels or well-being.

By incorporating Ginseng and Maca into your morning routine, you can naturally enhance your energy and productivity. These herbs offer a sustainable alternative to caffeine, providing a balanced boost that supports your body's overall health and resilience. Whether you're facing a busy day ahead or simply seeking to improve your morning vitality, Ginseng and Maca are excellent tools for achieving and maintaining high energy levels.

Ginseng and Maca for Sustained Energy

Ginseng and Maca, two powerful adaptogens, offer a natural way to boost energy levels and enhance overall vitality, making them perfect for inclusion in a morning routine aimed at increasing productivity and focus. Ginseng, particularly Siberian Ginseng (Eleutherococcus senticosus), is renowned for its ability to improve endurance and help the body manage stress more effectively. A daily intake of 200-400mg of Siberian Ginseng extract, standardized to contain at least 0.8 percent eleutherosides, the active compounds, can significantly contribute to sustained energy levels throughout the day. This specific dosage, taken ideally with breakfast in capsule form, leverages the adaptogenic properties of Ginseng to support the body's natural energy production mechanisms and stress response systems.

Maca (Lepidium meyenii), on the other hand, is a nutrient-dense root known for its remarkable nutritional profile, including essential vitamins, minerals, and amino acids that collectively support hormonal balance and energy metabolism. Incorporating 1-2 tablespoons of organic Maca powder into morning meals, such as smoothies or oatmeal, can provide a noticeable energy boost. The nutty flavor of Maca makes it a versatile addition to various recipes, enhancing not only the nutritional value but also the taste of breakfast dishes.

To effectively utilize Ginseng and Maca for sustained morning energy, consider the following detailed recommendations:

For Ginseng, the preferred method of consumption is in capsule form due to the convenience and precision in dosing. However, for those who enjoy the ritual of tea preparation, Ginseng tea can be an alternative. To prepare, steep 1-2 grams of dried Siberian Ginseng root in hot water for 10-15 minutes. Adjust the amount of Ginseng according to personal tolerance and desired effect, keeping in mind that starting with a lower dose and gradually increasing it can help assess individual sensitivity and effectiveness.

Maca powder can be easily blended into a variety of breakfast foods. For a simple yet energizing Maca smoothie, combine 1 tablespoon of Maca powder with 1 cup of almond milk, a handful of spinach, half a banana, and a tablespoon of almond butter. Blend until smooth for a nutritious and energizing start to the day. Alternatively, Maca powder can be stirred into oatmeal or yogurt, along with fruits and nuts for added texture and flavor.

When incorporating these adaptogens into your morning routine, it's crucial to consider timing and dosage. Taking Ginseng and Maca in the morning or early afternoon aligns with the body's natural rhythm, optimizing energy levels during the day while minimizing any potential impact on nighttime sleep patterns. Quality is also paramount when selecting Ginseng and Maca products. Opt for supplements and powders from reputable suppliers that provide organically certified herbs, ensuring purity and potency.

Listening to your body is essential when using adaptogens. While Ginseng and Maca are generally well-tolerated, individual responses can vary. Starting with a lower dose allows for monitoring of effects and adjustments as needed to find the optimal dosage that supports well-being without adverse effects.

By integrating Ginseng and Maca into the morning routine, individuals can experience a natural and sustained energy boost that supports productivity and focus throughout the day. These adaptogens, with their unique properties and nutritional benefits, offer a holistic approach to enhancing energy and vitality, aligning with the body's natural processes for optimal health and performance.

CHAPTER 2: MIDDAY PRODUCTIVITY ENHANCERS

Peppermint (Mentha piperita) and Rosemary (Rosmarinus officinalis) are two potent herbs that can significantly enhance midday productivity by improving mental alertness and cognitive function. Both herbs have been studied for their ability to increase concentration and memory, making them ideal for a midday boost. Here's how to incorporate these herbs into your daily routine for optimal productivity:

Peppermint Tea Preparation:

1. Boil 1 cup of water in a kettle.
2. Add 1 tablespoon of dried peppermint leaves to a tea infuser or teapot.
3. Pour the boiling water over the peppermint leaves and allow to steep for 5-7 minutes. The longer you steep, the stronger the flavor and benefits.
4. Remove the leaves and pour the tea into a cup. If desired, sweeten with honey or stevia for added flavor.

Rosemary Essential Oil Inhalation:

1. Add 3-5 drops of rosemary essential oil to a diffuser filled with water.
2. Turn on the diffuser and allow the aroma to fill the room. Inhaling rosemary essential oil can help enhance focus and clarity, especially during the midday slump.
3. Alternatively, place 1-2 drops of rosemary essential oil on a handkerchief or cotton ball and inhale deeply for a quick, invigorating effect.

Peppermint and Rosemary Desk Spray:

1. In a small spray bottle, combine ¼ cup of distilled water, 15 drops of peppermint essential oil, and 10 drops of rosemary essential oil.
2. Shake well to mix the oils with the water.
3. Lightly spray around your workspace to refresh the air and stimulate mental alertness. Avoid spraying directly onto electronic devices.

Growing Peppermint and Rosemary:

- Peppermint and rosemary can be easily grown in pots on a sunny windowsill. Both herbs prefer well-drained soil and at least 6-8 hours of direct sunlight daily.
- Regularly trim the peppermint and rosemary to encourage bushy growth and to prevent them from becoming leggy.
- Harvest peppermint leaves as needed for tea, and snip rosemary sprigs to use fresh or dry them for later use.

Incorporating Peppermint and Rosemary into Your Diet:

- Add fresh peppermint leaves to water or iced tea for a refreshing drink.
- Incorporate chopped rosemary into dishes such as roasted vegetables, soups, and bread for an aromatic flavor and cognitive boost.

Safety Precautions:

- While peppermint tea is generally safe for consumption, peppermint essential oil should be used externally and with caution, as it can be irritating to sensitive skin.
- Rosemary essential oil should also be used externally and in moderation. Pregnant women and individuals with epilepsy should avoid using rosemary essential oil.

By integrating peppermint and rosemary into your midday routine, you can naturally enhance your productivity and cognitive function. Whether through aromatic inhalation, enjoying a revitalizing tea, or utilizing a desk spray, these herbs offer a natural and effective way to stay focused and alert throughout the day.

Peppermint and Rosemary for Alertness

Peppermint (Mentha piperita) and Rosemary (Rosmarinus officinalis) stand out for their invigorating properties that can sharpen focus and enhance mental clarity, particularly valuable during the midday when energy levels tend to dip. The active compounds in peppermint, such as menthol, interact with the central nervous system to promote a sense of alertness and can temporarily alleviate mental fatigue. Similarly, rosemary contains 1,8-cineole, a compound shown to improve memory function and cognitive performance when its scent is inhaled.

To harness these benefits, incorporating peppermint and rosemary into a daily routine can be done through several methods, each tailored to fit seamlessly into various lifestyles and preferences. For a direct and potent approach, preparing a peppermint and rosemary tea provides a therapeutic dose of these herbs. Start by boiling water and then steeping a combination of fresh or dried peppermint leaves and a sprig of rosemary for about 5 to 7 minutes. This not only extracts the essential oils but also ensures the compounds responsible for enhancing alertness are preserved in the tea. Straining the leaves and adding a natural sweetener, like honey, can enhance the flavor profile of the tea while maintaining its cognitive benefits.

Another method to utilize the alertness-boosting properties of these herbs is through aromatherapy. Essential oils derived from peppermint and rosemary can be diffused in the workspace to create an environment conducive to focus and productivity. For those without a diffuser, adding a few drops of each oil to a small bowl of hot water can similarly disperse the aroma throughout the area. The inhalation of these scents has been linked to reduced feelings of frustration and an increased ability to concentrate on tasks.

For individuals on the go, creating a portable inhaler with these essential oils offers a quick and discreet way to invigorate the senses. This can be achieved by adding drops of peppermint and rosemary oils to a cotton wick and enclosing it in a portable inhaler tube. When feeling lethargic or in need of a mental boost, a few deep inhalations can provide immediate relief and a renewed focus.

Incorporating these herbs into the diet also contributes to sustained cognitive performance. Peppermint leaves can be added to salads or smoothies for a refreshing twist, while rosemary can be used as a seasoning for various dishes, from roasted vegetables to grilled meats. This not only infuses meals with flavor but also integrates the cognitive benefits of these herbs into daily nutrition.

It's important to note that while peppermint and rosemary are generally safe for consumption, their essential oils should be used with caution. Peppermint oil, for example, should be avoided by individuals with GERD (gastroesophageal reflux disease) as it can exacerbate symptoms. Similarly, pregnant women are advised to consult with a healthcare provider before using rosemary essential oil due to its potent effects.

By integrating peppermint and rosemary into one's daily routine through these methods, it's possible to naturally enhance mental alertness and productivity without relying on artificial stimulants. Whether through herbal teas, aromatherapy, dietary inclusion, or portable inhalers, these herbs offer a versatile and effective approach to combating midday lethargy and improving cognitive function.

CHAPTER 3: EVENING RECOVERY FOR ENERGY

For an effective evening recovery that ensures you wake up with renewed energy and vitality, incorporating **Reishi** (Ganoderma lucidum) and **Tulsi** (Ocimum sanctum), also known as Holy Basil, into your nightly routine can be transformative. These herbs are renowned for their adaptogenic properties, aiding in stress reduction and promoting a restful night's sleep, which is crucial for energy restoration.

Reishi, often referred to as the "Mushroom of Immortality," has been used for centuries in traditional Chinese medicine to support the immune system, reduce stress, and improve sleep quality. For evening use, Reishi can be taken in the form of a tea or supplement. To prepare Reishi tea, follow these steps:

1. Break down **Reishi mushroom slices** into smaller pieces to increase the surface area for extraction.
2. Add about **5 grams** of Reishi to **2 cups of boiling water**.
3. Reduce the heat and simmer for **1-2 hours**. The long simmering time is necessary to extract the active compounds from the tough mushroom.
4. Strain the tea and serve warm. For taste, consider adding a natural sweetener like honey or a slice of ginger.

Tulsi, also known as Holy Basil, is another powerful adaptogen that supports the body's stress response and promotes mental balance. Drinking Tulsi tea in the evening can help calm the mind and prepare the body for sleep. To make Tulsi tea:

1. Add **1-2 teaspoons** of dried Tulsi leaves to **1 cup of boiling water**.
2. Steep for **5-7 minutes**. This steeping time allows for the extraction of Tulsi's essential oils, which are responsible for its therapeutic effects.
3. Strain and enjoy the tea. You may add lemon or honey to enhance the flavor.

In addition to their individual benefits, combining Reishi and Tulsi can synergistically enhance their effects on stress reduction and sleep improvement. Consider alternating between Reishi and Tulsi tea each night or combining them for a powerful evening tonic.

For those preferring supplements, ensure you choose **high-quality, organic products** from reputable suppliers. The recommended dosage for Reishi extract is **300-500 mg** taken in the evening, while Tulsi supplements can be taken as directed on the product label, typically **300-400 mg**.

Practical Tips for Evening Recovery:
- Establish a routine by consuming your Reishi or Tulsi preparation at the same time each evening to help regulate your body's internal clock.
- Limit exposure to screens and bright lights after consuming your evening tonic to enhance its effects on sleep quality.
- Combine your herbal routine with other relaxing activities such as reading or meditation to further support relaxation and recovery.

By integrating Reishi and Tulsi into your evening routine, you're not only fostering a conducive environment for restful sleep but also nurturing your body's natural ability to recover and rejuvenate overnight. This holistic approach ensures you wake up feeling refreshed and energized, ready to tackle the day ahead with vitality.

Reishi and Tulsi for Relaxation

Reishi and Tulsi, two revered herbs in the realm of natural health, offer profound benefits for relaxation and recovery, especially when integrated into an evening routine to support energy restoration for the following day. These herbs work synergistically to enhance the body's resilience to stress and improve sleep quality, crucial components for maintaining productivity and vitality.

Reishi mushroom, known scientifically as Ganoderma lucidum, has been utilized for thousands of years in Eastern medicine for its adaptogenic properties, helping the body to manage stress and fostering a state of calm. To harness Reishi's benefits for relaxation and recovery, begin by sourcing high-quality, dried Reishi mushrooms. These can typically be found at health food stores or from reputable online suppliers. For evening recovery, a Reishi decoction is most effective. Measure approximately 5 grams of dried Reishi mushroom and add it to a pot containing about 500 milliliters of water. Bring the water to a boil, then reduce the heat and allow the Reishi to simmer gently for at least 60 minutes. This slow cooking process extracts the bioactive compounds responsible for Reishi's therapeutic effects. After simmering, strain the liquid to remove the mushroom pieces, resulting in a potent decoction. For taste, a slice of ginger or a dash of honey can be added. It's recommended to consume this Reishi decoction in the evening, about an hour before bedtime, to facilitate relaxation and enhance the quality of sleep.

Tulsi, also known as Holy Basil (Ocimum sanctum), is another adaptogen with a rich history of use in Ayurvedic medicine for its ability to mitigate stress and promote mental clarity. To prepare a Tulsi tea for evening recovery, start with fresh or dried Tulsi leaves. If using fresh leaves, a handful (approximately 10-15 leaves) is sufficient, whereas for dried Tulsi, one teaspoon will suffice. Boil 250 milliliters of water and pour it over the Tulsi leaves, allowing them to steep for about 5-7 minutes. The resulting infusion will have a fragrant aroma and a slightly spicy flavor. Tulsi tea can be enjoyed on its own or with a teaspoon of honey for added sweetness. Drinking Tulsi tea in the evening helps to calm the nervous system, reduce stress-induced insomnia, and support overall well-being.

For those seeking to integrate both Reishi and Tulsi into their evening routine for optimal relaxation and recovery, consider alternating between the two. For instance, one might choose to consume Reishi decoction on one night and Tulsi tea on the next, allowing the body to benefit from the unique properties of each herb. Additionally, both Reishi and Tulsi can be found in various supplement forms, including tinctures and capsules, offering a convenient alternative for those with time constraints. However, it's important to consult with a healthcare provider before adding any new supplements to your regimen, especially for individuals with existing health conditions or those taking medication.

Incorporating Reishi and Tulsi into the evening routine is a holistic approach to enhancing relaxation and recovery. These herbs not only support physical health by improving sleep quality and resilience to stress but also contribute to mental and emotional well-being, paving the way for a more productive and energetic tomorrow.

BOOK 38: SUSTAINABLE HOME APOTHECARY

CHAPTER 1: CREATING ZERO-WASTE HERBAL PRODUCTS

In the pursuit of a sustainable home apothecary, creating zero-waste herbal products is not only an environmentally friendly practice but also an enriching experience that connects us more deeply with the natural world. The key to achieving this lies in mindful sourcing, utilization, and processing of herbs.

Mindful Sourcing of Herbs: Begin by selecting organically grown herbs or, better yet, grow your own. This ensures that the herbs are free from pesticides and herbicides, which is better for both your health and the environment. For those herbs that you cannot grow or source locally, choose suppliers who prioritize sustainable practices.

Utilization of Every Part of the Herb: Many parts of an herb can be utilized, from leaf to root, in various preparations. For instance, after making a calendula infused oil, the remaining marc (the spent material) can be incorporated into homemade soaps or composted. This approach ensures that every part of the plant is honored and used to its fullest potential, minimizing waste.

Water Conservation in Herbal Preparations: When preparing decoctions or infusions, be mindful of water usage. Use only the amount of water necessary for the preparation to reduce waste. Additionally, water used for rinsing herbs can be repurposed to water plants in your garden, further reducing your ecological footprint.

Eco-friendly Packaging: Opt for reusable or compostable packaging for storing your herbal remedies. Glass jars, metal tins, and compostable bags are excellent choices that can be reused multiple times, significantly reducing the need for single-use plastics. Labeling can be done with paper or other biodegradable materials.

Energy-efficient Drying Methods: Drying herbs is a common preservation method in herbalism. To do this in an energy-efficient manner, utilize natural sunlight by hanging herbs in a dry, well-ventilated area or using solar dehydrators. These methods are not only gentle on the herbs, preserving their medicinal qualities, but also reduce energy consumption compared to electric dehydrators.

Creating Herbal Formulations with Minimal Waste: When creating tinctures, salves, or other herbal formulations, measure ingredients carefully to avoid excess. This not only conserves valuable herbal resources but also prevents the waste of other ingredients like oils, waxes, and alcohol.

Repurposing Leftover Ingredients: In the spirit of zero waste, find creative ways to repurpose any leftover ingredients. For example, beeswax remnants from making salves can be melted down to create new candles or used in other DIY projects. Alcohol from tincture making can be reused for cleaning purposes, provided it has not been compromised by toxic plants.

Composting: Finally, any organic waste that cannot be repurposed should be composted. This returns nutrients back to the earth and supports the health of your garden, creating a closed-loop system that mimics natural cycles.

By adopting these practices, you can significantly reduce waste in your home apothecary, contributing to the health of the planet while deepening your connection to the healing power of herbs.

CHAPTER 2: USING HERBAL BYPRODUCTS

Herbal byproducts, often overlooked, are a treasure trove of potential for sustainable practices within a home apothecary. The process of transforming these byproducts into valuable resources not only minimizes waste but also maximizes the utility of every herb in your collection. Here, we delve into specific methods and creative ideas for repurposing herbal byproducts, ensuring that you can implement these strategies effectively in your own sustainable home apothecary.

Herbal Pulp from Juicing or Infusions: After extracting juice or making infusions, the remaining herbal pulp contains fibers and a small amount of essential oils. This pulp can be dried and used as a mild exfoliant in homemade soaps or facial scrubs. To dry the pulp, spread it thinly on a baking sheet and place it in an oven set to the lowest possible temperature, leaving the door slightly ajar to allow moisture to escape. Check the pulp every 30 minutes until it's completely dried, which may take several hours depending on the moisture content.

Spent Herbs from Tinctures and Decoctions: Once you've pressed and strained your tinctures or decoctions, the spent herbs still have residual compounds that can be beneficial. These can be composted to enrich your garden soil, but another innovative approach is to use them as a natural dye for fabrics. Simmer the spent herbs in water to extract the remaining pigments, then strain. Soak natural fibers in this herbal dye for unique, eco-friendly textiles. Be sure to use a mordant, like alum, to fix the color to the fabric.

Herb-Infused Oils: After straining herb-infused oils, the leftover herbs can be gently warmed to release any remaining oil, which can then be collected and used for making salves or lip balms. The herb remnants, now mostly devoid of oil, can be incorporated into candles for a subtle aroma or added to compost.

Ash from Burning Herbs: If you use herbs for smudging or as incense, the ash that remains is a potent source of potassium and can be mixed into soil for potted plants or garden beds to promote plant health. Ensure the ash is cool and fully extinguished before use.

Herbal Tea Leaves: Used herbal tea leaves and bags can serve multiple purposes. They can be added directly to compost or used as a mulch around plants to retain moisture and deter pests. Additionally, soaking used tea leaves in water creates a mild, nutrient-rich plant feed that can be used for houseplants or garden plants.

Stems and Roots: Tougher parts of herbs, like stems and roots, that are not typically used in preparations can be boiled to create a cleaning solution for home use. Boil these parts in water, strain, and then add vinegar to the liquid. This solution can clean surfaces effectively and is especially good for glass.

Implementing these practices requires a shift in perspective, seeing value in what was previously considered waste. By adopting these methods, you not only contribute to a more sustainable and eco-friendly home apothecary but also deepen your connection to the natural world, understanding the full cycle of plant life and its myriad uses.

CHAPTER 3: SUSTAINABLE STORAGE AND ORGANIZATION

In the realm of creating a sustainable home apothecary, the organization and storage of herbs and herbal products play a pivotal role in maintaining the integrity and potency of your remedies while minimizing waste. The following strategies are designed to ensure that your herbal apothecary not only serves its purpose effectively but also aligns with eco-friendly practices.

Choose the Right Containers: Opt for glass jars with airtight lids for storing dried herbs and powders. Glass is inert, meaning it won't react with the herbs, and it's infinitely recyclable, making it a sustainable choice. Ensure the jars are of various sizes to accommodate different quantities of herbs, preventing waste from excess air space which can accelerate degradation. For labeling, use a chalk marker or reusable labels to easily update the contents as your inventory changes.

Maximize Freshness with Proper Placement: Store your jars in a cool, dark place away from direct sunlight and moisture. A cupboard or a pantry works well. This prevents the active compounds in the herbs from breaking down due to light and heat exposure. Consider installing a small dehumidifier in storage areas prone to dampness to protect against mold growth.

Implement a FIFO System: "First In, First Out" is a principle that ensures older stock is used before newer. Organize your herbs in a way that allows you to access the oldest jars first. This might mean placing newer jars at the back of the shelf or creating a rotating system where jars are moved forward as they are used.

Sustainable Herb Drying Racks: If you dry your own herbs, consider using a homemade drying rack made from reclaimed wood and mesh. This setup allows for adequate air circulation, which is crucial for preventing mold. Place the rack in a dry, well-ventilated area. Once the herbs are dry, store them immediately to preserve their quality.

Bulk Buying and Sharing: Purchase herbs in bulk to reduce packaging waste and share excess with friends or through community exchanges. This not only reduces waste but also fosters a sense of community and shared wellness. When buying in bulk, bring your own containers to the store if they allow it, further reducing plastic use.

Herb Gardens as Living Storage: Cultivate a small herb garden for the herbs you use most frequently. This living apothecary requires no packaging and ensures you have fresh herbs at your fingertips. Use compostable pots and natural pest control methods to keep your garden as sustainable as your indoor apothecary.

Digital Inventory Tracking: Keep a digital record of your herbs, including when they were acquired and their expected shelf life. This can help you use herbs while they are most potent and reduce waste from expired products. Apps designed for pantry management can be easily adapted for this purpose.

Repurpose and Recycle: When herbs are no longer viable for therapeutic use, find ways to repurpose them. Spent herbs can often be used for natural cleaning products, composted to enrich your garden soil, or even used as natural dye materials. Glass jars can be reused indefinitely for new batches of herbs or other household needs.

Community Resource Sharing: Engage with local herbalist communities to share resources like dehydrators, oil presses, or book resources. This not only reduces the need for each individual to purchase their own but also strengthens community ties and shared knowledge.

By meticulously selecting storage solutions, organizing your space to maximize the longevity of your herbs, and embracing community and sustainability at every step, your home apothecary can be a beacon of eco-consciousness and holistic wellness. These practices ensure that your herbal remedies are not only effective but also harmoniously aligned with the principles of sustainability and minimal environmental impact.

BOOK 39: HERBS FOR GRIEF AND EMOTIONAL LOSS

CHAPTER 1: HERBS FOR EMOTIONAL SUPPORT

In times of grief and emotional loss, turning to nature for solace and support can be incredibly healing. Herbs, with their subtle yet profound ability to balance and nurture, offer a gentle pathway towards emotional equilibrium. Here, we delve into specific herbs known for their supportive qualities during such tender times, focusing on how to incorporate them into daily routines for emotional support.

Lavender is renowned for its calming and soothing properties, making it an ideal herb for alleviating anxiety and promoting a sense of peace. To harness Lavender's benefits, consider adding a few drops of lavender essential oil to a diffuser in your living space or bedroom. This not only infuses the area with a serene aroma but also facilitates relaxation and better sleep. Alternatively, a lavender sachet placed under the pillow can help soothe the mind and ease into a restful night's sleep.

St. John's Wort, scientifically known as Hypericum perforatum, has been extensively studied for its potential to uplift the mood and combat mild to moderate depression. Its active compounds, including hypericin, appear to influence neurotransmitter activity in the brain, contributing to its mood-stabilizing effects. St. John's Wort can be consumed as a tea or in capsule form. For tea, steep one teaspoon of dried herb in a cup of boiling water for about 10 minutes. It's important to note that St. John's Wort may interact with certain medications, so consulting with a healthcare provider before use is crucial.

Holy Basil, or Tulsi, is revered in Ayurvedic medicine for its adaptogenic properties, helping the body and mind adapt to stress and fostering emotional resilience. Drinking a cup of Holy Basil tea can be a soothing ritual to start or end the day. To prepare, steep one tablespoon of fresh or dried Holy Basil leaves in hot water for about 5-8 minutes. The herb's natural compounds can help reduce stress and promote a sense of well-being.

Chamomile is another herb celebrated for its calming effects, particularly useful for those experiencing stress and insomnia during difficult times. A warm cup of chamomile tea before bed can help calm the nervous system and encourage a more peaceful sleep. Use two to three teaspoons of dried chamomile flowers per cup of boiling water, allowing it to steep for 10 minutes before straining and enjoying.

Ashwagandha, an adaptogen, supports the body's ability to manage stress and has been used in traditional medicine to strengthen the nervous system. Incorporating ashwagandha into your daily routine can be done through capsules or as a powder mixed into smoothies or warm milk. A typical dose ranges from 300-500 mg of the extract, taken with meals or as directed by a healthcare professional.

Incorporating these herbs into your daily routine requires mindfulness and consistency to observe their benefits fully. Whether choosing to integrate one or several of these herbs, it's essential to listen to your body and adjust accordingly. Each individual's response to herbs can vary, and what works for one may not work for another. Always start with lower doses to see how your body reacts and consult with a healthcare provider, especially if you are pregnant, nursing, or on medication. Through the mindful use of these herbs, one can find a natural pathway to healing and emotional support during times of grief and loss.

CHAPTER 2: ADAPTOGENS FOR RESILIENCE

Adaptogens are a unique class of herbs known for their ability to enhance the body's resilience to stress, both physical and emotional. These herbs work by modulating the release of stress hormones from the adrenal glands, helping the body to maintain optimal homeostasis. This balancing act is particularly beneficial during times of grief and emotional loss, where the body's stress response can be significantly heightened. For individuals navigating these challenging times, incorporating adaptogens into daily routines can offer a gentle support system, fostering long-term resilience and emotional stability.

Ashwagandha (Withania somnifera), often referred to as Indian ginseng, stands out for its stress-reducing properties. To harness its benefits, consider starting with a daily dose of 300-500 mg of ashwagandha root extract, ensuring it contains at least 5% withanolides for maximum efficacy. This adaptogen is particularly suited for reducing cortisol levels, enhancing mood, and supporting overall well-being.

Holy Basil (Ocimum sanctum), also known as Tulsi, is revered in Ayurvedic medicine for its holistic healing properties. For emotional balance and stress relief, brewing a tea from dried holy basil leaves can be especially comforting. Use 1-2 teaspoons of dried leaves per cup of boiling water, steeping for 5-10 minutes. Drinking this tea 2-3 times a day can help soothe the nervous system and promote a sense of calm.

Rhodiola Rosea is another powerful adaptogen with a long history of use in traditional medicine. It is particularly known for improving symptoms of burnout, which can include emotional exhaustion and reduced ability to cope with stress. The recommended starting dose is 100-300 mg of Rhodiola extract, standardized to contain 1% rosavins and 0.8% salidroside. Taking this supplement in the morning can help enhance energy levels and mental clarity throughout the day.

Schisandra Chinensis is a berry that has been used in Traditional Chinese Medicine to enhance resistance to stress and disease. Its adaptogenic properties can be beneficial for those experiencing emotional turmoil. Schisandra can be consumed as a dried berry, tea, or extract. A common dose is 1-3 grams of the dried berry or 100-300 mg of extract daily. This adaptogen is known for its hepatoprotective effects, supporting liver health, which can be particularly beneficial during times of stress.

Cordyceps (Cordyceps sinensis), a type of medicinal mushroom, offers unique benefits for energy and stamina, which can be depleted during periods of grief. The recommended dose for cordyceps is 1,000-3,000 mg per day of the mushroom extract. This adaptogen is also known for its antioxidant properties, supporting immune health and overall vitality.

Incorporating these adaptogens into your daily regimen requires mindfulness and patience. It's important to listen to your body and adjust dosages as needed, under the guidance of a healthcare professional, especially if you are taking other medications or have underlying health conditions. Additionally, combining adaptogens with a balanced diet, regular physical activity, and practices such as meditation and yoga can further enhance their benefits, supporting a holistic approach to healing and resilience during times of emotional loss.

CHAPTER 3: HERBAL RITUALS FOR EMOTIONAL HEALING

Creating rituals with herbs for emotional healing involves a series of steps that can help individuals process grief and emotional loss. These rituals can be personalized to fit one's emotional and spiritual needs, providing a sense of comfort and grounding. Here, we detail the process of setting up such rituals, focusing on the selection of herbs, preparation methods, and the creation of a sacred space for healing.

1. **Selecting Herbs for Emotional Healing**: Begin by choosing herbs known for their calming and soothing properties. Lavender, for its ability to reduce anxiety and induce calmness; chamomile, known for its soothing effects on the mind and body; and rose, which can help uplift the spirits and heal the heart. Ensure you source high-quality, organic herbs to maximize their therapeutic benefits.

2. **Preparing the Herbs**: For each herb selected, there are specific preparation methods to consider. For lavender and chamile, creating a tea is most beneficial. Use one teaspoon of dried herb per cup of boiling water, allowing it to steep for 10 minutes before straining. For rose, creating a rose water spray can be uplifting and refreshing. Simmer rose petals in water for 20 minutes, strain, and pour the liquid into a spray bottle.

3. **Creating a Sacred Space**: Choose a quiet, comfortable area where you won't be disturbed. You might want to include items that hold personal significance or evoke peace and serenity, such as photographs, stones, or crystals. Lighting a candle can also help to demarcate this space as sacred and dedicated to your healing process.

4. **Engaging in the Ritual**: Begin your ritual by setting an intention for your healing journey. This could be a silent affirmation or a written note that you keep within your sacred space. Sip the herbal tea slowly, allowing its warmth and flavor to soothe you. If using rose water, gently spray it around your space and on your face, breathing in its gentle fragrance.

5. **Meditation and Reflection**: While engaging with the herbs, take this time to meditate or reflect. You might focus on your breath, recite a mantra, or simply sit in silence, allowing yourself to feel whatever emotions arise without judgment. This is a time for self-compassion and acceptance.

6. **Closing the Ritual**: Once you feel the ritual is complete, take a moment to express gratitude for the healing journey you've embarked on. Extinguish the candle, signaling the end of your sacred time. You can repeat this ritual as often as needed, listening to your body and heart for guidance on frequency.

Remember, the power of these rituals lies not only in the herbs themselves but in the intention and mindfulness with which you engage in the process. Each step should be approached with care and respect, allowing the natural properties of the herbs to aid in your emotional healing journey.

BOOK 40: PRESERVING HERBAL KNOWLEDGE

CHAPTER 1: DOCUMENTING HERBAL TRADITIONS

In the realm of herbal traditions, the meticulous documentation of practices, recipes, and wisdom is paramount to preserving this invaluable knowledge for future generations. The process involves several critical steps, each requiring attention to detail and a commitment to accuracy.

Gathering Information: Start by compiling all available information on herbal practices, including oral traditions, written texts, and digital sources. Reach out to practitioners, healers, and herbalists who hold the knowledge passed down through generations. Record their insights, methods, and personal anecdotes that provide depth to the herbal practices.

Organizing Data: Once the information is collected, organize it systematically. Categories might include types of herbs, their uses, preparation methods, dosages, and regional variations in practices. Use a digital database to manage the information, ensuring it is easily searchable and can be updated over time.

Verifying Authenticity: It's crucial to verify the authenticity and accuracy of the information gathered. Cross-reference the collected data with reputable sources, scientific research, and historical texts. Engaging with experts in ethnobotany, traditional medicine, and pharmacognosy can provide validation and offer insights into the efficacy and safety of the documented remedies.

Ethical Considerations: Respect for the source of knowledge is essential. Obtain permission from indigenous communities and traditional healers before documenting and sharing their knowledge. Acknowledge their guardianship of the traditions and ensure that the documentation process does not exploit or misrepresent their cultural heritage.

Digital Preservation: Utilize digital tools for the preservation of herbal knowledge. Digital archives, databases, and online platforms can make the information accessible to a broader audience while safeguarding it against loss. Implement regular backups and use formats that are widely supported to ensure long-term accessibility.

Physical Documentation: In addition to digital methods, creating physical records such as printed books, manuscripts, and herbariums adds another layer of preservation. These tangible forms of documentation can be invaluable resources for researchers and practitioners and serve as historical artifacts for future generations.

Educational Outreach: Sharing the documented knowledge through educational programs, workshops, and publications can foster appreciation and understanding of herbal traditions. Collaborate with schools, universities, and community centers to integrate herbal wisdom into curriculums and public learning initiatives.

Community Involvement: Engage the community in the documentation process. Workshops, herb walks, and storytelling sessions can be powerful ways to gather information while involving the community in preserving its own heritage. This approach ensures the knowledge remains alive and relevant.

Legal and Ethical Publishing: Before publishing the documented knowledge, consider the legal and ethical implications. Ensure that intellectual property rights are respected and that the publication does not infringe on the rights of the individuals or communities involved. Seek legal advice to navigate copyright laws and intellectual property rights associated with traditional knowledge.

Sustainability Practices: Documenting herbal traditions also involves advocating for sustainable practices in the cultivation and harvesting of medicinal plants. Include guidelines for ethical sourcing, conservation efforts, and sustainable agriculture practices to ensure the longevity of herbal resources.

By adhering to these detailed steps, the documentation of herbal traditions can be conducted with the respect, accuracy, and integrity it deserves. This meticulous approach ensures that the wisdom of herbal practices is preserved, accessible, and continues to enrich the lives of future generations, fostering a deeper connection to the natural world and its healing powers.

CHAPTER 2: TEACHING HERBAL WISDOM TO CHILDREN

Teaching herbal wisdom to children involves a hands-on, interactive approach that caters to their innate curiosity and desire to explore the world around them. The goal is to instill a deep appreciation for nature and an understanding of the benefits of herbs in a way that is engaging, fun, and educational. Here are detailed steps and recommendations for introducing children to herbal wisdom:

1. **Start with a Garden Tour**: Begin by taking children on a tour of a garden, whether at home, a community garden, or a local botanical garden. Point out various herbs, discussing their names, smells, and colors. Encourage children to gently touch and smell the herbs, fostering a sensory connection. For example, guide them to rub a mint leaf between their fingers and inhale deeply to experience its refreshing scent.

2. **Herb Planting Activity**: Engage children in planting their own herbs. Provide small pots, organic potting soil, and herb seeds such as basil, parsley, or chives, which are easy to grow and care for. Demonstrate how to fill a pot with soil, plant the seeds according to the packet instructions, and water gently. Discuss the importance of sunlight and water for plant growth, recommending placing the pots in a sunny window and establishing a regular watering schedule.

3. **Crafting Herbal Sachets**: Guide children in making their own herbal sachets. Supply dried lavender, chamomile, or rose petals, small cloth bags or squares of fabric, and ribbons. Show them how to fill the fabric with a mix of dried herbs and secure it with a ribbon. Explain how these sachets can be used to scent drawers or as a natural way to help relax at bedtime.

4. **Cooking with Herbs**: Introduce children to the culinary uses of herbs through simple cooking activities. Choose easy recipes like making pesto with fresh basil or sprinkling chopped parsley over homemade soup. Involve children in the process of picking the herbs, washing them, and adding them to the dish, highlighting the flavor enhancement herbs provide.

5. **Herbal Art Projects**: Incorporate herbs into art projects to stimulate creativity. One idea is to make herbal sun prints on construction paper using a variety of herb leaves. Arrange the leaves on the paper, set it in the sun for a few hours, and then remove the leaves to reveal the prints. Discuss the unique shapes and textures of different herb leaves.

6. **Storytime with Herbal Themes**: Select books that incorporate plants or herbs into their stories. Read together, then discuss the herbal elements of the story, such as the use of a specific herb for healing or the role of plants in the ecosystem. This can help children understand the significance of plants beyond their physical appearance.

7. **Herbal Tea Party**: Host a herbal tea party, allowing children to choose from safe, child-friendly herbs like chamomile or mint. Show them how to steep the herbs in hot water to make tea, and discuss the calming or refreshing properties of each. Serve the tea with honey or lemon to taste, and enjoy a conversation about the different flavors.

8. **Nature Walks and Herb Identification**: Take children on nature walks in areas where wild herbs grow. Equip them with a simple field guide to help identify common herbs. Teach them to observe but not pick wild plants, emphasizing respect for nature and the importance of conservation.

9. **Herbal First Aid Basics**: Introduce basic herbal remedies for minor issues like scrapes or bug bites. Demonstrate how to apply lavender oil for a calming effect or aloe vera gel for skin soothing. Stress the importance of seeking adult supervision when using herbs for health purposes.

10. **Create an Herb Journal**: Encourage children to keep an herb journal where they can draw pictures of herbs, write down their names, and note their uses or any interesting facts they learn. This can be a fun way for them to document their herbal learning journey.

By engaging children in these activities, you can foster a lifelong interest in herbal wisdom and natural living. The hands-on experiences help children to learn by doing, making the knowledge more impactful and likely to be remembered. It's important to supervise all activities, especially those involving the consumption or topical application of herbs, to ensure safety.

CHAPTER 3: DIGITAL TOOLS FOR HERBAL PRESERVATION

In the realm of herbal preservation, leveraging digital tools can significantly enhance the accuracy, accessibility, and longevity of herbal knowledge. The following outlines a comprehensive approach to utilizing digital platforms and technologies for the effective preservation of herbal traditions.

Digital Databases and Libraries: Establish a centralized digital repository to store extensive information on herbs, including their scientific names, common names, uses, preparation methods, and dosages. This database should allow for easy searching, categorizing, and updating of information. Utilize database software that supports multimedia entries, enabling the inclusion of photos, videos, and audio recordings that can illustrate harvesting techniques, plant identification, and preparation methods.

Cloud Storage Solutions: Implement cloud storage services to ensure that the digital archive is backed up in real-time and accessible from anywhere. This redundancy is crucial for preserving the integrity of the data against physical disasters or technological failures. Services like Google Drive, Dropbox, or Microsoft OneDrive offer scalable solutions that can grow with the database.

Mobile Applications: Develop a mobile app that provides easy access to the herbal database. This app can serve as a field guide for plant identification, a reference for herbal remedies, and a platform for community contributions to the database. Incorporate features such as image recognition to help users identify plants in the wild and a forum for sharing experiences and advice.

Social Media Platforms: Utilize social media to share knowledge, updates, and discussions related to herbal practices. Platforms like Instagram, YouTube, and Facebook can host educational content, live Q&A sessions, and community discussions. These platforms can also facilitate the formation of a global community of herbal enthusiasts who can contribute to and benefit from the shared knowledge.

E-Learning Platforms: Create online courses and webinars that offer structured learning paths for individuals at various levels of herbal knowledge. These courses can range from introductory topics on herbal medicine to advanced studies on phytochemistry and ethnobotany. Platforms like Teachable, Udemy, or Coursera provide the infrastructure needed to host these courses and track learner progress.

Digital Newsletters and Blogs: Regularly publish newsletters and blog posts that delve into specific aspects of herbal medicine, such as spotlighting individual herbs, sharing seasonal remedies, or discussing the latest research findings. This content can help keep the community engaged and informed while driving traffic to the digital database and e-learning courses.

Interactive Webinars and Workshops: Host live webinars and workshops that allow for real-time interaction between experts and learners. These sessions can cover a wide range of topics, from hands-on demonstrations of herbal preparation techniques to discussions on the cultural significance of certain plants. Utilize webinar platforms that support interactive features like polls, Q&A sessions, and breakout rooms for smaller group discussions.

Virtual Reality (VR) and Augmented Reality (AR) Experiences: Explore the use of VR and AR to create immersive learning experiences. For example, a VR application could simulate a walk through a forest, teaching users how to identify and harvest various medicinal plants. Similarly, an AR app could overlay information about the medicinal properties of plants when a user points their smartphone camera at them.

Online Forums and Discussion Boards: Establish online forums where practitioners, students, and enthusiasts can ask questions, share experiences, and offer advice. These forums can be organized by topic, such as plant identification, herbal preparation, or health conditions, facilitating focused discussions and knowledge exchange.

Digital Preservation Policies: Develop and implement policies that ensure the ethical use, sharing, and preservation of digital herbal knowledge. This includes securing permissions from contributors, respecting indigenous knowledge and intellectual property rights, and adhering to data privacy laws.

By integrating these digital tools and strategies, the preservation of herbal knowledge can be significantly enhanced, ensuring that this invaluable wisdom remains accessible and relevant for future generations. The key to success lies in the careful planning, execution, and ongoing management of these digital resources, coupled with a commitment to fostering a global community of herbal knowledge sharing.

Made in United States
Troutdale, OR
01/09/2025

27797276R00177